Pharmacognosy and Phytotherapy

Pharmacognosy and Phytotherapy

Editor: Kendall Jefferson

FOSTER ACADEMICS
www.fosteracademics.com

www.fosteracademics.com

FOSTER ACADEMICS

Cataloging-in-Publication Data

Pharmacognosy and phytotherapy / edited by Kendall Jefferson.
p. cm.
Includes bibliographical references and index.
ISBN 978-1-63242-836-3
1. Pharmacognosy. 2. Materia medica, Vegetable. 3. Herbs--Therapeutic use.
4. Medicinal plants. 5. Botany, Medical. I. Jefferson, Kendall.
RS160 .P43 2019
615.321--dc23

Foster Academics,
118-35 Queens Blvd., Suite 400,
Forest Hills, NY 11375, USA

ISBN 978-1-63242-836-3 (Hardback)

Contents

Preface VII

Chapter 1 **Characterization of alkaloid constitution and evaluation of antimicrobial activity of *Solanum nigrum* using gas chromatography mass spectrometry (GC-MS)** **1**
Huda Jasim, Ameera Omran Hussein, Imad Hadi Hameed and Muhanned Abdulhasan Kareem

Chapter 2 **Separate and co-administration of *Amaranthus spinosus* and vitamin C modulates cardiovascular disease risk in high fat diet-fed experimental rats** **18**
Abayomi S. Faponle, Adeleke Atunnise, Bukunola O. Adegbesan, Olugbenga O. Ogunlabi, Kuburat T. Odufuwa and Emmanuel O. Ajani

Chapter 3 **Pharmacological properties of *Pomaria sandersonii, Pentanisia prunelloides* and *Alepidea amatymbica* extracts using *in vitro* assays** **26**
Muleya, E., Ahmed, A. S., Sipamla, A. M., Mtunzi, F. M. and Mutatu, W.

Chapter 4 **Palliative treatment of cancer in resource poor settings: Traditional medicine perspective** **34**
Florence Dushimemaria and Davis R. Mumbengegwi

Chapter 5 **Ethnobotanical survey of healing medicinal plants traditionally used in the main Moroccan cities** **41**
Messaoudi Moussi, Filali, H., Tazi, A. and Hakkou, F.

Chapter 6 **Biochemical analysis of *Origanum vulgare* seeds by fourier-transform infrared (FT-IR) spectroscopy and gas chromatography-mass spectrometry (GC-MS)** **60**
Huda Jasim Al-Tameme, Imad Hadi Hameed, Salah Ali Idan and Mohammed Yahya Hadi

Chapter 7 **Analgesic and anti-inflammatory effects of the ethanol extract of *Elytraria marginata* Vahl (whole plant) in Wistar rats** **77**
J. S. Ashidi, O. J. Ojetola, P. I. Aziba and E. O. Ajaiyeoba

Chapter 8 **Herbal medicines use among diabetic patients in Oriental Morocco** **83**
Zayneb Alami, Hayat Aynaou, Bouchra Alami, Youssef Hdidou and Hanane Latrech

Chapter 9 **Evaluation of the anthelmintic activity of pumpkin seeds (*Cucurbita maxima*) in mice naturally infected with *Aspiculuris tetraptera*** **91**
Erol Ayaz, Cengiz Gökbulut, Hamit Coşkun, Arzu Türker, Şeyda Özsoy and Kübra Ceylan

Chapter 10 **Phytochemical analysis of *Urtica dioica* leaves by fourier-transform infrared spectroscopy and gas chromatography-mass spectrometry** **96**
Huda Jasim Al-Tameme, Mohammed Yahya Hadi and Imad Hadi Hameed

Chapter 11 **Phytochemical studies and thin layer chromatography of leaves and flower extracts of *Senna siamea lam* for possible biomedical applications** 111
Ismail Adamu Hassan, Idris Abdullahi Nasiru, Amina Muhammed Malut, Ibrahim Abdulkadir S. and Audu Sani Ali

Chapter 12 **Design and optimisation of novel Huperzine a analogues capable of modulating the acetylcholinesterase receptor for the management of Alzheimer's disease** 120
Sara Bonavia and Claire Shoemake

Chapter 13 **Antiprotozoal and cytotoxic activities, and the acute toxicity of extracts from of *Brucea sumatrana* Roxb. (Simaroubaceae) leaves collected** 130
Cimanga R. Kanyanga, Tshodi M. Ehata, Nsaka S. Lumpu, Kikweta C. Munduku, Mbenza A. Phuati, Kambu O. Kabangu, Cos, P., Maes, L., Apers, S., Vlietinck, A. J. and Pieters, L.

Chapter 14 **Analysis of bioactive chemical compounds of *Aspergillus niger* by using gas chromatography-mass spectrometry and fourier-transform infrared spectroscopy** 140
Imad Hadi Hameed, Lena Fadhil Hamza and Sabreen A. Kamal

Chapter 15 **Hepatoprotective effects of the decoction and macerated leaves of *Rhamnus alaternus* L. on rats exposed to carbon tetrachloride** 172
Abdelkrim Berroukche, Khaled Kahloula, Miloud Slimani, Imane Denai and Kheira Ammour

Chapter 16 **Preliminary screening of anti-inflammatory effect of phytochemicals on chemotaxis of human neutrophils** 182
Uthayashanker R. Ezekiel and Rita M. Heuertz

Chapter 17 **Analysis of bioactive chemical compounds of *Euphorbia lathyrus* using gas chromatography-mass spectrometry and Fourier-transform infrared spectroscopy** 188
Azhar Abduameer Sosa, Suhaila Husaein Bagi and Imad Hadi Hameed

Chapter 18 **Determination of metabolites products by *Penicillium expansum* and evaluating antimicobial activity** 206
Lena Fadhil Hamza, Sabreen A. Kamal and Imad Hadi Hameed

Chapter 19 **New pentacyclic triterpene ester and flavone glycoside from the biologically active extract of *Carduus pycnocephalus* L.** 233
Wafaa H. B. Hassan, Hanan M. Al-Youssef, Latifa AL-Shammari and Rehab H. Abdallah

Permissions

List of Contributors

Index

Preface

This book aims to highlight the current researches and provides a platform to further the scope of innovations in this area. This book is a product of the combined efforts of many researchers and scientists, after going through thorough studies and analysis from different parts of the world. The objective of this book is to provide the readers with the latest information of the field.

The sub-specialty of pharmacy concerned with the study of the medicinal drugs derived from plants and other natural sources is called pharmacognosy. It involves the study of the physical, biological and chemical properties of drugs, as well as the search of new drugs from natural sources. The alternative and pseudoscientific practices of using unrefined plant or animal extracts for the purpose of treatment is called phytotherapy. Herbal medicines are used to treat patients suffering from chronic conditions or diseases like ashtma, cancer, diabetes, etc. This book traces the progress of pharmacognosy and phytotherapy, and highlights some of their key concepts and applications. It strives to provide a fair idea about these disciplines and to help develop a better understanding of the latest advances within these fields. This book includes contributions of experts, which will provide innovative insights into these fields.

I would like to express my sincere thanks to the authors for their dedicated efforts in the completion of this book. I acknowledge the efforts of the publisher for providing constant support. Lastly, I would like to thank my family for their support in all academic endeavors.

Editor

Characterization of alkaloid constitution and evaluation of antimicrobial activity of *Solanum nigrum* using gas chromatography mass spectrometry (GC-MS)

Huda Jasim[1], Ameera Omran Hussein[2], Imad Hadi Hameed[1]* and Muhanned Abdulhasan Kareem[2]

[1]Department of Molecular Biology, Babylon University, Hilla City, Iraq.
[2]Babylon University, Centre of Environmental Research, Iraq.

In this study, the alkaloid compounds of *Solanum nigrum* have been evaluated. The chemical compositions of the leaf methanol extract of *S. nigrum* were investigated using Gas chromatography-mass specroscopy (GC-MS). GC-MS analysis of *S. nigrum* alkaloid leaf methanol extract revealed the existence of the cyclopentasiloxane-decamethyl, L-proline, ethylester, 2-ethyl-1-butanol, methyl ether, cyclopentasiloxane-ocamethyl, betanedioic acid, hydroxyl, diethyl, ester, 1.1.3.3.5.5.7.7-octamethy-l-7-(2methyl-propoxy) tetrasiloxane-1, dodecanoic acid, 3-hydroxy-, ethyl ester, cyclopentasiloxane-ocamethyl, dodecanedoic acid, bistert-butyldimethylsilyl ester, 2-pyrrolidinecarboxylic acid-5-oxo, ethyl ester, 1-dodecanamine, N.N-dimethyl, cyclooctasiloxane, hexadecamethyl, 5-keto-2, 2-dimethylheptanoic acid, ethyl ester, cyclodecasiloxane, eicosamethyl, 9.12.15-octadecatrienoic acid, octadecanoic acid, octadecenal, 9-octadecenamide, octadecane, 3-ethyl-5-(ethylbutyl), N-acetyl-L-tryptophan ethyl ester, ethyl iso-allocholate, phthalic acid, di(2-propylpentyl)ester and 17-(1.5-Dimethylhexyl)-10. 13-dimethyl-2.3.4.7.8.9.10.11. 12.13.14.15.16.17-tetradecahydro-1H. Alkaloids extract from leaf of *S. nigrum* were assayed for *in vitro* antibacterial activity against *Escherichia coli*, *Proteus mirabilis, Staphylococcus aureus, Pseudomonas aerogenosa* and *Klebsiella pneumonia* using the diffusion method in agar. The zone of inhibition was compared with different standard antibiotics. The diameters of inhibition zones ranged from 0.8 to 2.01 mm for all treatments.

Key words: Alkaloids, antibacterial activity, gas chromatography-mass specroscopy (GC-MS) analysis, *Solanum nigrum*.

INTRODUCTION

Plants are rich source of secondary metabolites with interesting biological activities (Koduru et al., 2006). Several plant products have been shown to exert a protective role against the formation of free radicals and playing a beneficial role in maintaining disease condition (Ajitha et al., 2001). *Solanum nigrum* is a common weed in gardens, fields and waste-land throughout the country (up to 1500 m altitude) (Figure 1). It is found in Baghdad,

*Corresponding author. E-mail: imad_dna@yahoo.com.

Basrah, Kut, Tal-Kaif, and Sulaimaniya.Leaves of *S. nigrum* contain solanin; solanidin are poisonous to cattle, sheep, horses and goat. The effects of poison are necrosis, paralysis, salivation, vomiting and diarrhoea. The medicinal value of drug plants is due to the presence of some chemical substances in the plant tissues which produce a definite physiological action on the human body. These chemicals include alkaloids, flavanoids, glucosides, tannins, gums, resins, essential oils, fatty oils, carbon compounds, hydrogen, oxygen, nitrogen salts of some chemicals, etc. Very few of these chemicals are toxic also (Haraguchi et al., 1999; Sashikumar et al., 2003).

The photochemicals with adequate antibacterial activity will be used for the treatment of bacterial infections (Iwu et al., 1999; World Health Organization, 2002; Purohit and Vyas, 2004; Krishnaraju et al., 2005). Successful extraction is largely dependent on the type of solvent used in the extraction procedure. The most often tested extracts are water extract as a sample of extract that is primarily used in traditional medicine and extracts from organic solvents, such as methanol, as well as ethyl acetate, acetone, chloroform, and dichlormethane. Diffusion and dilution method are two types of susceptibility test used to determine the antibacterial efficacy of plant extracts. Diffusion method is a qualitative test which allows classification of bacteria as susceptible or resistant to the tested plant extract according to the size of diameter of the zone of inhibition (Alves et al., 2000; Palombo and Semple, 2001; Uzun et al., 2004; Cos et al., 2006; Ncube et al., 2008; Stanojević et al., 2010). Considering the high economical and pharmacological importance of secondary plant metabolites, industries are deeply interested in utilizing plant tissue culture technique for large scale production of these substances (Misawa, 1994). The aim of this study is to assess the antibacterial activity of alkaloids extracts from the leaves of *S. nigrum*, which can be the basis for the synthesis of new antibiotics. This is because of increase in the emergence of bacterial strains resistant to multiple clinical disease.

MATERIALS AND METHODS

Collection and preparation of plant

In this research, the leaves were dried at room temperature for 13 days and when properly dried the leaves were powdered using clean pestle and mortar, and the powdered plant was size reduced with a sieve. The fine powder was then packed in airtight container to avoid the effect of humidity and then stored at room temperature.

Extraction and identification of alkaloids

The powdered leaves (2 g) were boiled in a water bath with 20 ml of 5% sulphuric acid in 50% ethanol. The mixture was cooled and filtered. A portion was reserved. Another portion of the filtrate was put in 100 ml of separating funnel and the solution was made alkaline by adding two drops of concentrated ammonia solution. Equal volume of chloroform was added and shaken gently to allow the layer to separate. The lower chloroform layer was run off into a second separating funnel. The ammoniacal layer was reserved. The chloroform layer was extracted with two quantities each of 5 ml of dilute sulphuric acid. The various extracts were then used for the following test.

Mayer's test

To the filtrate in test tube I, 1 ml of Mayer's reagent was added drop by drop. Formation of a greenish coloured or cream precipitate indicates the presence of alkaloids (Evans, 2002).

Dragendoff's test

To the filtrate in test tube II, 1 ml of Dragendoff's reagent was added drop by drop. Formation of a reddish-brown precipitate indicates the presence of alkaloids (Evans, 2002).

Wagner's test

To the filtrate in tube III, 1 ml of Wagner's reagent was added drop by drop. Formation of a reddish-brown precipitate indicates the presence of alkaloids (Evans, 2002).

Gas chromatography-mass specroscopy (GC-MS) analysis

GC-MS analysis of the methanol extract of *S. nigrum* was carried out using a Clarus 500 Perkin- elmer (Auto system XL) Gas Chromatograph equipped and coupled to a mass detector Turbo mass gold-Perkin Elmer Turbomass 5.1 spectrometer with an Elite-1 (100% Dimethyl poly siloxane), 30 m × 0.25 mm ID × 1 μm of capillary column. For GC-MS detection, an electron ionization system was operated in electron impact mode with ionization system operated in electron impact mode with ionization energy of 70 eV. The instrument was set to an initial temperature of 110°C, and maintained at this temperature for 2 min. At the end of this period, the oven temperature was raised up to 280°C, at the rate of an increase of 5°C/min, and maintained for 9 min. Helium gas (99.999%) was used as carrier gas at a constant flow rate of 1 ml/min, and an injection volume of 2 μl was employed (split ratio of 10:1). The injector temperature was maintained at 250°C, the ion-source temperature was 200°C, the oven temperature was programmed at 110°C (isothermal for 2 min), with an increase of 100°C/min to 200°C, then 5°C/min to 280°C, ending with a 9 min isothermal at 280°C. Mass spectra were taken at 70 eV; a scan interval of 0.5 s and fragments from 45 to 450 Da. The solvent delay was 0 to 2 min and the total GC-MS running time was 36 min. The samples were injected in split mode as 10:1. Mass spectral scan range was set at 45 to 450 (m/z). The mass detector used in this analysis was Turbo-Mass Gold-Perkin Elmer and the software adopted to handle mass spectra and chromatograms was a Turbo-Mass ver 5.2.

Measurement of antibacterial activity

The antibacterial activity of alkaloids was determined using agar well diffusion method. Wells of 5 mm diameter were punched in the agar medium with sterile cork borer and filled with plant alkaloid extract. Standard antibiotics, penicillin, kanamycin, cefotoxime, streptomycin and refampin (1 mg/ml) were also tested for their antibacterial activity. The plates were incubated at 370°C for

Table 1. Compounds present in the leaves extract of *Solanum nigrum* using GC-MS analysis.

Serial No.	Phytochemical compound	Formula	Molecular weight	Exact mass	Structure
1	Cyclopentasiloxane. decamethyl	$C_{10}H_{30}O_5Si_5$	370	370.093956	Figure 3
2	L-Proline, ethylester	$C_7H_{13}NO_2$	143	143.094628	Figure 4
3	2-Ethyl-1-butanol, methyl ether	$C_7H_{16}O$	116	116.1201153	Figure 5
4	Cyclopentasiloxane. ocamethyl	$C_8H_{24}O_4Si_4$	296	296.075165	Figure 6
5	Betanedioic acid , hydroxyl,diethyl, ester	$C_8H_{14}O_5$	190	190.084124	Figure 7
6	1.1.3.3.5.5.7.7-Octamethy-l-7-(2methyl-propoxy) tetrasiloxane-1	$C_{12}H_{34}O_5Si_4$	370	370.14833	Figure 8
7	Dodecanoic acid, 3-hydroxy-, ethyl ester	$C_{14}H_{28}O_3$	244	244.203845	Figure 9
9	Dodecanedoic acid. Bistert-butyldimethylsilyl ester	$C_{24}H_{50}O_4Si_2$	458	458.324762	Figure 10
10	2-Pyrrolidinecarboxylic acid-5-oxo, ethyl ester	$C_7H_{11}NO_3$	157	157.073894	Figure 11
11	1-Dodecanamine, N.N-dimethyl	$C_{14}H_{31}N$	213	213.24565	Figure 12
12	Cyclooctasiloxane, hexadecamethyl	$C_{16}H_{48}O_8Si_8$	592	592.15033	Figure 13
13	5-keto-2, 2-dimethylheptanoic acid, ethyl ester	$C_{11}H_{20}O_3$	200	200.141245	Figure 14
14	Cyclodecasiloxane, eicosamethyl	$C_{20}H_{60}O_{10}Si_{10}$	740	740.187912	Figure 15
15	9.12.15-Octadecatrienoic acid	$C_{18}H_{30}O_2$	278	278.22458	Figure 16
16	Octadecanoic acid	$C_{18}H_{36}O_2$	284	284.27153	Figure 17
17	Octadecenal	$C_{18}H_{34}O$	266	266.260965	Figure 18
18	9-Octadecenamide	$C_{18}H_{35}NO$	281	281.271864	Figure 19
19	Octadecane, 3-ethyl-5-(ethylbutyl)	$C_{26}H_{54}$	366	366.422552	Figure 20
20	N-Acetyl-L-tryptophan ethyl ester	$C_{15}H_{18}N_2O_3$	274	274.131742	Figure 21
21	Ethyl iso-allocholate	$C_{26}H_{44}O_5$	436	436.318874	Figure 22
22	Phthalic acid, di(2-propylpentyl)ester	$C_{24}H_{38}O_4$	390	390.27701	Figure 23
23	17-(1.5-Dimethylhexyl)-10. 13-dimethyl-2.3.4.7.8.9.10.11. 12.13.14.15.16.17-tetradecahydro-1H	$C_{27}H_{46}O$	386	386.354866	Figure 24

The negative control was added without adding the cultures to know the sterile conditions. Then Petri dishes were placed in the refrigerator at 4°C or at room temperature for 1 h for diffusion, then incubate at 37°C for 24 h. Observation was done on zone of inhibition which produced different antibiotics. Measurement was done using a scale and the average of two diameters of each zone of inhibition was recorded.

RESULTS AND DISCUSSION

GC-MS analysis of alkaloid compound clearly showed the presence of twenty three compounds. The alkaloid compound, formula, molecular weight and exact mass are as shown in Table 1. The GC-MS chromatogram of the 23 peak of the compounds detected are as shown in Figure 2. Chromatogram GC-MS analysis of the methanol extract of *S. nigrum* showed the presence of twenty three major peaks and the components corresponding to the peaks were determined as follows. The first setup peaks were determined to be cyclopentasiloxane-decamethyl (Figure 3). The second peaks were indicated to be L-proline, ethylester (Figure 4). The next peaks was considered to be 2-ethyl-1-butanol, methyl ether, cyclopentasiloxane-ocamethyl, betanedioic acid, hydroxyl, diethyl, ester, 1.1.3.3.5.5.7.7-Octamethy-l-7-(2methyl-propoxy) tetrasiloxane-1, dodecanoic acid, 3-hydroxy-, ethyl ester, cyclopentasiloxane-ocamethyl, dodecanedoic acid, bistert-butyldimethylsilyl ester, 2-pyrrolidinecarboxylic acid-5-oxo, ethyl ester, 1-dodecanamine, N.N-dimethyl, cyclooctasiloxane, hexadecamethyl, 5-keto-2, 2-dimethylheptanoic acid, ethyl ester, cyclodecasiloxane,

Table 2. Zone of inhibition (mm) of test bacterial strains to alkaloid leaf extracts of *Solanum nigrum* (L.) and standard antibiotics.

Alkaloid antibiotic	*K. pneumonia*	*P. aeruginosa*	*S. aureus*	*P. mirabilis*	*E. coli*
Alkaloid	1.8±0.42	1.4±0.59	1.9±0.61	2.01±0.51	1.7±0.62
Kanamycin	0.8±0.3	0.5±0.4	0.6±0.2	0.4±0.1	0.9±0.1
Cefotoxime	1.3±0.5	1.5±0.1	1.2±0.1	1.2±0.6	1.2±0.3
Penicillin	1.1±0.2	1±0.5	1±0.4	1±0.2	1.6±0.1
Streptomycin	1.2±0.3	1.1±0.3	1.3±0.5	1.7±0.2	1.3±0.6
Rifampin	1.1±0.1	1.1±0.1	1.2±0.5	0.6±0.1	0.8±0.2

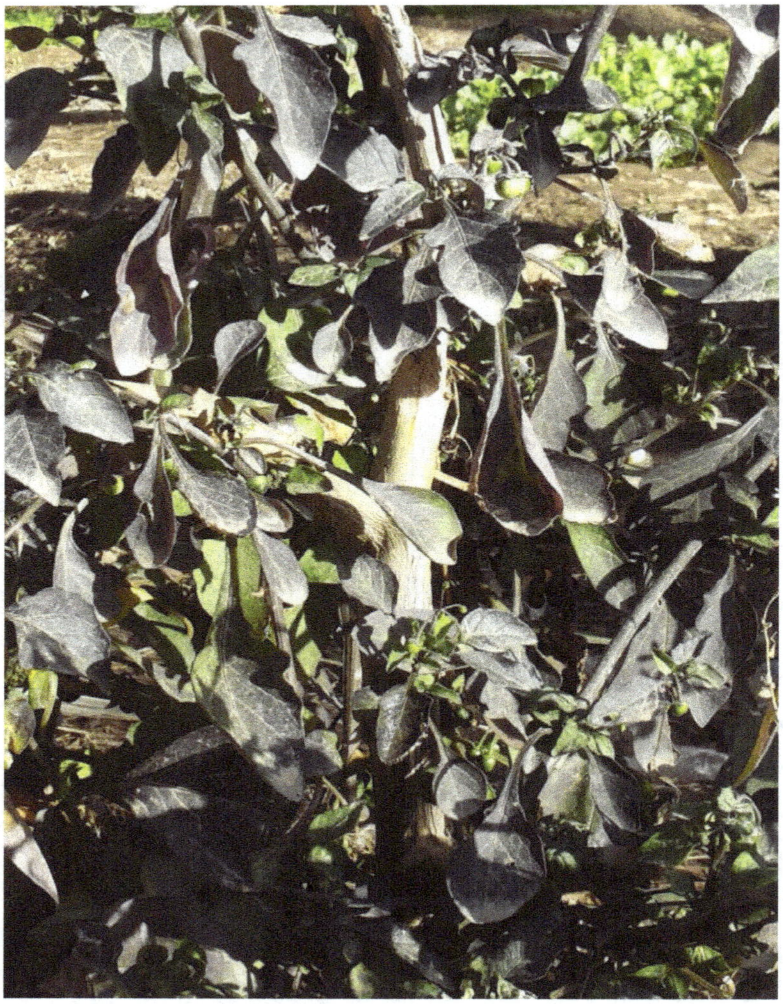

Figure 1. Leaves of *Solanum nigrum*.

eicosamethyl, 9.12.15-octadecatrienoic acid, octadecanoic acid, octadecenal, 9-octadecenamide, octadecane, 3-ethyl-5-(ethylbutyl), N-Acetyl-L-tryptophan ethyl ester, ethyl iso-allocholate, phthalic acid, di(2-propylpentyl)ester and 17-(1.5-Dimethylhexyl)-10. 13-dimethyl-2.3.4.7.8.9.10.11.12.13.14.15.16.17-tetradecahydro-1H (Figures 5 to 23). Among the identified phyto-compounds are the property of anti-oxidant and antimicrobial activities (Stainer et al., 1986; Singh et al., 1998; Prescott et al., 1999; Kumar et al., 2001; Purohit and Vyas, 2004; John and Senthilkumar, 2005; Venkatesan et al., 2005; Santh et al., 2006; Sazada et al., 2009). Plant based antimicrobials have enormous therapeutic potential as they can serve the

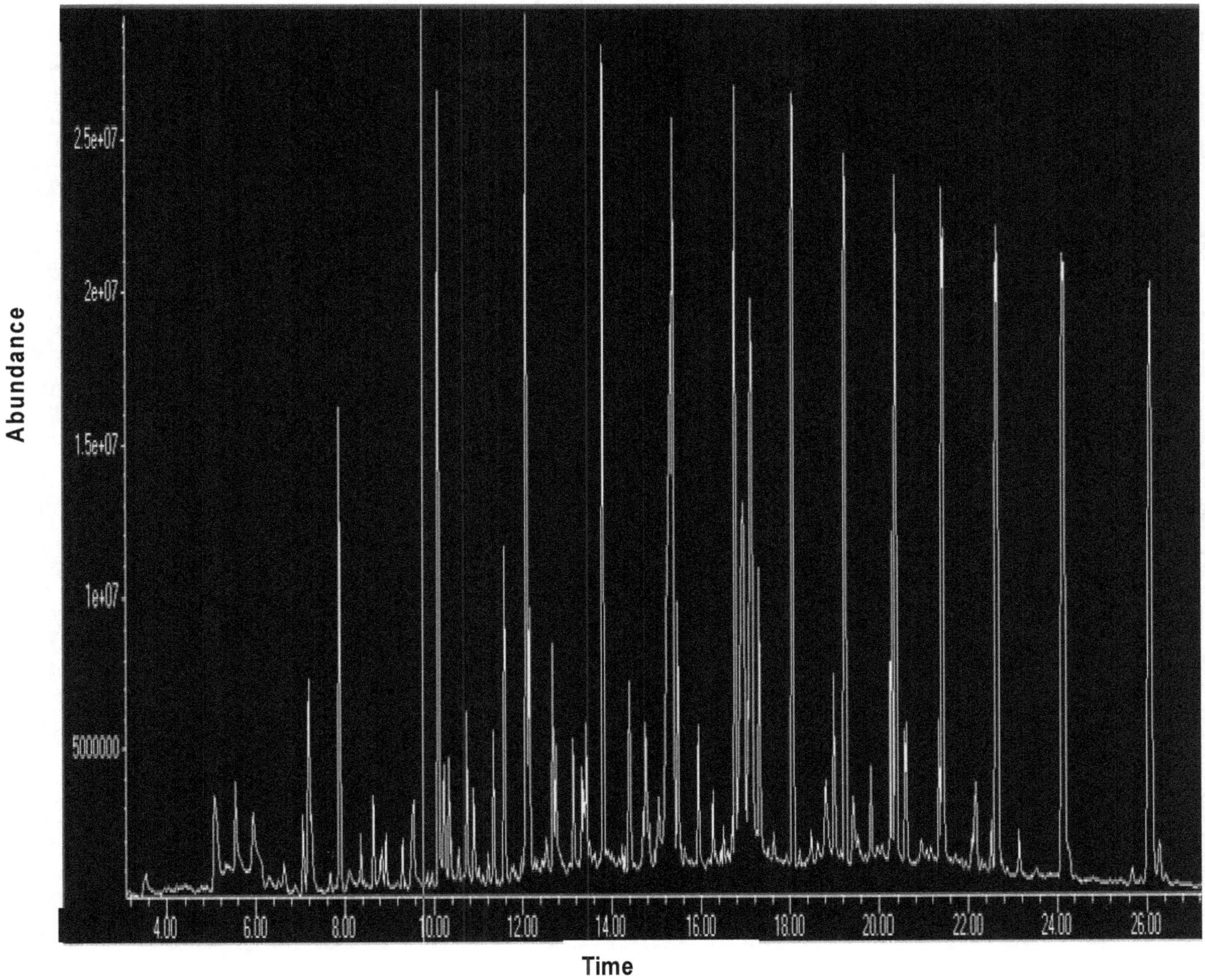

Figure 2. GC-MS Profile of leaves extract of *Solanum nigrum*.

purpose with lesser side effects. Continued further exploration of plant derived antimicrobials is needed today.

The results of the antimicrobial activity of the extracts of leaves of *S. nigrum* are as shown in Table 2. It was observed that the sensitivity tests show the effect of crude extracted alkaloids from seeds and roots of different bacterial strains, giving varying diameters depending on the tested strains.

The clear zone of growth inhibition was noted around the well due to diffusion of alkaloid compound. The diameter of the zone denotes the relative susceptibility of the test microorganism to a particular antimicrobial. The obtained results of the crude extracts were compared with the standard antibiotics such as penicillin, kanamycin, cefotoxime, streptomycin and refampin. All the tested organisms are highly sensitive to the methanol leaf extract (1.4 to 2 mm) than the standard antibiotics which showed more or less activity (0.4 to 1.7 mm).

The presence of antimicrobial substances in the higher plants is well established. Plants have provided a source of inspiration for novel drug compounds as plants derived medicines have made significant contribution towards human health (Walton and Brown, 1999). Further works on the types of phytoconstituents and purification of individual groups of bioactive components can reveal the exact potential of the plant to inhibit several pathogenic microbes. *S. nigrum* is the most potent plant against pathogenic microorganisms. However, further studies are needed, including toxicity evaluation and purification of active antibacterial constituents from *S. nigrum* extracts looking toward a pharmaceutical use.

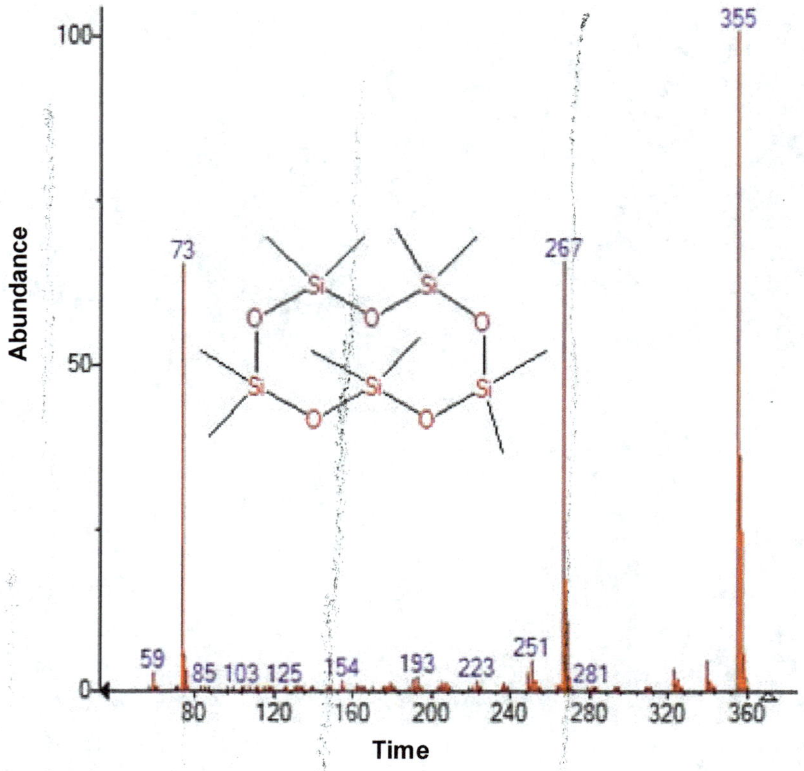

Figure 3. Structure of cyclopentasiloxane-decamethyl present in the leaves extract of *Solanum nigrum* using GC-MS analysis.

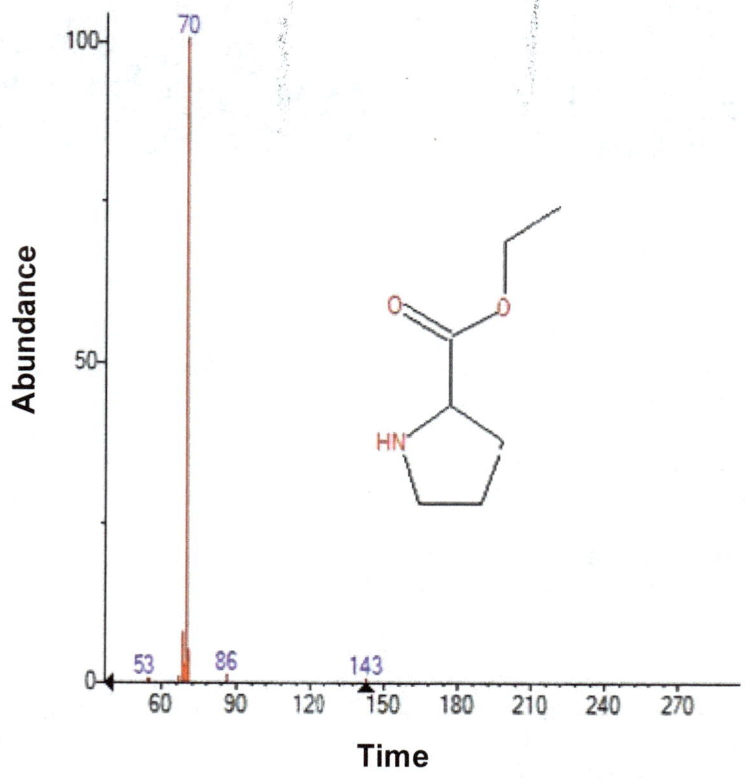

Figure 4. Structure of L-Proline, ethylester present in the leaves extract of *Solanum nigrum* using GC-MS analysis.

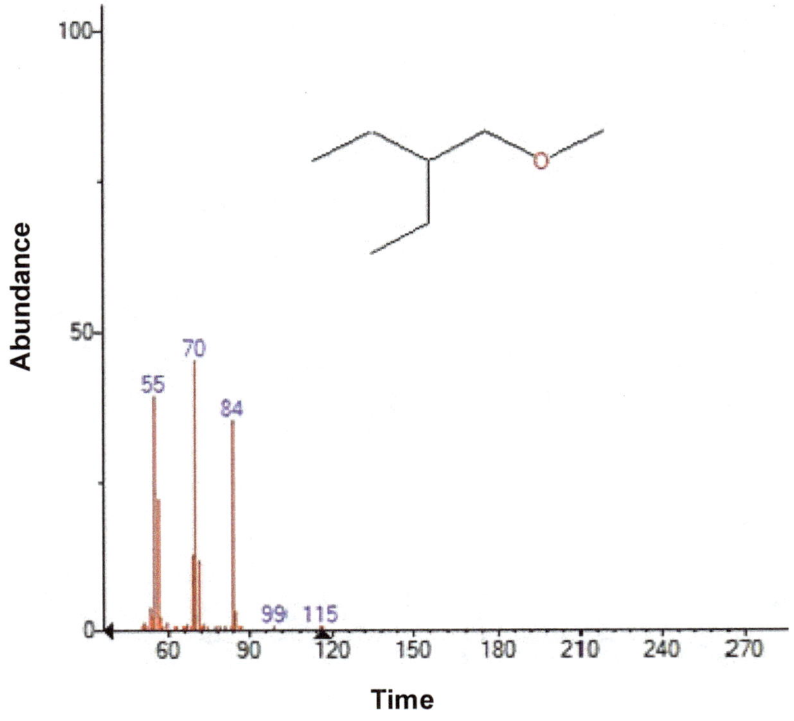

Figure 5. Structure of 2-ethyl-1-butanol, methyl ether present in the leaves extract of *Solanum nigrum* using GC-MS analysis.

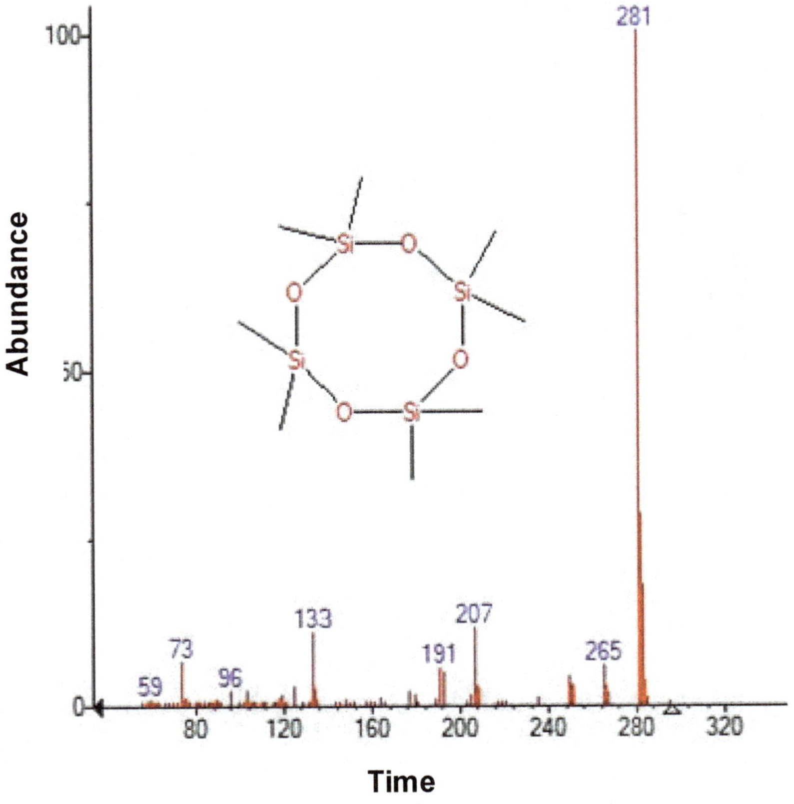

Figure 6. Structure of cyclopentasiloxane-ocamethyl present in the leaves extract of *Solanum nigrum* using GC-MS analysis.

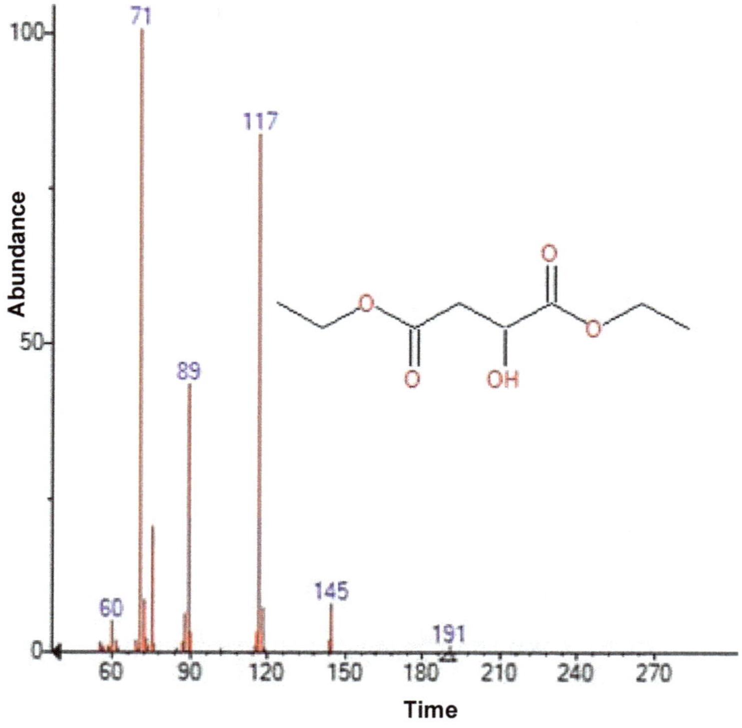

Figure 7. Structure of betanedioic acid, hydroxyl, diethyl, ester present in the leaves extract of *Solanum nigrum* using GC-MS analysis.

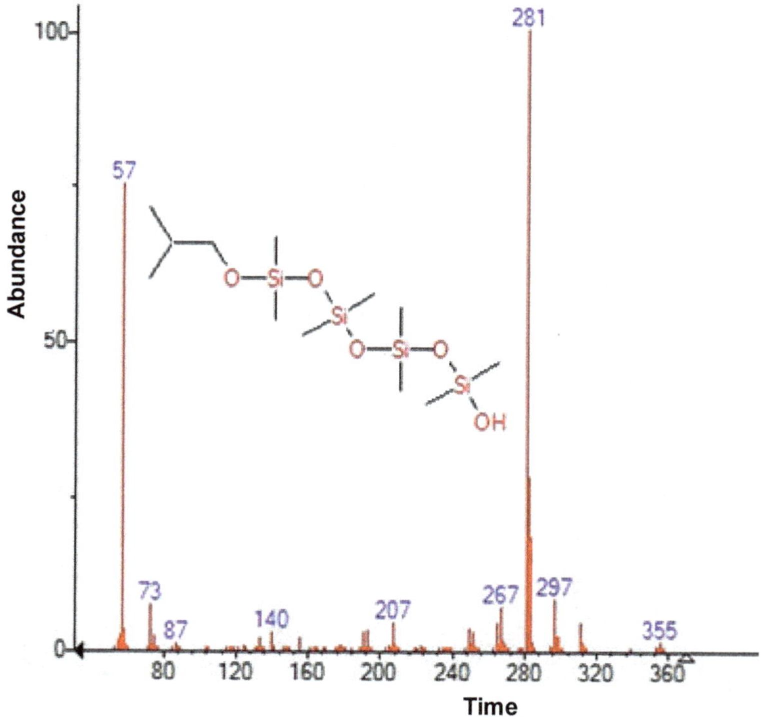

Figure 8. Structure of 1.1.3.3.5.5.7.7-Octamethy-l-7-(2methyl-propoxy) tetrasiloxane-1 present in the leaves extract of *Solanum nigrum* using GC-MS analysis.

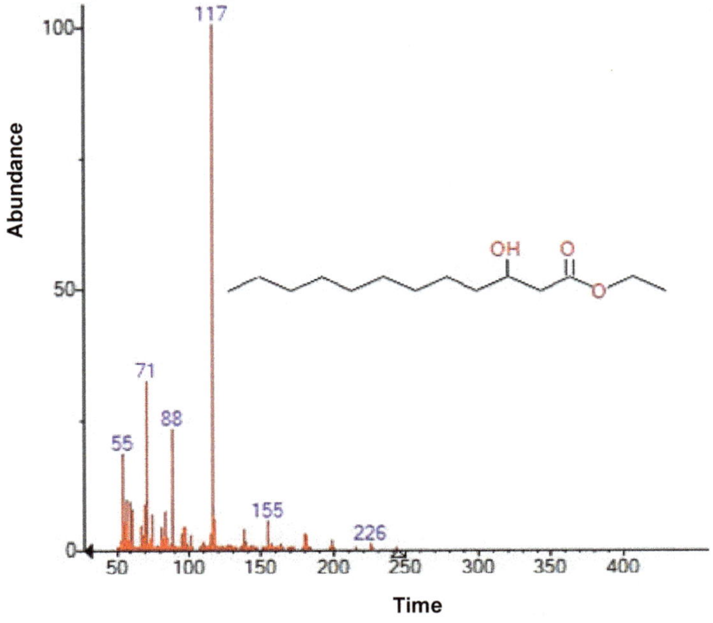

Figure 9. Structure of dodecanoic acid, 3-hydroxy-, ethyl ester present in the leaves extract of *Solanum nigrum* using GC-MS analysis.

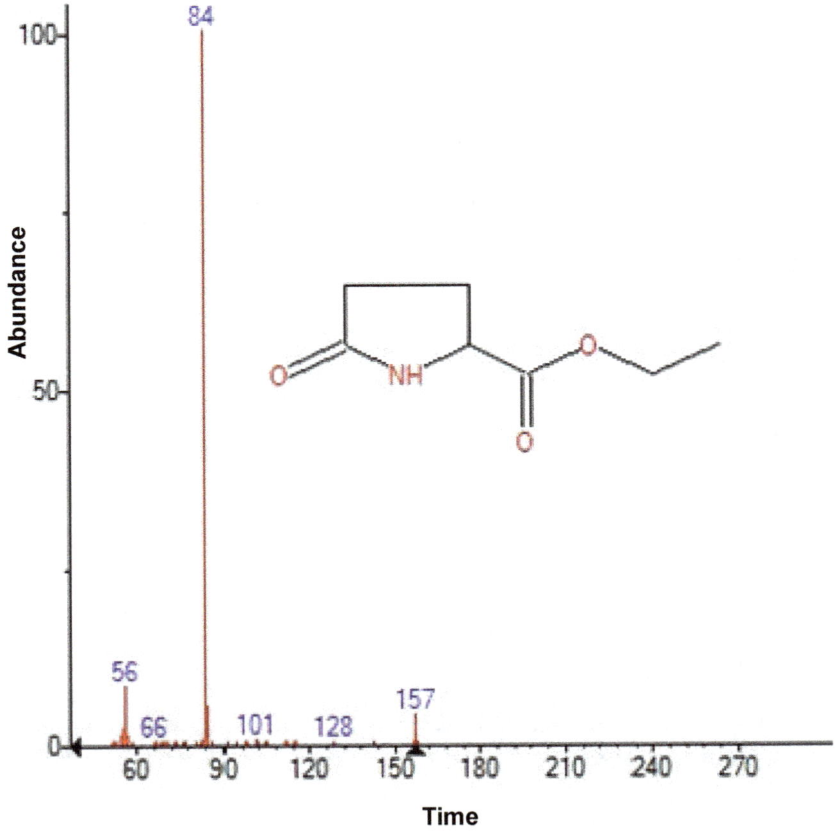

Figure 10. Structure of 2-pyrrolidinecarboxylic acid-5-oxo, ethyl ester present in the leaves extract of *Solanum nigrum* using GC-MS analysis.

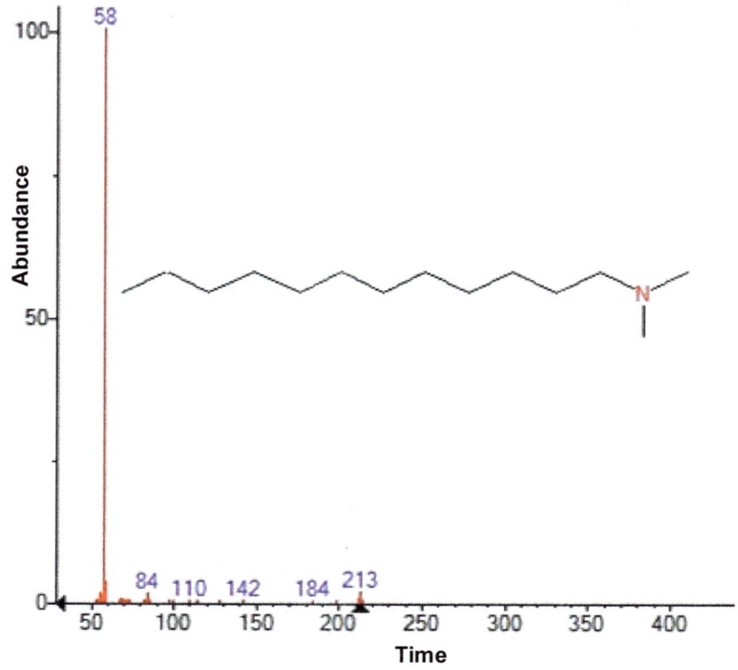

Figure 11. Structure of 1-dodecanamine, N.N-dimethyl present in the leaves extract of *Solanum nigrum* using GC-MS analysis.

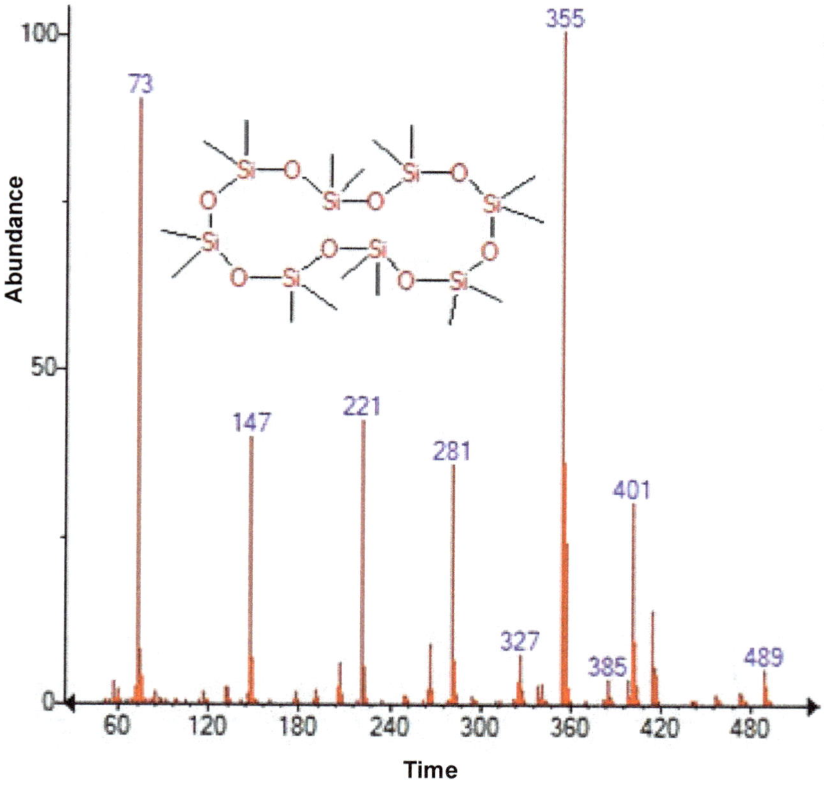

Figure 12. Structure of cyclooctasiloxane, hexadecamethyl present in the leaves extract of *Solanum nigrum* using GC-MS analysis.

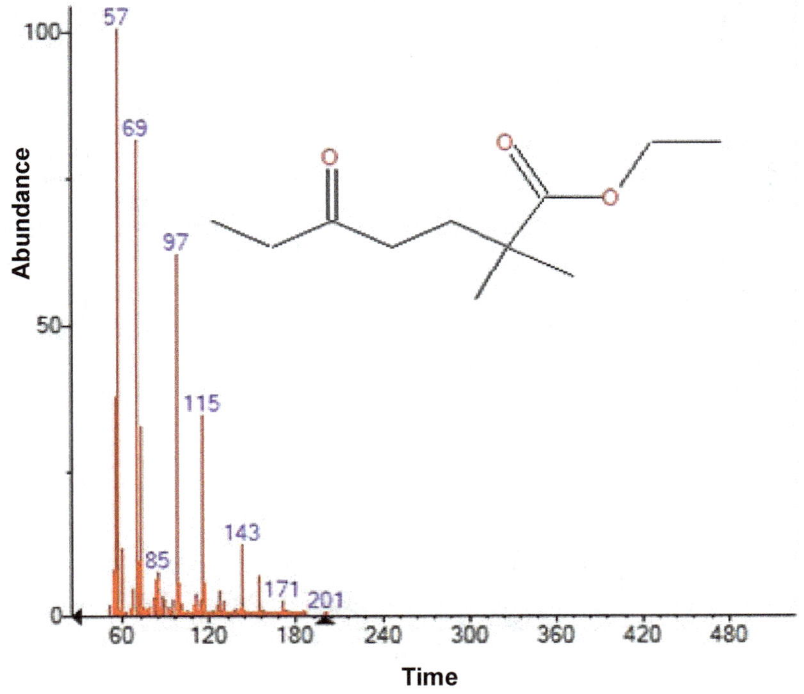

Figure 13. Structure of 5-keto-2, 2-dimethylheptanoic acid, ethyl ester present in the leaves extract of *Solanum nigrum* using GC-MS analysis.

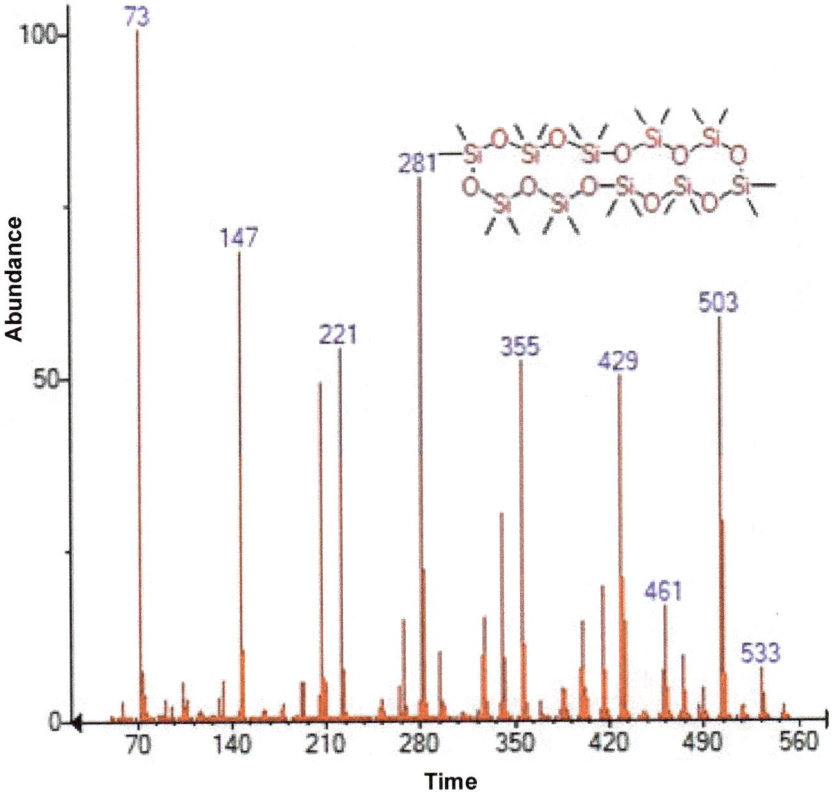

Figure 14. Structure of cyclodecasiloxane, eicosamethyl present in the leaves extract of *Solanum nigrum* using GC-MS analysis.

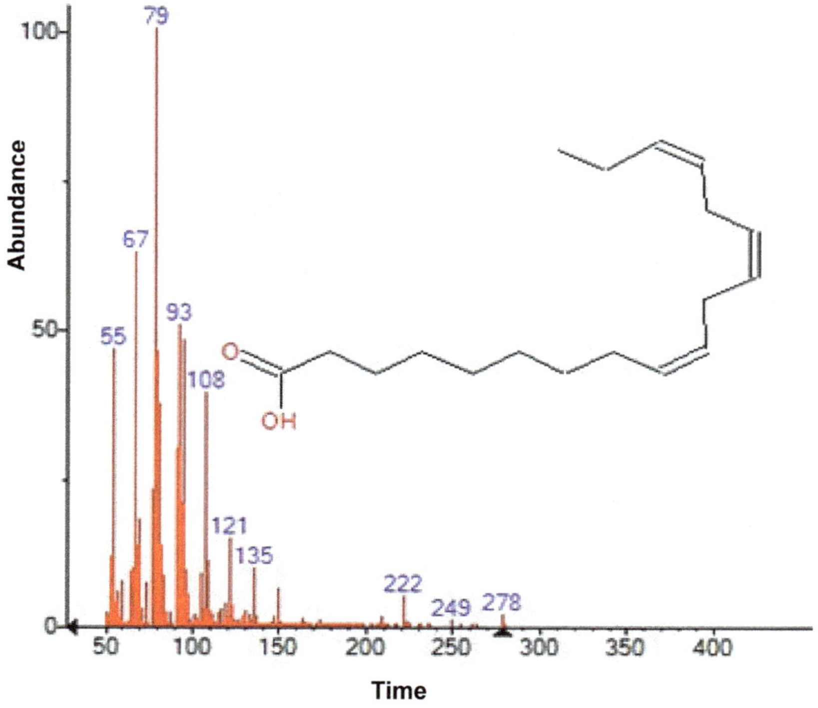

Figure 15. Structure of 9.12.15-octadecatrienoic acid present in the leaves extract of *Solanum nigrum* using GC-MS analysis.

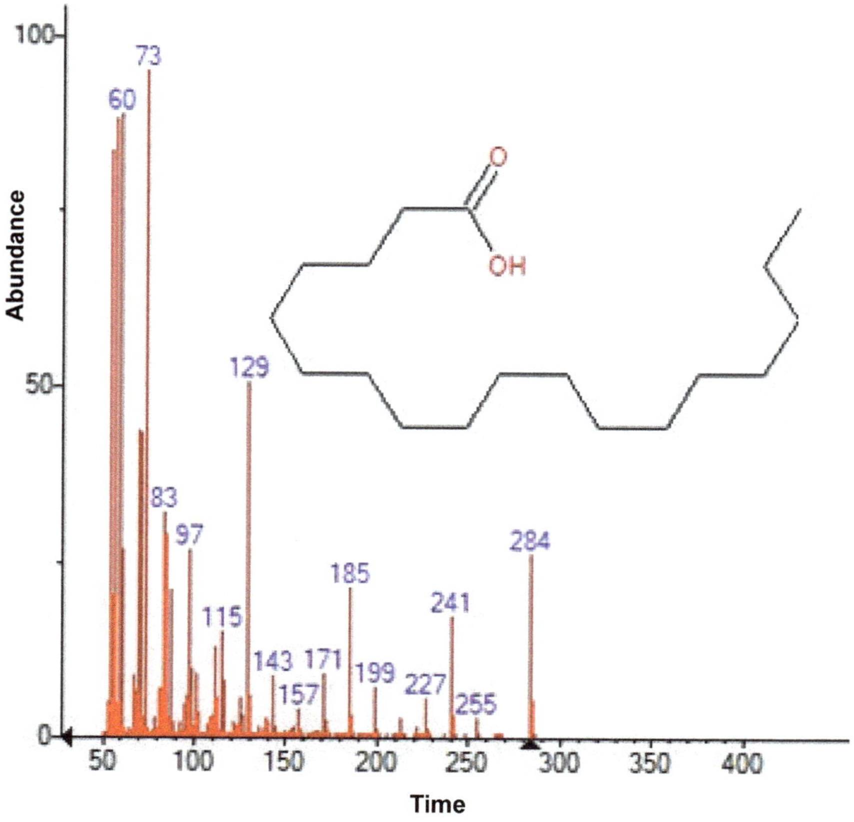

Figure 16. Structure of octadecanoic acid present in the leaves extract of *Solanum nigrum* using GC-MS analysis.

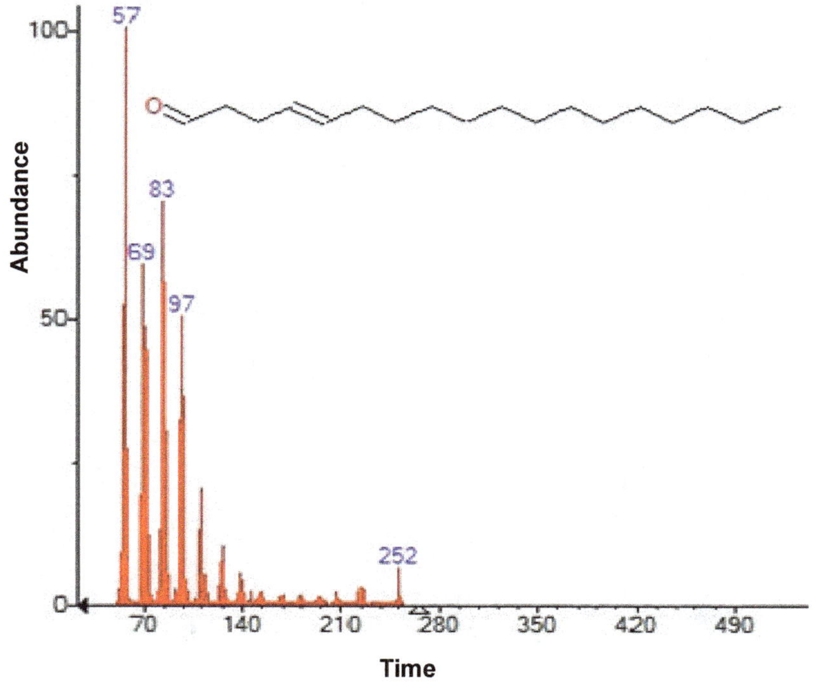

Figure 17. Structure of octadecenal present in the leaves extract of *Solanum nigrum* using GC-MS analysis.

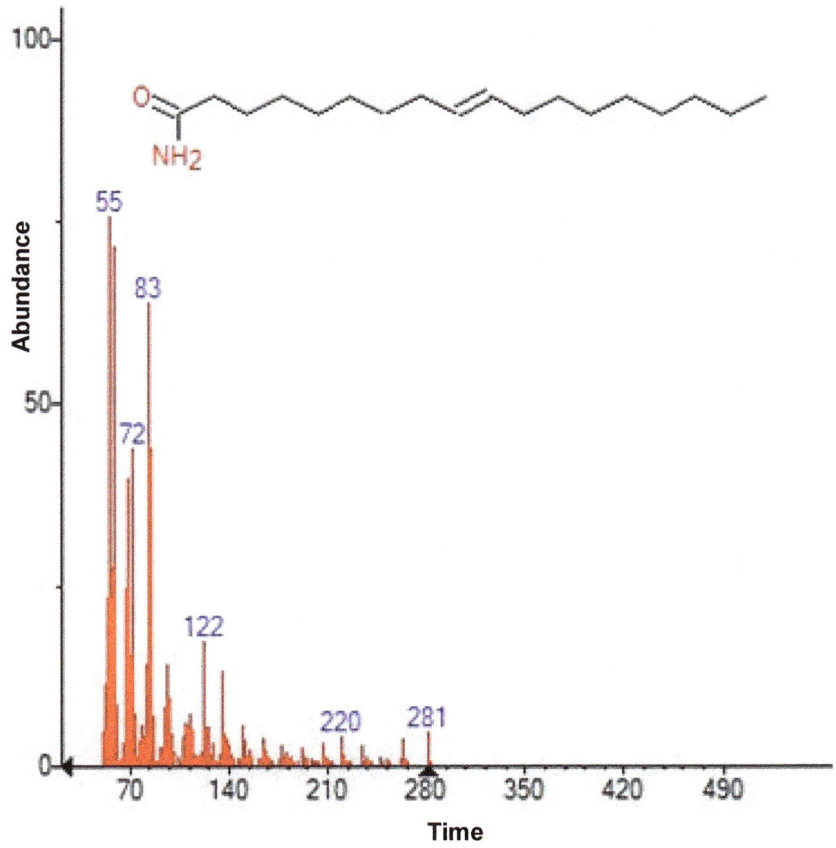

Figure 18. Structure of 9-octadecenamide present in the leaves extract of *Solanum nigrum* using GC-MS analysis.

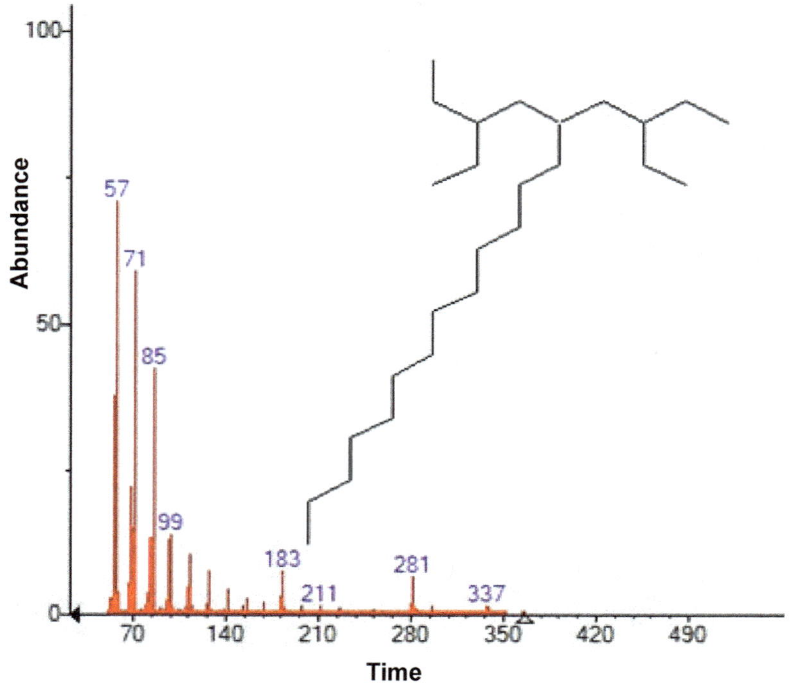

Figure 19. Structure of octadecane, 3-ethyl-5-(ethylbutyl) present in the leaves extract of *Solanum nigrum* using GC-MS analysis.

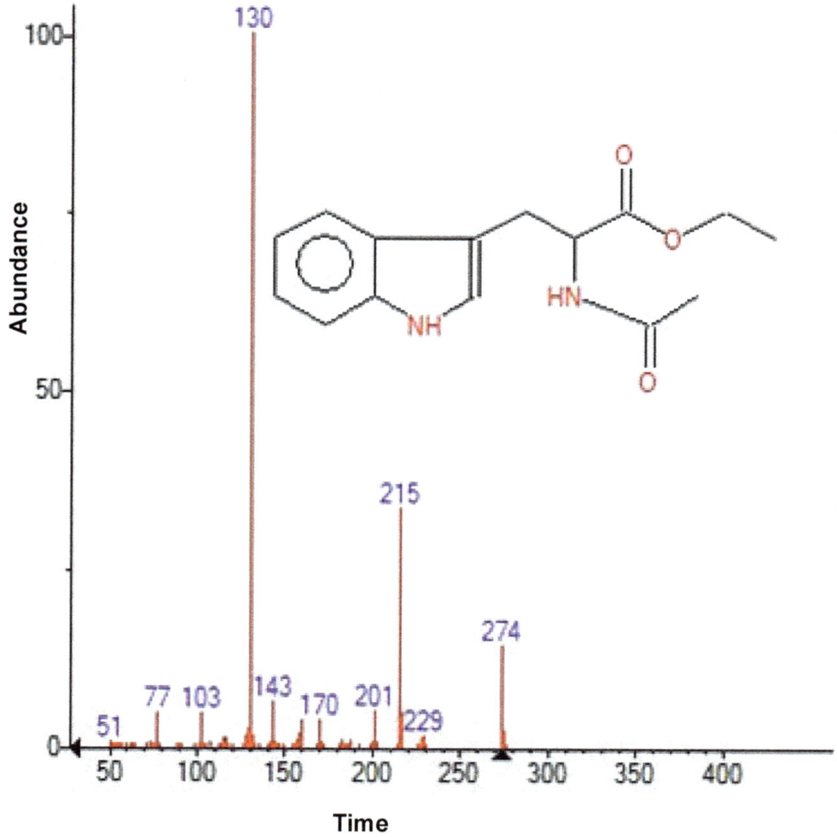

Figure 20. Structure of N-acetyl-L-tryptophan ethyl ester present in the leaves extract of *Solanum nigrum* using GC-MS analysis.

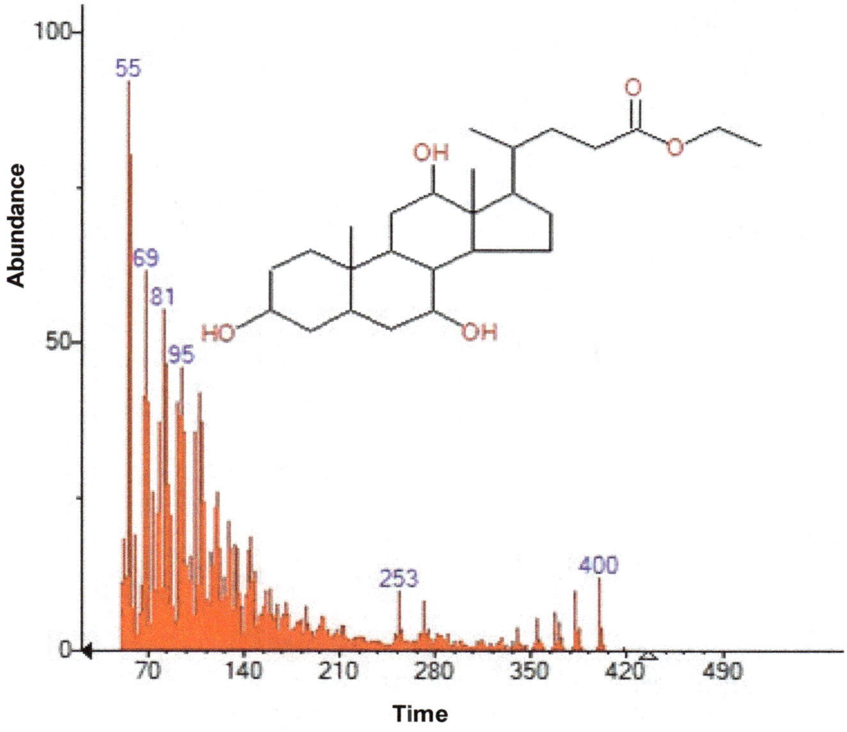

Figure 21. Structure of ethyl iso-allocholate present in the leaves extract of *Solanum nigrum* using GC-MS analysis.

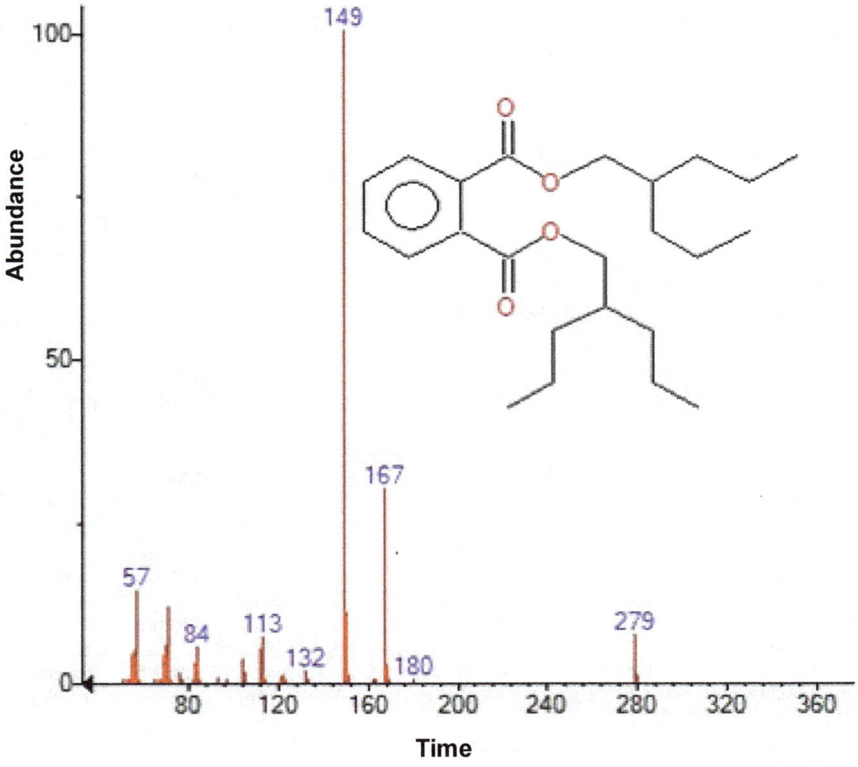

Figure 22. Structure of phthalic acid, di(2-propylpentyl)ester present in the leaves extract of *Solanum nigrum* using GC-MS analysis.

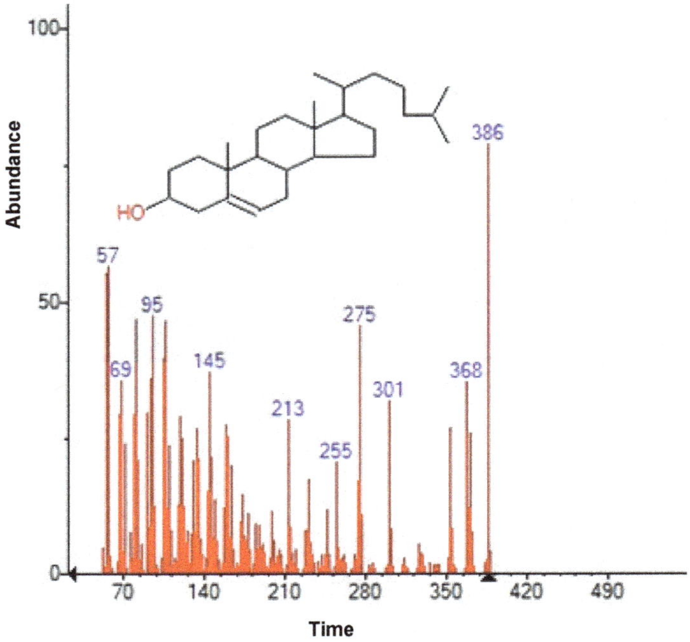

Figure 23. Structure of 17-(1.5-Dimethylhexyl)-10. 13-dimethyl-2.3.4.7.8.9.10.11. 12.13.14.15.16.17-tetradecahydro-1H present in the leaves extract of *Solanum nigrum* using GC-MS analysis.

Conclusion

Twenty three chemical alkaloids constituents have been identified from ethanolic extract of the *S. nigrum* by GC-MS. *In vitro* antibacterial evaluation of *S. nigrum* forms a primary platform for further phytochemical and pharmacological investigation for the development of new potential antimicrobial compounds.

ACKNOWLEDGEMENT

The authors thank Dr. Abdul-Kareem Al-Bermani, Lecturer, Department of Biology, for valuable suggestions and encouragement.

REFERENCES

Ajitha M, Rajanarayana K 2001. Role of oxygen free radicals in human disease. Indian Drugs.38:545-554.

Alves TM, Silva AF, Brandão M, Grandi TS, Smânia E, Smânia Júnior A, Zani C (2000). Biological Screening of Brazilian Medicinal Plants. Memórias do Instituto. Oswaldo Cruz 95:(3)367-373.

Cos P, Vlietinck AJ, Berghe DV, Maes L (2006). Anti-infective potential of natural products: How to develop a stronger in vitro proof-of-concept. J. Ethnopharmacol. 106(3) 290-302.

Evans WC (2002). Trease and Evans Pharmacognosy, 15th edition. WB Saunders Company Ltd, London. Pp. 137-139,230-240.

Haraguchi H, Kataoka S, Okamoto S, Hanafi M, Shibata K (1999). Antimicrobial triterpenes from Ilex integra and the mechanism of antifungal action. Phytother. Residence 13:151-156.

Iwu MW, Duncan AR, Okunji CO (1999). New antimicrobials of plant origin. In: Janick J (ed.), Perspectives on New Crops and New Uses. Alexandria, VA: ASHS Press. pp. 457-462.

John Britto S, Senthilkumar S (2005). Antibacterial activity of Solanum incanum L. leaf extracts. Asian J. Microbiol. Biotech. Environ. Sci. 3:65-66.

Koduru S, Grierson DS, Afolayan AJ (2006). Antimicrobial Activity of *Solanum aculeastrum*. Pharm. Biol. 44:266-283.

Krishnaraju AV, Rao TV, Sundararaju D (2005). Assessment of bioactivity of Indian medicinal plants using Brine shrimp (*Artemia salina*) lethality assay. Int. J. Appl. Sci. Eng. 2:125-134.

Kumar VP, Shashidhara S, Kumar MM, Sridhara BY (2001). Cytoprotective role of Datura Stramonium against gentamicin-induced kidney cell (vero cells) damage in vitro. Fitoterapia 72:481-486.

Misawa M (1994). Plant tissue culture. An alternative for production of useful metabolities. FAO Agriculture Services Bulletin, Rome. No. 108

Ncube NS, Afolayan AJ Okoh AI (2008). Assessment techniques of antimicrobial properties of natural compounds of plant origin: current methods and future trends. Afr. J. Biotechnol. 7(12):1797-1806.

Palombo EA, Semple SJ (2001). Antibacterial activity of traditional Australian medicinal plants. J. Ethnopharmacol. 77(2-3):151-15.

Prescott LM, Harley JP, Klein DN (1999). Microbiology 4th ed. Bistin: The McGraw-Hill Companies Inc. pp. 685.

Purohit SS, Vyas SP (2004). Medicinal plants cultivation a scientific approach including processing and financial guidelines. 1st edition. Publishers Agrobios, Jodhpur, India. pp. 1-3.

Santh RT (2006). Antibacterial activity of *Adhatoda vasica* leaf extract. Asian J. Microbiol. Biotech. Environ. Sci. 8(2):287-289.

Sashikumar JM, Remya M, Janardhanan K (2003). Antimicrobial activity of ethno medicinal plants of Nilgiri biosphere reserve and Western Ghats. Asian J. Microbiol. Biotechnol. Environ. Sci. 5:183-185.

Sazada S, Arti V, Ayaz AR, Fraha J, Mukesh K (2009). Preliminary

phytochemical analysis of some important medicinal and aromatic plants. 3(5-6):188-195.
Singh SK, Saroj K, Tirupathi UJ, Singh AK, Singh RH (1998). An antimicrobial principle from *Speranhtus indicus*. Int. J. Crude Drug 26:235-239.
Stainer RY, Ingraham JL, Wheelis ML (1986). General Microbiology, 5th ed. London: The MacMillan Press Ltd.
Venkatesan M, Vishwanathan MB, Ramesh N, Lakshmanaperumalsamy P (2005). Antibacterial potential from Indian *Suregada angustifolia*. J. Ethnopharmacol. 99(3):349-52.
Stanojević D, Čomić L, Stefanović O (2010). In vitro synergy between Salvia officinalis L. and some preservatives. Cent. Eur. J. Biol. 5 (4) 491-495.
Uzun E, Sariyar G, Adsersen A, Karakoc B, Otük G, Oktayoglu E, Pirildar S (2004). Traditional medicine in Sakarya Province (Turkey) and antimicrobial activities of selected species. J. Ethnopharmacol. 95(2-3):96-287.
Walton J, Brown DE (1999). Chemical from plants, perspectines on plant secondary products. Imperial College Press London UK. 2-5
World Health Organization (2002). WHO Traditional medicine strategy 2002-2005, World Health Organization.

2

Separate and co-administration of *Amaranthus spinosus* and vitamin C modulates cardiovascular disease risk in high fat diet-fed experimental rats

Abayomi S. Faponle[1], Adeleke Atunnise[1], Bukunola O. Adegbesan[1], Olugbenga O. Ogunlabi[1], Kuburat T. Odufuwa[1] and Emmanuel O. Ajani[2*]

[1]Department of Biochemistry, Faculty of Basic Medical Sciences, Ikenne Campus, Obafemi Awolowo College of Health Sciences, Olabisi Onabanjo University, Ago-Iwoye, Nigeria.
[2]Phytomedicine, Toxicology and Drug Development Laboratory, Department of Biosciences and Biotechnology, Kwara state University, Malete, P. M B. 1530, Ilorin, Nigeria.

Report indicates that global death from cardiovascular diseases is more than any other diseases hence research is being intensified to provide scientific data in support of the use of traditional plants for its management. In this study, the efficacy of *Amaranthus spinosus* on lipid disorder occasioned by dietary regimen supplemented with lard and its role in oxidative stress was compared with vitamin C. Forty adult male rats randomized into 5 groups of 8 each were used. Group 1 was the control, while groups 2, 3, 4 and 5 were placed on lard supplemented diet. Leaf extract of *A. spinosus* was administered to rats in groups 3 while group 4 was co-administered with *A. spinosus* and vitamin C. Group 5 was administered with vitamin C alone. The extract was administered at a dose of 250 mg/kg while vitamin C was administered at a dose of 10 UI/kg. All administrations were performed orally as a single dose continuously for 28 days. High fat diet increased malondialdehyde concentration but reduced the concentrations of glutathione (GSH) and the activities of catalase and superoxide dismutase in the heart. It also increased plasma cholesterol, triglyceride, low density lipoprotein (LDL) and very low density lipoprotein (VLDL) cholesterol but lowered high density lipoprotein (HDL) cholesterol concentration. Although, no significant alterations were observed in the cholesterol and triglyceride levels of the heart, there was a significant increase in the atherogenic indices of plasma. Separate and combined administration of *A. spinosus* and vitamin C reverses these unfavorable alterations. The effect of separate administration of *A. spinosus* was also observed in the study to compare effectively with its combined administration with vitamin C. Based on this study, *A. spinosus* may be useful as a base medicine for the management of cardiovascular diseases (CVD) related disorder.

Key words: Atherogenic index, *Amaranthus spinosus,* cardiovascular risk, herbal medicine, high-fat diet, lipoprotein.

INTRODUCTION

Cardiovascular diseases (CVDs) are a class of pathologies involving the heart or blood vessels (arteries, capillaries, and veins). They refer to any disease that affects the cardiovascular system, mainly cardiac diseases, vascular diseases of the brain and kidney, and peripheral arterial disease (Ursula et al., 2014). Reported data (Sydney et al., 2012) indicated that an estimated 17.5 million people died from CVDs in 2012, representing 31% of all global deaths. Of these deaths, an estimated 7.4 million were due to coronary heart disease and 6.7 million were due to stroke and the number is expected to grow to 23.6 million by 2030 (World Health Organization (WHO), 2015). This report is supported by data from previous studies (Ignarro et al., 2007; Burta et al., 2008; Norozi et al., 2011).

Obesity, high blood pressure, insulin resistance, and aging are associated with the development of CVDs (De Marchi et al., 2013). Other important factors are diet, lifestyle, environmental, genetic and epigenetic interactions (Haslam and James, 2002). These factors reflect complex pathological processes in which oxidative stress caused by reactive oxygen species (ROS) plays a pivotal role. Oxidative stress represents an imbalance between reactive oxygen species (ROS) production and the cellular antioxidant defense system. In stress conditions, ROS levels increase, and because of their high reactivity, participate in a variety of chemical reactions. They are involved in cell damage, necrosis and apoptosis via oxidation of lipids, proteins and DNA (Elahi et al., 2009) and provoke also endothelial dysfunction, infiltration and activation of inflammatory cells (Hulsmans et al., 2012). Oxidative stress has been noted to play a central role in the pathogenesis of atherosclerosis and thus a critical feature in atherogenesis (Lee et al., 2012). An increased generation of ROS in the vascular wall and a reduction of nitric oxide (NO) bioavailability lead to endothelial dysfunction in atherogenesis (Lee et al., 2012; Channon and Guzik, 2012). ROS cause damage to cellular structures within the vascular wall, and trigger several redox-sensitive transcriptional pathways, shifting the cell towards a proatherogenic transcriptomic profile.

Increasing evidence indicates that certain natural products can influence the aetiology, progression and treatment of CVD (Osadolor et al., 2005; Amadou et al., 2009; Zuchi et al., 2010; Sahebkar, 2013) and this may occur by modifying risk factors such as obesity, dyslipidaemia as well as factors involved in systemic inflammation, oxidative stress and thrombosis (Parikh et al., 2005; Napoli et al., 2007). The role of dietary fat in health has been under intensive research during the past decades (Ursula et al., 2014). Many observational studies reported that the total amount of dietary fat has only a minor or no effect on the risk of lifestyle diseases such as CVD, type 2 diabetes mellitus (T2DM), and cancer or the level of the risk factors of these diseases, or markers (abdominal adiposity, blood pressure (BP), serum lipid profile, and insulin sensitivity) (Food and Agriculture Organization (FAO), 2010). However, the quality of fat has been shown to have a significant effect on serum lipid profile and blood pressure (BP) (Uusitupa et al., 2013) as well as endothelial function and low-grade inflammation, and these has been shown to affect the risk of CVD (Graham et al., 2007; FAO, 2010; Astrup et al., 2011; Lopez-Garcia et al., 2004; Uusitupa et al., 2013). Current studies are focused at investigating certain neutraciticals with potential to reduce cardiovascular disease risk by improving plasma lipid profile (Cinzia et al., 2010; Norata et al., 2013; Sahebkar et al., 2014).

Amaranthus spinosus L. (prickly amaranthus or water leaf) is known among the Yoruba tribe of Nigeria as "efo tete" or "tete eleegun". It is a medicinal plant under the family of Amaranthaceae and an annual or perennial herb native to Tropical America (Bagepalli et al., 2010). The plant grows in cultivated areas as well as in waste places. The leaves are stacked and alternate (Debiprasad et al., 2013). Medicinal uses of *A. spinosus* as reported in the literatures (Bagepalli et al., 2010; Debriprasad et al., 2013) include: diuretic, stomach disorder, peptic ulcer and anemia (leaf infusion); gonorrhea, eczema and menorrhea (root paste). In some traditional homes in Nigeria, the plant is being used as analgesic, antipyretic, laxative, diuretic, anti-snake venum and antidiabetic.

Although the plant is very popular in the traditional medicine in Nigeria as anti-diabetic and anti- lipidemic agent suggesting that it may be a good agent in the management of cardiovascular diseases, but scientific evidence is lacking in support of this use. The aim of this study therefore is to provide scientific data to validate the use of the plant in the management of cardiovascular disorders and oxidative stress and compare its efficacy with that of vitamin C.

MATERIALS AND METHODS

Preparation of plant extract

Fresh leaves of *A. spinosus* were collected from a local garden in Ikenne, Nigeria in July, 2013. The plant materials were

*Corresponding author. E-mail: emmanuel.ajani@kwasu.edu.ng or ajaniimman@gmail.com.

authenticated at the Department of Plant Science, Faculty of Science, Olabisi Onabanjo University, Nigeria. A voucher number Ars 013 NF was assigned and voucher specimen was thereafter deposited at the Herbarium. Twenty (20) grams of the powderedsample was macerated with 100 ml 70% methanol, filtered, concentrated using rotary evaporator (Yamato Scientific RE301A- W, Tokyo) and lyophilized with Hull brand (SP Scientific Series, USA) freeze-drier. Stock solution was prepared by dissolving the dried extracts in distilled water and was stored at -20°C until used.

Animal handling

Forty male Wistar strain rats, weighing between 150 and 220 g self-reed at the Animal holding, Faculty of Basic Medical Sciences, Olabisi Onabanjo University, Ikenne, Nigeria were used in the study. The animals were kept under ambient condition and were allowed to acclimatize for a week while being fed with standard rat chow (obtained from Animal Care Nig. Ltd) and water *ad libitum*. Experimental animals were handled appropriately as outlined by the guidelines of Experimental Animals Ethics Code of the Faculty of Basic Medical Sciences, Olabisi Onabanjo University, Nigeria. The protocol conforms to the guidelines of the National Institute of Health for laboratory animal care and use (NIH, 2011), and in accordance with the principles of good laboratory procedure (WHO, 1998). The rats were randomly assigned in to 5 groups of 8 rats each. The rats were then treated as follows:

Group 1: Normal control (standard rat chow),
Group 2: Test control (high dietary fat),
Group 3: Test I (high dietary fat and administered with *A. spinosus*, extract),
Group 4: Test II (high-fat fat and administered with *A. spinosus* extract + vitamin c),
Group 5: Test III (high dietary fat and administered with vitamin c).

High fat diet was prepared by supplementing the normal rat chow with 15% lard (Chi et al., 1982). All the rats were fed with their respective diet *ad libitum*. The extract and vitamin C were administered orally using oral intubator at a dose of 250 mg kg^{-1} and 10 UI kg^{-1}, respectively. All administrations were carried out once daily for 28 consecutive days.

Preparation of organ homogenate and blood sample

After the administration of last dose, the rats were fasted for 12 h and then anesthetized in a closed jar of cotton-soaked diethyl ether. Blood was withdrawn from the rats by cardiac puncture after which they were sacrificed by cervical dislocation. The blood samples were collected in heparinized bottles and the heart excised, weighed and stored in buffered petri-dishes before being homogenized in phosphate buffer (pH 7.3) (Paul et al., 2013). Afterwards, blood samples and heart homogenates were centrifuged and supernatant collected for biochemical analyses.

Biochemical assay

Assay for catalase and superoxide dismutase activities was according to the previously described methods of Sinha (1972) and Marklund and Marklund (1974), respectively. Lipid peroxidation was assessed by determining the malondialdehyde as decribed by Varshney and Kale (1990). Reduced glutathione was measured by the method of Beutler et al. (1963). Heart lipid was extracted using the method of Folch et al. (1957). Randox™ diagnostic kits (Randox Laboratories, U.K.) was then used for estimation of the lipid content. Cholesterol and triglyceride were determined enzymatically (Belcher et al., 1991). HDL-cholesterol (HDL-C) was estimated by the HDL precipitant method (Bachorik and Albers, 1996). VLDL-cholesterol (VLDL-C) and LDL-cholesterol (LDL-C) were calculated using Friedewald et al. (1972) formula. Atherogenic index of plasma (AIP) was calculated using the formula of Abot et al. (1998) and coronary risk ratio (CRR) was obtained by the method of Allard et al. (1994).

VLDL-C = Serum triglyceride/2.2,
LDL-C = Total serum cholesterol-Total serum triglycerides/5-Total serum HDL-C,
AIP = Total serum triglycerides/Total serum HDL-C,
CRR = Total cholesterol/HDL-C.

Statistical analysis

Statistical package for social sciences (SPSS) *v*20.0 software package was used for data processing. Data analyses were done with one-way analysis of variance (ANOVA) and level of significance tested at $p \leq 0.05$ with Duncan multiple range test (DMRT).

RESULTS

When compared with the normal control, the result of the lipid peroxidation and antioxidant status (Table 1) showed that increased dietary fat significantly ($p \leq 0.05$) raised the level of malondialdehyde (MDA) in the rat and lowered significantly the level of reduced GSH and catalase activity. Separate administration of *A. spinosus* and vitamin C and when co-administered into rats placed on high dietary fat prevented increase in the level of heart MDA and significantly raised the level of reduced GSH and catalase activity. Although the catalase activity of rats placed on vitamin C (61.59 ± 2.09) was not different from that of those treated with *A. spinosus* (61.09 ± 1.47) and that which was co- administered with vitamin C and *A. spinosus* (65.94 ± 2.17), the level of reduced GSH of rats placed on vitamin C alone (25.97 ± 1.18) was observed to be lower than that of rats placed on *A. spinosus* (29.02 ± 1.58) and that of rats co-administered with vitamin C and *A. spinosus* (28.71 ± 1.18). No significant ($p \geq 0.05$) difference was observed in the superoxide dismutase (SOD) activity of the treated groups when compared among each other and the activities were also not significantly different from that of the control groups. No significant alteration was observed in the total cholesterol and triglyceride level of the heart both with high fat diet and when vitamin C and *A. spinosus* were either separately administered or co-administered to rats placed on high fat diet (Table 2).

Result of plasma lipid profile (Table 3) indicates that

Table 1. Effects of treatment on heart oxidative status.

Group	Treatment	MDA (nmol MDA/g tissue)	Catalase (µg/mg protein) ×10^3	SOD (ng/mg protein) × 10^3	Reduced GSH (µg/g tissue) × 10^3
1 (Normal control)	SRF	5.21 ± 0.19^{a}	54.61 ± 4.45^{a}	3.30 ± 0.01^{a,b}	28.13± 1.16^{a}
2 (Test Control)	HF	6.56 ± 0.08^{b}	25.15 ± 2.90^{b}	3.33 ± 0.00^{b}	22.20 ± 0.46^{b}
3 (Test 1)	HF + AS	5.21 ± 0.08^{a}	61.09 ± 1.47^{c}	3.25 ± 0.02^{a}	29.02 ± 1.58^{a}
4 (Test 2)	HF +As + VC	5.26 ± 0.12^{a}	65.94 ± 2.17^{c}	3.30 ± 0.01^{a,b}	28.71 ± 1.18^{a}
5 (Test 3)	HF + VC	4.56 ± 0.04^{c}	61.59 ± 2.09^{c}	3.32 ± 0.01^{b}	25.97 ± 0.85^{c}

Results presented are mean ± SEM (n=8). Mean values were compared using one-way ANOVA. Level of significance was evaluated using Duncan's multiple range test (DMRT). Value in the same column with similar superscript are not significantly different (p>0.05) from each other. SRF = Standard Rat Feed, HF = High fat diet, AS= *Amaranthus spinosus*, VC = Vitamin C, MDA = Malondialadehyde, SOD = Superoxidedismutase and GSH = Reduced glutathione.

Table 2. Effect of treatment on the heart cholesterol and protein level.

Group	Treatment	Cholesterol (mmol/L)	Triglyceride (mmol/L)	Total protein (mg/dl)
1 (Normal control)	SRF	89.70 ± 3.47^{a}	54.50 ± 0.93^{a}	5.88 ± 0.33^{a}
2 (Test control)	HF	88.70 ± 3.47^{a}	56.17 ± 2.55^{a}	5.46 ± 0.09^{a}
3 (Test 1)	HF + AS	86.90 ± 3.05^{a}	51.79 ± 3.58^{a}	5.20 ± 0.19^{a}
4 (Test 2)	HF + As + VC	82.00 ± 4.64^{a}	57.46 ± 3.27^{a}	5.17 ± 0.18^{a}
5 (Test 3)	HF + VC	87.60 ± 6.99^{a,}	57.17 ± 1.08^{a}	5.22 ± 0.12^{a}

Results presented are mean ± SEM (n=8). Mean values were compared using one-way ANOVA. Level of significance was evaluated using Duncan's multiple range test (DMRT). Value in the same column with similar superscript are not significantly different (p>0.05) from each other. SRF = Standard Rat Feed, HF = High fat diet, AS= *Amaranthus spinosus*, VC = Vitamin C, MDA = Malondialadehyde, SOD = Superoxidedismutase, GSH = Reduced glutathione.

increased dietary fat significantly raised both the total cholesterol concentration (224.56 ± 9.03 mmol/L) and plasma triglyceride concentration (101.30 ± 6.68 mmol/L) significantly ($p \leq 0.05$) above the normal control (133.94 ± 0.95 mmol/L) concentration. Separate treatment with *A. spinosus* and vitamin C and their co-administration prevented this increase. The result also indicates that when separately administered, the concentration of plasma cholesterol of rats treated with vitamin c (158.18 ± 4.08 mmol/L) was significantly higher than that of the rat treated with *A. spinosus* (138.21 ± 0.42 mmol/L), but when co-administered, the plasma cholesterol concentration (126.81 ± 1.24 mmol/L) was lower than that of the rat treated with *A. spinosus* alone. No significant difference was observed in the plasma triglyceride concentration of rat treated with *A. spinosus* alone (67.48 ± 0.96 mmol/L) and that which was co-administered with *A. spinosus* and vitamin C (66.08 ± 4.03 mmol/L). The observed triglyceride concentration in both groups though lower than that of the group placed on high dietary fat without subsequent treatment (101.30 ± 6.68 mmol/L) was significantly higher ($p \leq 0.05$) than the normal control value (58.96 ± 0.36mmol/L). Separate administration of vitamin C also reduced the plasma triglyceride level below that of rats placed on high fat diet without treatment, however, the observed value of 92.16 ± 3.70 mmol/L was still higher than that of the group treated with *A. spinosus*.

Table 3 also indicates that high fat diet significantly ($p \leq 0.05$) increased the plasma LDL-cholesterol above the normal control value but lowered the plasma HDL-Cholesterol significantly ($p \leq 0.05$). There was no significant difference in LDL- concentration for all treatments. The observed plasma HDL-cholesterol concentration of rat separately treated with vitamin C and *A. spinosus* (73.29 ± 0.56 and 86.88 ± 5.41 mmol/L, respectively) were not different from each other and were also not different from that of rats co-administered with *A. spinosus* and vitamin C (74.75 ± 1.26 mmol/L) and the normal control value (79.19 ± 0.77 mmol/L). However, the observed values in all these groups of rats were significantly ($p \geq 0.05$) higher than that of the rats placed on high fat diet but without treatment (30.87 ± 0.04 mmol/L). The result of VLDL- cholesterol concentration followed the same pattern, however the observed VLDL-cholesterol concentration of 23.14 ± 1.03 mmol/L in rats treated with vitamin C alone was significantly higher than that of the rats treated with *A. spinosus* (13.51 ± 0.05

Table 3. Effect of treatment on plasma lipid profile.

Group	Treatment	Cholesterol (mmol/L)	Triglyceride (mmol/L)	LDL-cholesterol (mmol/L)	HDL-cholesterol (mmol/L)	VLDL-cholesterol (mmol/L)
1 (Normal control)	SRF	133.94 ± 0.95^{a}	58.96 ± 0.36^{a}	31.95 ± 1.48^{a}	79.19 ± 0.77^{a}	13.10 ± 0.07^{a}
2 (Test control)	HF	224.56 ± 9.03^{b}	101.30 ± 6.68^{b}	42.43 ± 1.21^{b}	30.87 ± 0.04^{b}	22.09 ± 1.01^{b}
3 (Test 1)	HF + AS	138.21 ± 0.42^{a}	67.48 ± 0.96^{c}	33.84 ± 5.51^{b}	86.88 ± 5.41^{a}	13.51 ± 0.05^{a}
4 (Test 2)	HF + As + VC	126.81 ± 1.24^{c}	66.08 ± 4.03^{c}	38.85 ± 0.82^{b}	74.75 ± 1.26^{a}	13.29 ± 0.61^{a}
5 (Test 3)	HF + VC	$158.18 \pm 4.08^{d,}$	92.16 ± 3.70^{b}	38.46 ± 4.23^{b}	73.29 ± 0.56^{a}	23.14 ± 1.03^{b}

Results presented are mean ± SEM (n=8). Mean values were compared using one-way ANOVA. Level of significance was evaluated using Duncan's multiple range test (DMRT). Value in the same column with similar superscript are not significantly different ($p>0.05$) from each other. SRF = Standard Rat Feed, HF = High fat diet, AS = *Amaranthus spinosus*, VC = Vitamin C, MDA = Malondialadehyde, SOD = Superoxidedismutase, GSH = Reduced glutathione.

mmol/L) alone and that of rats co-administered with *A. spinosus* and vitamin C (13.29 ± 0.61 mmol/L).

Table 4 shows that high fat diet significantly ($p \geq 0.05$) increased the atherogenic indices (atherogenic risk index of plasma, AIP and coronary risk ratio, CRR). However, in rats placed on high fat diet and separately treated with *A. spinosus,* the AIP (0.81 ± 0.01) and CRR (1.60 ± 0.03) were not significantly different ($p \geq 0.05$) from those of the normal control value (0.77 ± 0.01 and 1.68 ± 0.01, respectively). Similarly, the observed AIP (0.89 ± 0.05) and CRR (1.70 ± 1.10) in rats co administered with *A spinosus* and vitamin C, were not different from that of the normal control value. Although the AIP and CRR was reduced during treatment with vitamin C alone (when compared with the normal control value), the observed values were significantly higher than those observed in the normal control group.

DISCUSSION

Cardiovascular disease is currently one of the world's leading causes of death (Ikewuchi and Ikewuchi, 2009). One of the major risk factors for the development of cardiovascular disease is dyslipidemia (American Diabetic Association, 2004; Shen, 2007). Dyslipidemia usually involve elevated plasma levels of triglycerides, total cholesterol, LDL and VLDL-cholesterol and a low level of HDL-cholesterol (Howard, 1987; Lekin and Lipsky, 2003; American Diabetic Association, 2004). Our result indicates that lard is a dietary fat capable of predisposing to cardiovascular disease. This is indicated by increased plasma cholesterol, triglyceride, LDL-cholesterol and VLDL-cholesterol and a reduce HDL-cholesterol observed in the study when rats were placed on lard supplemented diet. Lard is an animal fat which contains saturated fatty acid. Over the years, studies had reported an association between intake of dietary saturated fatty acids (SFA) and serum cholesterol levels (Mensink et al., 2003; Lukas and George, 2014) Therefore, any nutritional and pharmacologic intervention that improves or normalizes abnormal lipid metabolism may be useful in reducing the risk of cardiovascular diseases. Data from our study thus support this assertion.

Presently, several drugs are available for the management of dyslipidemia. However, there is renewed interest in the use of herbal products (Mudhaffar, 2013; Assmann et al., 2008). This is partly due to the perceived safety of herbal drug and poverty level particularly among the rural populace. Report from the present study indicates that *A. spinosus* leaves contain phytochemicals capable of ameliorating symptoms of cardio-vascular disease. Rats treated with the extract while subsisting on high fat diet showed a reduced level of triglyceride, plasma total cholesterol, plasma LDL-cholesterol and VLDL-cholesterol and an increased level of plasma HDL-cholesterol when compared with those not treated with the extract. A high plasma triglyceride level is both an independent and synergistic risk factor for cardiovascular diseases (Dobiasova, 2004; McBride, 2007) and is often associated with hypertension, abnormal lipoprotein metabolism, obesity, insulin resistance and diabetes mellitus (Ostlund and Lin, 2007; McBride, 2007).

Our study demonstrated a reduction in triglyceride level occasioned by *A. spinosus* in rats

Table 4. Effect of Treatment on Atherogenic and Coronary Risk Indices.

Group	Treatment	AI	CRR
1 (Normal control)	SRF	0.77 ± 0.01	1.68 ± 0.01
2 (Test control)	HF	3.45 ± 0.05	7.45 ± 0.12
3 (Test 1)	HF + AS	0.81 ± 0.01	1.60 ± 0.03
4 (Test 2)	HF + AS + VC	0.89 ± 0.05	1.70 ± 0.10
5 (Test 3)	HF + VC	1.26 ± 0.06	2.16 ± 0.05

Results presented are mean ± SEM (n=8). Mean values were compared using one-way ANOVA. Level of significance was evaluated using Duncan's multiple range test (DMRT). Value in the same column with similar superscript are not significantly different (p>0.05) from each other. SRF = Standard Rat Feed, HF = High fat diet, AS = *Amaranthus spinosus*, VC = Vitamin C, MDA = Malondialadehyde, SOD = Superoxidedismutase, GSH = Reduced glutathione, AI = Atherogenic Index, CRR: Coronary Risk Index.

placed on high fat diet. We also observed that along with triglyceride and total cholesterol, *A. spinosus* also caused significant reduction in plasma LDL-cholesterol and VLDL-cholesterol and an increase in LDL-cholesterol, suggesting that it is a potent agent in reducing risk of cardiovascular disease. This is in conformity with reports from previous study which indicated that an elevated LDL-cholesterol concentration in plasma is atherogenic (Rang et al., 2005; Lichtennstein et al., 2006; Martirosyan et al., 2007), whereas, a high HDL-cholesterol level is cardioprotective (Miller and Miller, 1977; Assmann et al., 2008).

Atherogenic indices are powerful indicators of the risk of heart disease and have been successfully used as an additional index when assessing cardiovascular (CV) risk factors: the higher the value, the higher the risk of developing cardiovascular disease and *vice versa* (Frohlich and Dobiasova, 2003; Dobiasova, 2004; Brehm et al., 2004; Takasaki, 2005). AIP values of −0.3 to 0.1 are associated with low, 0.1 to 0.24 with medium and above 0.24 with high CV risk (Dobiasova, 2006). Observation from our study indicates that high fat diet increases atherogenic indices (AI and CRR) suggesting that high fat diet predisposes to cardiovascular diseases. *A. spinosus* was observed to significantly reduce atherogenic indices (CRR and AIP). The effect produced by separate administration of the extract was not different from that observed with co-administration of the extract and vitamin C. Although separate administration of vitamin c was also observed in our study to also reduce atherogenic indices, the effect was however not as pronounced as it was with *A. spinosus*. In an attempt to be able to investigate the role of oxidative stress in the development of CVD and the possible mechanism by which *A. spinosus* ameliorates the disorder, we assessed the oxidative status of the heart during treatment. Result from the study indicate that rats placed on high fat diet showed increased MDA level, decreased catalase activity and decrease reduced glutathione concentration. Administration of *A. spinosus* during treatment however prevented increase in malondialdehyde level and also boosted the antioxidant status. Thus, this suggests that the extract is capable of reducing oxidative stress induced by high dietary fat.

The imbalance between ROS production and the cellular antioxidant defense system resulting from oxidative stress has been implicated in cell damage, necrosis and apoptosis via oxidation of lipids, proteins and DNA (Elahi et al., 2009) and provoke also endothelial dysfunction, infiltration and activation of inflammatory cells (Hulsmans et al., 2012). Studies have reported that oxidative stress has a central role in the pathogenesis of atherosclerosis and that it is indeed a critical feature in atherogenesis (Liao et al., 1994; Elahi et al., 2009; Lee et al., 2012). An increased generation of ROS in the vascular wall and a reduction of nitric oxide (NO) bioavailability lead to endothelial dysfunction in atherogenesis (Lee et al., 2012). ROS cause damage to cellular structures within the vascular wall, and trigger several redox-sensitive transcriptional pathways, shifting the cell towards a proatherogenic transcriptomic profile. Animal models of atherosclerosis demonstrate the involvement of ROS in atherosclerosis by the accumulation of lipid peroxidation products (Liao et al., 1994). This is supported by the report from our study when we observed increased MDA level with increased fat diet. ROS and reactive nitrogen species (RNS) produced by the endothelium promote oxidative modification of low density lipoprotein in the phase that precedes the transfer into the subendothelial space of the arterial wall, where they initiate atherosclerosis (Stocker and Keaney, 2004). Data from our study thus suggest that *A. spinosus* contains bioactive component which has antioxidative potential and thus is able to mop up these ROS and prevent subsequent damage to the cellular macromolecules.

Studies on the stem bark extract of *A. spinosus* identified the betalains isolated from the bark of the plant as amaranthin, isoamaranthine, hydroxycinnamates, rutin, quercetin and kaempferol glycosides (Stintzing et al., 2004; Ashok et al., 2008). Betalains are well known for their antioxidant, anticancer, antiparasitosis and antiviral properties (Hussain et al., 2008). Our study thus suggests the antioxidant properties of *A. spinosus* as a basis for its cardioprotective effect. This agrees with previous reports on cardiovascular protective effect of *Vaccinium meridionale* (Yasmin et al., 2013), *Phyllanthus emblica* and *Piper rostratum* (Wattanpitayakul et al., 2005) and methanolic extract of *Amaranthus viridis* (Saravanan et al., 2013).

Conclusion

Our study showed antihyperlipidaemic effect of *A. spinosus*, indicating a possible protective mechanism of the plant against the development of atherosclerosis and coronary heart disease in high fat fed rat. The study also lends support to the antioxidative potential of the plant and suggests that this is the mechanism by which it serves as a cardioprotective agent. Provided animal to human extrapolation is allowed, our result suggests that the plant may be recommended as base medicine for use in managing cardiovascular diseases and in the development of drug against cardiac related disorder.

REFERENCES

Abot RD, Wilson PWB, Castelli WP (1998). HDL-cholesterol, total cholesterol screening and myocardial infarction. Arteriosclerosis 8:207-211.

Allard JP, Royall D, Kurian R, Muggh R, Jeejeebhoy KN (1994). Effects of β-Carotene supplementation on lipid peroxidation in human. Am. J. Clin. Nutr. 59:884-890.

Amadou IS, Yong-Hui S, Sun J, Guo-Wei L (2009). Fermented soybean products: Some methods, antioxidants compound extraction and their scavenging activity. Asian J. Biochem. 4:68-76.

American Diabetic Association (2004). Dyslipidemia management in adults with diabetes. Diabetes Care 27:S68-S71

Ashok KBS, Lakshman K, Chandrasekhar KB, Saleemulla K, Narayana SVB (2008). Estimation of rutin and quercetin in *Amaranthus spinosus* L. Asian J. Chem. 20:1633-1635.

Assmann GH, Schulte H, Funke E, Eckardstein A (2008). The emergence of triglycerides as a significant independent risk factor in coronary artery disease. Eur. Heart J. 19 (suppl M):M8-M14.

Astrup AJ, Dyerberg J, Elwood P, Hermansen K, Hu FB, Jakobsen MU (2011). The role of reducing intakes of saturated fat in the prevention of cardiovascular disease: where does the evidence stand? Am. J. Clin. Nutr. 93:684-688.

Bachorik PS, Albers JJ (1996). Precipitation methods for quantification of lipoproteins. In: Methods in Enzymology, Albers JJ and Segrest JP (eds), Academic Press, Orlando,129 (Part B) pp. 78-100.

Bagepalli SAK, Kuruba L, Jayaveera KN, Devangam SS, Avalakondarayappa AK, Bachappa M. Antioxidant and antipyretic properties of methanolic extract of *Amaranthus spinosus* leaves. Asian Pac. J. Trop. Med. 3(9):702-706.

Belcher JD, McNamara JR, Grinstead GF, Rifai N, Warnick GR, Bachorik P, Frantz I (1991). Measurement of cholesterol concentration. In: Methods for Clinical laboratory Measurements of Lipid and Lipoprotein Risk Factors. Rifai N, Warnick GR (eds) AACC Press, Washington pp. 75-86.

Beutler EO, Duron D, Kelly BM (1963). Improved method for the determination of blood glutathione. J. Lab. Clin. Med. 61:882-888.

Brehm AG, Pfeiler B, Pacini G, Vierhapper H, Roden M (2004). Relationship between serum lipoprotein ratios and insulin resistance in obesity. Clin. Chem. 50:2316-2322.

Burta OF, Tirlea OL, Quadri SM (2008). Phytotherapy in cardiovascular diseases: from ethnomedicine to evidence based medicine. J. Biol. Sci. 8:242-247.

Channon KM, Guzik TJ (2012). Mechanisms of superoxide production in human blood vessels: relationship to endothelial dysfunction, clinical and genetic risk factors. J. Physiol. Pharmacol. 53:515-524.

Cinzia Z, Giuseppe A, Thomas FL, Ulf L (2010). Nutraceuticals in cardiovascular prevention: lessons from studies on endothelial function. Cardiovasc. Ther. 28:187-201

Debiprasad GM, Prasenjit G, Tanaya R, Prasanta KM (2013). Anti peptic ulcer activity of the leaves of *Amaranthus spinosus* Lin rats. Mint. J. Pharm. Med. Sci. 1:52-53.

De Marchi E, Baldassari F, Bononi A, Wieckowski MR, Pinton P (2013). Oxidative Stress in Cardiovascular Diseases and Obesity: Role of p66Shc and Protein Kinase C. Oxid. Med. Cell. Longev. 2013: 564961.

Dobiasova M (2006). AIP-atherogenic index of plasma as a significant predictor of cardiovascular risk: from research to practice. Vnitr. Lek. 52:64-71.

Dobiasova M (2004). Atherogenic index of plasma: Theoretical and practical implications. Clin. Chem. 50:1113-1115.

Elahi MM, Kong YX, Matata BM (2009). Oxidative stress as a mediator of cardiovascular disease. Oxid. Med. Cell. Longev. 2:259-269.

FAO (2010). Fats and fatty acids in human nutrition. Report of an expert consultation. 10–14 November 2008, Geneva. FAO Food and Nutrition Paper 91. Rome: Food and Agricultural Organisation of the United Nations.

Folch JM, Less M, Sloanestanley GH (1957). A simple method for the isolation and purification of total lipid from animal tissues. J. Biol. Chem. 226:497-501.

Friedewald WT, Levy RI, Fredrickson DS (1972). Estimation of the concentration of low density lipoprotein cholesterol in plasma, without use of the preparative ultracentrifuge. Clin. Chem. 18:499-502.

Frohlich J, Dobiásová M (2003). Fractional Esterification Rate of Cholesterol and Ratio of Triglycerides to HDL-Cholesterol Are Powerful Predictors of Positive Findings in Coronary Angiography. Clin. Chem. 49:1873-1880.

Graham I, Atar D, Borch-Johnsen K,Boysen G,Burell G, Cifkova R (2007). European guidelines on cardiovascular disease prevention in clinical practice: full text. Fourth Joint Task Force of the European Society of Cardiology and other societies on cardiovascular disease prevention in clinical practice (constituted by representatives of nine societies and by invited experts). Eur. J. Cardiovasc Prev. Rehabil. 14 (Suppl 2):S1-113.

Howard BV (1987). Lipoprotein metabolism in diabetes mellitus. J. Lipid Res. 28:613-628.

Hulsmans MED, Van N, Holvoet P (2012). Mitochondrial reactive oxygen species and risk of atherosclerosis. Curr. Atheroscler. Rep. 14:264-276.

Hussain ZG, Amresh S, Satyawan R, Chandana VR (2008). Hepatoprotective activity of *Amarnathus spinosus* in experimental animals. Food Chem. Toxicol. 46:3419-3421.

Ignarro L, Balestrier ML, Napol C (2007). Nutrition, physical activity and cardiovascular disease: an update. Cardiovasc. Res. 73:326-340.

Ikewuchi CJ, Ikewuchi CC (2009). Alteration of Plasma Lipid Profiles and Atherogenic Indices by *Stachytarpheta jamaicensis* L. (Vahl). Clin. Chem. 18:499-502

Lee RM, Margaritis KM, Channon M, Antoniades C (2012). Evaluating oxidative stress in human cardiovascular disease: methodological aspects and considerations. Curr. Med. Chem. 19:2504-2520.

Lekin JB, Lipsky MS (2003). American Medical Association Complete Medical Encyclopedia. Random House References: New York pp. 154-159

Liao FA, Andalibi JH, Qiao H, Allayee AM, Fogelman M, Lusis AJ, (1994). Genetic evidence for a common pathway mediating oxidative stress, inflammatory gene induction, and aortic fatty streak formation in mice. J. Clin. Invest. 94:877-884.

Lichtennstein AH, Appel LJ, Brands M, Carnethon M, Daniels S, Franklin B, Kris-Etherton P, Harris WS, Howard B, Karanja M, Lefevre M, Rudel L, Sacks F, van Horn L, Winston M, Wylie-Rosett J, Franch HA (2006). Diet and Lifestyle Recommendations Revision 2006. A Scientific Statement from the American Heart Association Nutrition Committee. Circulation 114:82-96.

Lopez-Garcia EMB, Schulze JE, Manson J, Meigs B, Albert CM, Rifai N (2004). Consumption of (n-3) fatty acids is related to plasma biomarkers of inflammation and endothelial activation in women. J. Nutr. 134:1806-1811.

Lukas SH, Georg H (2014). Dietary fatty acids in the secondary prevention of coronary heart disease: a systematic review, meta-analysis and meta-regression. BMJ 4:4-11.

Marklund S, Marklund G (1974). Involvement of the superoxide anion radical in the autoxidation of pyrogallol and a convenient assay for superoxide dismutase. Eur. J. Biochem. 47:469-474.

Martirosyan DM, Miroshnichenko LA, Kulokawa SN, Pogojeva AV, Zoloedov VI (2007). Amaranth oil application for heart disease and hypertension. Lipids Health Dis. 6:1-8.

McBride PE (2007). Triglycerides and Risk for Coronary Heart Disease. Curr. Atheroscler. Rep. 10(5):386-90.

Mensink RP, Zock PL, Kester AD (2003). Effects of dietary fatty acids and carbohydrates on the ratio of serum total to HDL cholesterol and on serum lipids and apolipoproteins: a meta-analysis of 60 controlled trials. Am. J. Clin. Nutr. 77:1146-1155.

Miller GJ, Miller NE (1977). Plasma high density lipoprotein concentration and development of ischaemic heart disease. Lancet 1:16-18.

Mudhaffar SK (2013). Atherogenic Index of Plasma (AIP) As a Parameter in Predicting Cardiovascular Risk in Males Compared To the Conventional Dyslipidemic Indices (Cholesterol Ratios). Karbala J. Med. 6:123-127.

Napoli CL, Aderiye OBL, Akele O (2007). Hypocholesterolemia activity of nono in albino rats. Int. J. Dairy Sci. 2:393-397.

NIH (2011). Guide for Care and Use of Laboratory Animals. 11th Edition. National Academies Press, Washington, DC. pp. 43-48.

Norata GD, Ballantyne CM, Catapano AL (2013). New therapeutic principles in dyslipidaemia: focus on LDL and Lp(a) lowering drugs. Eur. Heart J. 34:1783-1789.

Osadolor HB, Orhue NEJ, Nwokocha CR (2005). Serum Lipids and Lipoproetins Profile in Hypertensive Patients Reporting for Treatment at Central Hospital, Benin City, Nigeria. Int. J. Med. Sci. 5(4):284-288

Ostlund RE Jr., Lin X (2007). Regulation of cholesterol absorption by phytosterols. Curr. Atheroscler. Rep. 8:487-491

Parikh P, McDaniel MC, Ashen MD, Muller JI, Sorentuib M (2005). Diets and carbohydrate diseases: An evidence based assessment. J. Am. Cardiol. 45:1379-1387.

Paul S, Ghosh D, Ghosh AK, Mitra E, Dey M, Chattopahyya A (2013). Lead induces oxidative stress in rat heart and liver tissue homogenates: an *in vitro* study. J. Cell Tissue Res. 13:3829-3837.

Rang HP, Dale MM, Ritter JM, Moore PK(2005). Pharmacology. 5th ed. Elsevier: India. pp. 229-235.

Sahebkar A (2013). Why it is necessary to translate curcumin into clinical practice for the prevention and treatment of metabolic syndrome? Biofactors 39:197-208.

Sahebkar A, Chew GT, Watts GF (2014). Recent advances in pharmacotherapy for hypertriglyceridemia. Prog. Lipid. Res. 56:47-66

Saravanan G, Ponmurugan P, Sathivavathi M, Vadivukkarasi S, Sengottuvelu S (2013). Cardioprotective activity of Amaranthus viridis Linn: effect on serum marker enzymes, cardiac troponin and antioxidant system in experimental myocardial infarcted rats. Int. J. Cardiol. 165:494-498.

Shen GX (2007). Lipid disorders in diabetes mellitus and current management. Curr. Pharmaceut. Anal. 3:17-24.

Sydney CS, Amy C, Roberto F, David R, Holmes S, Susanne L, Diana VM, Johanna R, Ralph L, Sacco H, Kathryn T, David AW, William AZ (2012). Our Time: A Call to Save Preventable Death From Cardiovascular Disease (Heart Disease and Stroke). J. Am. Coll. Cardiol. 60:2342-2348.

Sinha AK (1972). Colorimetric assay of catalase. Anal. Biochem. 47: 389-394.

Stintzing FC, Kammerer D, Schieber A, Hilou A, Nacoulma O, Carle R (2004). Betacyanins and phenolic compounds from *Amaranthus spinosus* L., and *Boerhaavia erecta*. Z. Naturforsch C. 59:1-8.

Stocker R, Keaneyn JF (2004). Role of oxidative modifications in atherosclerosis. Physiol. Rev. 84:1381-1478.

Takasaki Y (2005). Serum Lipid Levels and Factors Affecting atherogenic Index in Japanese Children. J. Physiol. Anthropol. Appl. Human Sci. 24:511-515.

Ursula S, Lotte L, Tine T, Thorhallur I, Haldorsson R, Matti U, Wulf B (2014). Effect of the amount and type of dietary fat on cardiometabolic risk factors and risk of developing type-2 diabetes, cardiovascular disease, and cancer: a systematic review. Food Nutr. Res. 58:25145-25152

Uusitupa MK, Hermansen H, Savolainen MJ, Schwab U, Kolehmainen M, Brader L (2013). Effects of an isocaloric healthy Nordic diet on insulin sensitivity, lipid profile and inflammation markers in metabolic syndrome – a randomized study (SYSDIET). J. Intern. Med. 274:52-66.

Varshney R, Kale RK (1990). Effects of calmodulin antagonists on radiation-induced lipid peroxidation in microsomes. Int. J. Radiat. Biol. 58:33-43.

Wattanpitayakul SK, Chularojnontri L, Herunsale A, Charuchongkolwongse S, Niumsakul S, Bauer JA (2005). Screening of antioxidants from medicinal plants for cardioprotective effect against doxorubicin toxicity. Basic Clin. Pharmacol. Toxicol. 96:80-87

WHO (1998). Basic OECD principles of GLP. World Health Organization, Geneva, Switzerland. 70-79.

WHO (2015). Global action plan for the prevention and control of NCDs 2013-2020. WHO fact sheet. No 317.

Yasmin EL, Juliana F, Luisa FG, Benjamín R, José LR, Guillermo S, Susana M (2013). Antioxidant Activity and Cardioprotective Effect of a Nonalcoholic Extract of *Vaccinium meridionale* Swartz during Ischemia-Reperfusion in Rats. Evid-Based. Compl. Altern. Med. 516727-516737.

Zuchi C, Ambrosio G, Lüscher TF, Landmesser U (2010). Nutraceuticals in cardiovascular prevention: lessons from studies on endothelial function. Cardiovasc Ther. 28:187-201.

Pharmacological properties of *Pomaria sandersonii, Pentanisia prunelloides* and *Alepidea amatymbica* extracts using *in vitro* assays

Muleya, E.[1, 2]*, Ahmed, A. S.[2], Sipamla, A. M.[1], Mtunzi, F. M.[1] and Mutatu, W.[3]

[1]Department of Chemistry, Vaal University of Technology, P. Bag 021, Vanderbijlpark, 1900, South Africa.
[2]Phytomedcine Programme, University of Pretoria, P. Bag X04, 0110, Onderstepoort, South Africa.
[3]Midlands State University, P. Bag 9055, Gweru, Zimbabwe.

The antimicrobial, anti-inflammatory and free radical scavenging activities of root crude acetone extracts and fractions of different polarities from *Pomaria sandersonii* (Fabaceae), *Pentanisia prunelloides* (Rubiaceae) and *Alepidea amatymbica* (Apiaceae) were determined using *in vitro* assays. The antioxidant properties of extracts and fractions were assessed by reduction of 2, 2´-azinobis (3-ethylbenzothiazoline)-6-sulfonic acid and 2, 2-di (4-*tert*-octylphenyl)-1-picrylhydrazyl radicals which was measured by changes in absorbance using an ultraviolet-visible spectrophotometer. Anti-inflammatory activity of the plant extracts against 15 soybean lipoxygenase enzyme was measured by monitoring the change in absorbance at 234 nm after incubation of 15-LOX with linoleic acid (134 µM) as substrate. The anti-microbial activities were determined by measuring the minimum inhibitory concentrations using a serial dilution microplate method with terazolium violet as a growth indicator. The minimal inhibitory concentration (MIC) value of the dichloromethane (DCM) and ethyl acetate fractions (1 mg/ml) of *P. sandersonii* was 80 µg/ml in each case against *Staphylococcus aureus* and *Escherichia coli*. The inhibition activity of 15 soybean lipoxygenase enzyme by the crude extracts at concentration of 25 µg/ml was 97% for *P. sandersonii*, 79% for *P. prunelloides* and 55% for *A. amatymbica*. This indicates that extracts for these plants can be used as dietary supplements in the management of inflammation related conditions.

Key words: Extract, fraction, anti-inflammatory, antibacterial, anti-oxidant, antifungal, antioxidant.

INTRODUCTION

The pathogenic bacteria associated with some diseases in many communities/settlements in South Africa include *Escherichia coli* (gastroenteritis); *Enterococcus faecalis* (endocarditis), *Pseudomonas aeruginosa* (inflammation, sepsis in the lungs, urinary tract and kidneys) and *Staphylococcus aureus* (tonsillitis, scarlet fever, minor skin infections, impetigo, boils, abscesses and scalded skin syndrome) (Hamer, 2007). Some of the fungal pathogens also associated with diseases in the community include *Candida albicans,* which are important

*Corresponding author. E-mail: e_muleya@yahoo.co.uk.

opportunistic yeast involved in oropharyngeal and genital candidiasis (Pfaller and Diekemer, 2004). *Aspergillus fumigatus* is implicated in causing a range of diseases called aspergillosis whose symptoms include cough, fever, wheezing, skin sore and vision problems (Walsh et al., 2008).

In Zululand of South Africa, the use of medicinal plants for prevention and cure of different ailments is well established as part of their cultural heritage. *Alepidea amatymbica* Eckl. & Zeyh. (Apiaceae) is one of the most important species used as medicinal plant in KwaZulu-Natal (KZN) of South Africa and Lesotho (van Wyk, 2008). The rhizomes and roots of *A. amatymbica* (known as Ikhathazo) are used for the treatment of colds and chest complaints (Watt and Breyer, 1962). The plant is used in treating gastrointestinal disorder, respiratory tract infection, hypertension and constipation (Hutchings, 1989). The antimicrobial, cyclooxygenase-1 and 2, genotoxicity (Mulaudzi et al., 2009) and antiplasmodial activity (Clarkson et al., 2004) of *A. amatymbica* root extracts have been reported before. Phytochemical investigation of the root and aerial part of the plant revealed the presence of ent-9, (11)-dehydro-16-kauren-19-oic acid, ent-16-kauren-19-oic acid (Rustaiyan and Sadjadi, 1987) which may be the active compounds. Kaurenoic acid isolated from *Helichrysum krausii* is active against *S. aureus*, *Bacillus cereus*, *Bacillus subtilis* (MIC 10 µg/ml), *Escherichia coli* and *S. marcescens* (1 to 10 µg/ml) (Bremner and Meyer, 2000). However, there is no report on antioxidant activities of extracts and fractions from *A. amatymbica.*

Pentanisia prunelloides (Kotzeh ex Eckl & Zeyh.) Walp. (Rubiaceae) also features as a prominent medicinal plant for treating ailment associated with inflammation, microbial infection, muscular contraction stomach pain haemorrhoids, snakebite and rheumatism in Zulu traditional medicine (Hutchings et al., 1996). Boiled grated dried bulb is usually taken orally to stop vomiting and diarrhoea in children (Bisi-Johnson et al., 2009). Anti-microbial, cytotoxicity and cyclooxygenase-1 enzyme inhibitory activity of the plant has been reported (Jager et al., 1996). Root and leaf extracts of *P. prunelloides* inhibit COX-1 and the viral replication of the influenza A virus (Yff et al., 2002). Pharmacological investigation of the plant has led to the isolation of palmitic acid as the anti-microbial agent (Yff et al., 2002). *Pomaria sandersonii* (Fabacea) (Harv) B. B. Simpson and G. P. Lewis is also used in Zulu traditional medicine for pain, inflammation and anti-haemolytic activity (Dlamini personal communication). It is endemic to South Africa, grows in the Eastern Cape, KwaZulu- Natal region. It is on the red list of South African plants (Raimondo et al., 2009). This is the first time of recording the ethno pharmacological use of the plant in southern Africa. There is no scientific report on the biological activities of extracts from *P. sandersonii.*

The aim of this study was to scientifically validate the traditional use of *P. prunelloides* (Rubiaceae), *P. sandersonii* (Fabaceae) and *A. amatymbica* (Apiaceae) in treating infections and oxidative stress relating to inflammation. Therefore, this work focuses on the antibacterial, antifungal, antioxidant (DPPH and ABTS radical scavenging assays) and anti-inflammatory activity of the crude extracts and their fractions of different polarities.

MATERIALS AND METHODS

Plant selection and collection

An ethnobotanical survey based on verbal interviews conducted with nine traditional healers of Mabandla village of Umzimkhulu Local Municipality, Kwa-Zulu Natal, South Africa (30° 15′ 45″ S, 29° 55′ 15″ E) for plants used traditionally in the treatment of infectious and inflammatory diseases was carried out. The plants listed in Table 1 were identified and collected with the help of Mr. Sanoyi Paulos Dlamini the head of traditional healers from the village. Authentication of plants was done at South Africa National Biodiversity Institute, Pretoria and their voucher specimens are maintained at Pretoria National Botanical Garden.

Plant treatment

Plant root and bulb materials collected from Mabandla village, Kwa-Zulu Natal, were washed, air dried at room temperature for three weeks and ground to powder using a Lasec Polymix PX-MFC 90D grinder. Dried plant pulverised material was stored in glass containers in a cool dry place. Crude extracts were made by shaking fine ground plant powder (200 g) in a ratio of 1 g to 10 ml acetone for 6 h followed by filtering (Eloff, 1998a). Excess solvent was recovered on a rotary vapour until the extract was concentrated. Concentrated slurry was dried at room temperature in the fume hood under an air stream. The crude dried plant extract was stored at 4°C until it is required for biological assays.

Liquid-liquid extraction (fractionation)

Dried crude acetone extracts were re-constituted in 200 ml of 70% acetone and extracted sequentially with hexane followed by dichloromethane, ethyl acetate, acetone and methane. The residual water fraction was dried in a conventional oven at 50°C for 96 h. Absolute methanol was added every 24 h to prevent the growth of fungi. The dried water fractions were extracted with acetone and methanol successively to produce fractions of different polarities. Filtered fractions were concentrated on a rotary evaporator and then air dried at room temperature under a fan. The dried fractions were weighed and results are recorded in Table 2.

Quantitative evaluation of the biological activities of the plant extracts

Minimum inhibitory concentrations (MIC)

Minimum inhibitory concentrations of the crude extracts and fractions were determined by twofold serial dilution using 96-well microtitre plate against *S. aureus* (ATCC 29213), *P. aeruginosa* (ATCC 27853), *E. faecalis* (ATCC 29212) and *E. coli* (ATCC 25922). Tetrazolium violet was used as a growth indicator (Eloff, 1998b). In brief, 100 µL distilled water was placed in each of the wells using a multichannel micropipette. Thereafter, 100 µL of extract (10 mg/ ml) was added to the first well of column and serially diluted to prepare

Table 1. Ethnopharmacological information of the plant use in this study.

Botanical name/traditional names	Voucher number	Traditional medicinal use
Alepidea amatymbica Eckl. & Zeyh (Apiaceae) (Ikhathazo(isiZulu) Losoko,(Sesotho)	2116-0	Colds, influenza, stomach and respiratory ailments, rheumatism and wounds (Somova et al., 2001; Stafford et al., 2004; Van Staden et al., 2009).
Pentanisia prunelloides, Klotzeh ex Eckl & Zeyh.) Walp. (Rubiaceae) (Isicimamlilo (isiZulu)	1200-1	Root extract is used to treat aches and pains Kaidoo, T. L. (1997)
Pomaria sandersonii (P.s.) (Harv) B. B. Simpson & G.P. Lewis (Fabaceae) (Istholwane (isiZulu)	14806-0	Root extract is used for post natal care for mothers after child birth for fast recovery Traditional healer, Mabandla Village, Umzimkulu, Kwa-Zulu Natal, South Africa (2009).

Table 2. The percentage yield of the crude extracts and fractions of the plants.

Plant species	Crude	H	DCM	ET	AC	METH	W
P. sandersonii	7.818±0.78	0.64±0.06	31.33±3.10	16.34±1.60	23.77±2.20	25.18±2.50	-
A. amatymbica	7.65±0.76	31.14±3.10	41.31±4.10	0.91±0.09	0.84±0.08	23.73±2.37	-
P. prunelloides	5.05±0.49	1.15±0.12	0.82±0.08	-	9.83±0.10	7.05±.08	80.81±8.00

C= crude extract, H= hexane fraction, DCM= dichloromethane fraction, ET = ethyl acetate fraction, AC = acetone fraction and METH= methanol fraction, W= Water fraction.

a concentration range between 5.0 and 0.04 mg/ml in the first well and last well respectively. The solvent blank (negative control) and antibiotic (gentamicin for bacteria and amphotericin B for fungi) were included as positive control. From an overnight culture of bacteria grown in diluted Mueller Hinton broth, 100 µL of relevant bacteria dispensed into each well and incubated at 37°C for 18 to 24 h before adding 40 µl (0.2 mg/ml) of iodonitrotetrazolium violet, Sigma (INT) solution. Colour change was noted after 30, 60, and 120 min to determine the lowest concentration which inhibited growth (MIC). MIC of the crude extracts and fractions against *Candida albicans* and *A. fumigatus* were determined using the above-mentioned serial dilution assay with some modifications (Masoko et al., 2005). Fungal stock was prepared using Sabouraud dextrose broth instead of Mueller Hinton broth used for bacteria culture. All measurements were performed in triplicate.

DPPH anti-oxidant assay

For DPPH anti-oxidant assay, using 96 well plates and a VERSAmax™ tunable microplate reader (Labotech), 40 µl of 0,5 mg/ml plant extract and fraction were determined by a twofold serial dilution in 160 µl of 0.0025% of DPPH (total volume 200 µl), methanol (negative control) or trolox (positive control). After 30 min, the absorbance was measured at 516 nm wavelength. Methanol was used as negative control and trolox (2.5 to 0.5 mg/ml) was used as positive control. The free radical DPPH˙ scavenging (reduction) was calculated from the equation: Activity (% of DPPH reduction) = $\{(A - A_x) / A\} \times 100\%$, where A is absorbance of DPPH solution with methanol, A_x is absorbance of a DPPH solution with a tested fraction solution or trolox (positive control). All measurements were performed in triplicate.

ABTS$^{\bullet+}$ Scavenging assay

The ABTS$^{\bullet+}$ radical cation was prepared by mixing 7 mM ABTS stock solution and incubating for 12 to16 h in the dark at room temperature until a steady absorbance was obtained to indicate that the reaction was complete. Plant extracts and fractions (40 µL of 0.5 mg/ml) were mixed with 160 µL of the ABTS$^{\bullet+}$ radical cation (total volume 200 µl) in a 96-well microtitre plate. Absorbance of the mixture was read at 734 after six minutes using VERSAmax™ tunable microplate reader (Labotech). Methanol was used as negative control and trolox (25 to 0.5 g/ml) was used as positive control. All measurements were performed in triplicate.

Lipoxygenase inhibition

Inhibitory activity of the plant extracts against 15-soybean lipoxygenase (15-LOX) enzyme was evaluated according to Malterud and Rydland (2000) in borate buffer (0.2 M, pH 9.00). Increase in absorbance at 234 nm was read 5 min at interval of 30 s after addition of 15-LOX, using linoleic acid (134 µM) as substrate. The final enzyme concentration was 167 µg/ml. Test substances were added as dimethyl sulfoxide (DMSO) solutions (final DMSO concentration of 1.6%) while DMSO alone was added in control experiments. The enzyme solution was kept on ice, and controls were measured at intervals throughout the experimental periods to ensure that the enzyme activity was constant. All measurements were performed in triplicate.

RESULTS

Yield

The yields of the crude methanol extracts and fractions of various polarities were presented in Table 2. The highest percentage yield of 7.82% was from *P. sandersonii* but had the lowest hexane fraction yield of 0.64%. *A. amatymbica* extract had the highest fraction of non-polar

Table 3. Free radical scavenging activity of the crude extract and fractions of varied polarities (µg/ml).

Sample	*Pomaria sandersonii*		*Alepidea amatymbica*		*Pentanisia prunelloides*	
	DPPH (EC_{50})	ABTS (EC_{50})	DPPH (EC_{50})	ABTS (EC_{50})	DPPH (EC_{50})	ABTS (EC_{50})
Cr	5.6±0.71	3.24±0.13	7.68±0.59	1.27±0.16	68.89±9.21	213.66±35.00
H	3.58±0.44	11.31±3.70	19.82±1.74	152.00±22.45	111.93±10.55	3987.33±372.75
DCM	2.93±0.14	7329±117.53	36.25±3.33	1.75±1.02	98.62±6.55	28.68±9.46
ET	-	88.76±3.50	13.51±1.03	-	12.49±0.42	1.10±0.26
Ac	70.62±5.38	102.40±15.44	4.17±0.37	5.96±0.82	5.36±1.05	0.08±0.03
Met	2.61±0.07	0.19±0.04	31.34±2.00	-	4.08±0.65	2.72±1.77

Cr = crude extract, H = hexane fraction, DCM = dichloromethane fraction, ET = ethyl acetate fraction, Ac = acetone fraction, Met = methanol fraction, Positive standards: trolox = 0.04±0.001, ascorbic acid = 0.04±0.001

constituents (72%) that were hexane and DCM soluble. *P. prunelloides* had the highest water soluble component of 80% yield.

Antimicrobial activities

The minimum inhibitory concentrations of the crude methanol extracts and fractions of various polarities were presented in Figures 2 to 4. The antimicrobial activities of *A. amatymbica* crude extract and fractions were moderate to good against the bacterial and fungi tested with MICs ranging from 160 to 625 µg /ml. The crude extracts and fractions of *P. prunelloides* had weak (160 to 320 µg /ml) antibacterial activity (Figure 4). The anti-fungal activity was low at 625 µg /ml for the crude extract and fractions from *P. prunelloides*. The crude extract and fractions of *P. sandersonii* displayed good antimicrobial activity with MICs ranging from 20 to 1250 µg /ml (Figure 3). Dichloromethane and ethyl acetate fractions of *P. sandersonii* had MIC of 80 µg /ml against *S. aureus, E. coli* and *P. aeruginosa* which is comparable to the activities of the antibiotic standard gentamycin. The fractions had good activity against *E. faecalis* with MIC of 40 µg /ml. The dichloromethane, acetone and methanol fractions of the *P. sandersonii* also had good antifungal inhibitory activity (20 µg /ml) against C. *albicans* and *A. fumigatus* (Figure 3).

Antioxidant and lipoxygenase inhibitory activity

Pentanisia prunelloides

The EC_{50} values for hexane, DCM and acetone *P. prunelloides* fractions indicated that they were more reactive with $DPPH^{•}$ radical while there was a comparable activity with both radicals with the methanol fractions with EC_{50} of 2.619 µg/ml for $DPPH^{•}$ and µg/ml for $ABTS^{•+}$ radicals (Table 3). The lipoxygenase inhibitory activity of 79% indicates high anti-inflammatory activity.

Pomaria sandersonii

All the plant extracts and fractions used in this study displayed some anti-radiative activity although, the crude extract $DPPH^{•}$ and $ABTS^{•+}$ for *P. sandersonii* displayed the highest activity compared to all of the plant's samples. DCM fraction was more reactive towards $ABTS^{•+}$ displaying activity of 0.19 µg/ml compared to the methanol extract which had $DPPH^{•}$ displaying activity of 2.61 µg/ml (Table 3). The hexane fraction was more active againist $DPPH^{•}$ compared to the reaction with $ABTS^{•+}$ radical. The crude extract of *P. sandersonii* had a high lipoxygenase inhibitory activity of 97% at concentration of 25 µg/ml.

Alepidea amatymbica

The DCM fractions of *A. amatymbica* also displayed different activities towards the two radicals. EC_{50} values for the crude and acetone fractions were 4.17µg/ml towards $DPPH^{•}$ and 5.96µg/ml towards $ABTS^{•+}$ respectively. The lipoxygenase inhibitory activity of 55% at concentration of 25 µg/ml indicated moderate anti-inflammatory activity for *A. amatymbica.* The results indicate that the *A. amatymbica* fractions contain antioxidants.

DISCUSSION

Our results demonstrated biological activities of the methanolic crude extracts, hexane, dichloromethane, ethyl acetate and acetone fractions obtained from *A. amatymbica, P. prunelloides* and *P. sandersonii* which are used to manage inflammation related conditions. The plants exhibited antibacterial, anti-inflammatory and anti-oxidative properties.

The antimicrobial activity (MIC) of the extracts was determined using the broth microdilution method based on the principle of contact of a test organism to a series of dilutions of test substance. The crude extract and fractions (hexane, dichloromethane, ethyl acetate) of *A. amatymbica* (Figure 1) displayed good to moderate (160 to 320 µg/ml) anti-bacterial activity against all the organisms tested, however, the methanol fraction

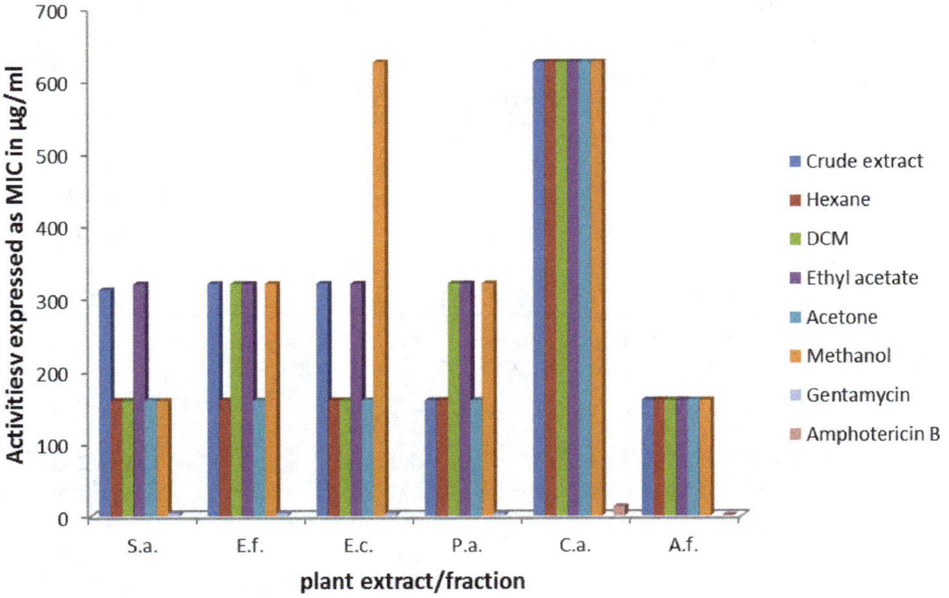

Figure 1. Antimicrobial activities of *Alepedia amatymbica* crude extracts and fractions of different polarities as indicated by solvent used: S.a .= *Staphylococcus aureus*, E.f .= *Enterococcus faecalis*, E.c. = *Escherichia coli*, P.a. = *Pseudomonas aeruginosa*, C.a. = *Candida albicans*, A.f .= *Aspergillus fumigatus.* Gentamycin and amphotericin B were the positive standards.

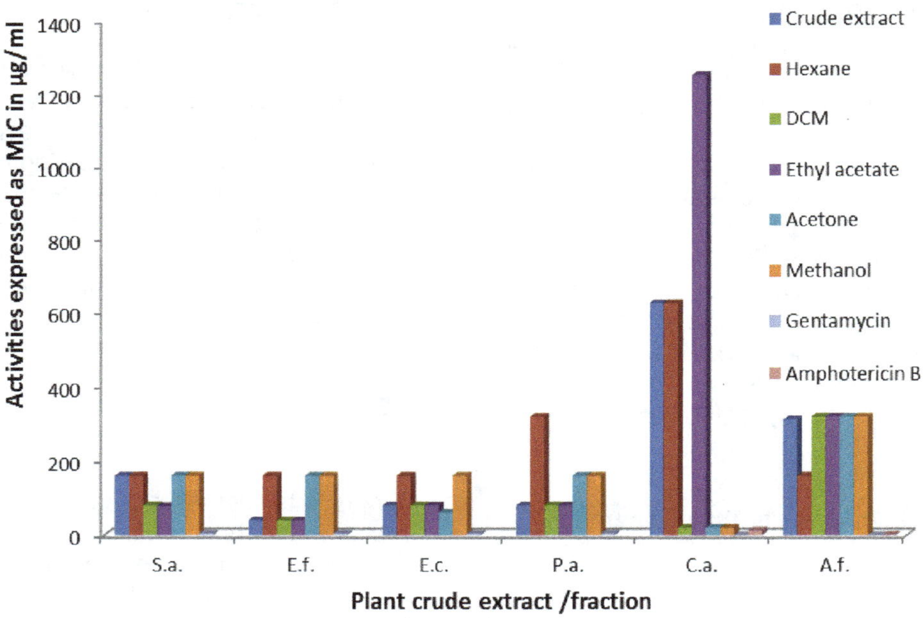

Figure 2. Antimicrobial activities of *Pomaria sandesonni* crude extracts and fractions of different polarities as indicated by solvent used: S.a .= *Staphylococcus aureus*, E.f .= *Enterococcus faecalis*, E.c. = *Escherichia coli*, P.a. = *Pseudomonas aeruginosa*, C.a. = *Candida albicans*, A.f .= *Aspergillus fumigatus*. Gentamycin and amphotericin B were the positive standards.

showed a lower MIC (625 µg/ml) against *E coli.* The activity of the *A. amatymbica* extract and fractions against *C. albicans* was also low (MIC = 625 µg/ml). In a related study, Mulaudzi et al. (2009) reported lower anti-bacterial and anti-fungal activities of polar root extracts and fractions (water and ethanol) from *A. amatymbica.* The

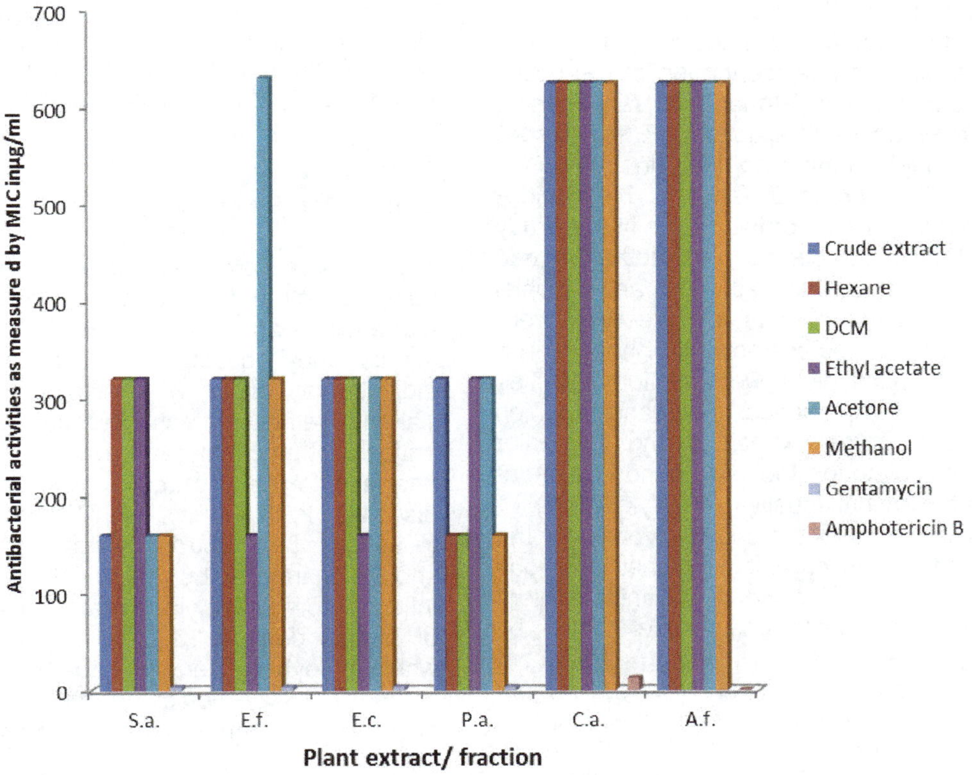

Figure 3. Antimicrobial activities of *Pentanisia prunelloides* crude extracts and fractions of different polarities as indicated by solvent used: *S.a .= Staphylococcus aureus*, *E.f .= Enterococcus faecalis, E.c. = Escherichia coli, P.a. = Pseudomonas aeruginosa, C.a. = Candida albicans, A.f .= Aspergillus fumigatus.* Gentamycin and amphotericin B were the positive standards.

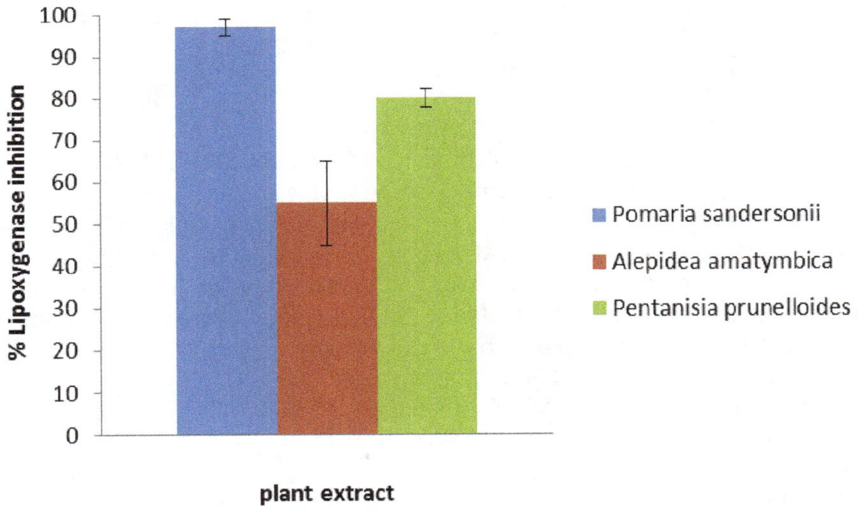

Figure 4. Percentage inhibition of 15-soybean lipoxygenase enzyme by the crude extracts at concentration of 25 µg/ml (n=3).

antimicrobial activity of *P. Prunelloides* (Figure 3), which is used traditionally for the treatment of dysmenorrhoea, was good to moderate (160 to 320 µg/ml). Anti-bacterial activity of the *P. prunelloides* acetone fraction was low displaying MIC of 625 µg/ml against *E. faecalis*. Yff et al. (2002), also reported a similar investigation, that anti-bacterial activity of the water, ethanol and ethyl acetate extracts from *P. prunelloides* root had low bacterial growth inhibition (0.39 to 12.5 mg/ml). The low activity values in some of the extracts tested in this study could be due to the impure form and/ or low concentration of the active compound(s) in the extracts (Rabe and Van Staden, 1997). DCM and ethyl acetate fractions of *P. sandersonii* (Figure 2) displayed highest inhibitory activities (80 µg /ml in each case) against *S. aureus, E. faecalis, E. coli* and *P. aeruginosa* compared to the other two plants in this study. The more polar fractions (acetone and methanol) had good anti-candidal activity (MIC= 20). The antimicrobial activity of the three plant extracts and fractions were more significant in the non-polar fractions of hexane and dichloromethane. The relatively higher inhibitory activities could be attributed to the presence of terpenoids which had been detected in crude extracts during an earlier qualitative test study, although the compounds have not been isolated and tested individually (Van Wyk , 2008).

Inflammation is an important process involved in the defence mechanisms of an organism against infectious and other deleterious stimuli. However, inflammatory responses to infectious agents can evade control by immuno-regulatory mechanisms. Existing treatment protocols for such inflammation-driven diseases remain less than optimal. In this study, ethanol crude extract of *A. amatymbica* rhizome had 50% LOX inhibition (Figure 4). Although, Mulaudzi et al. (2009) reported that the petroleum ether, DCM and ethanol extracts of *A. amatymbica* rhizome has 90% inhibitory COX-2 activity. The difference in activity could be due to the difference of LOX enzymes and methods used in determining the anti-inflammatory property of the plant. *P. prunelloides* had high 15-LOX inhibitory activity (79%) with EC_{50} value of 15.98 mg/L. The more polar leaf extracts of *P. prunelloides* earlier reported had good COX-1 inhibitory activity (leaf water extract = 74%, root water extract =74%) (Yff et al., 2002). Methanol crude extract of *P. sandersonii* was the most active with 97% LOX inhibitory activity. This is consistent with the fact that the fraction, being the most polar is also rich in polyphenols which are responsible for the anti-inflammatory activity.

Oxidative stress plays a significant role in the pathogenesis of infectious and inflammatory disease. The crude extracts, and more polar fractions of ethyl acetate, acetone and methanol soluble from the three plants have appreciable antioxidant activity. Acetone crude leaf extract, DCM and Ethyl acetate fractions of *P. sandersonii* had higher $ABTS^{\bullet+}$ scavenging ability compared to corresponding reaction with the DPPH radical. *P. sandersonii* samples (crude and fractions) were the most active against $ABTS^{\bullet+}$ (1.274 to 5.973 µg/ml) compared to all the plants studied (Table 3), except for the hexane fraction which displayed low activity (111.93µg/ml for DPPH) and (3987.33µg/ml for ABTS).

The low activity in the hexane fraction could attribute the possible absence of polyphenols in the non-polar fraction as compared to the high activities displayed by the more polar fractions rich in polyphenols. This is the first time reporting biological activities of *P. sandersonii* and are compared with the two relatively more well-known South African medicinal plants.

Conclusion

This study revealed that while medicinal plants still play a very vital role in the primary health care of the people of Mabandla village, Zululand, South Africa, the three plants in this study possess significant biological activities as indicated by the *in vitro* assays that were carried out. Taken together, the anti-infectious, anti-inflammatory and antioxidant mechanisms may help to develop better novel pharmacological drugs for various degenerative diseases. In this study, 15-LOX from soybean was used to assess the *in vitro* inhibitory activity. These findings should therefore be cautiously applied to the anti-inflammatory activity in humans because the mechanism of human derived 15 LOX may be different from that which is soybean derived. Other enzymes such as COX-1 and COX-2 should be studied to obtain a more accurate assessment of anti-inflammatory activity of the plants. These medicinal plants have demonstrated broad spectra of activity that might help to discover new pharmacological compounds which could serve as agents for human and animal health maintenance. The results obtained in this study also validate the traditional use of these plants to manage infectious and inflammation related disorders, however, *in vivo* studies are still necessary to completely validate the claims leading to isolation and characterisation of active compounds.

ACKNOWLEDGEMENTS

The authors acknowledge the University of Pretoria Phytomedicine programme, Vaal University of Technology for funding the study, Traditional healers of Mabandla Village, Kwa-Zulu Natal, South Africa and Midlands State University, Gweru Zimbabwe.

REFERENCES

Bisi-Johnson MA, Obi CL, Kambizi L, Nkomo M (2009). A survey of indigenous herbal diarrhoeal remedies of O.R. Tambo district, Eastern Cape Province, South Africa. Afr. J. Biotech. 9(8), 1245-1254.

Bremner PD, Meyer JJM (2000). Prenyl-butyrylphloroglucinol and kaurenoic acid: two antibacterial compounds from *Helichrysum kraussii*. S. Afr. J. Bot. 66:115-117.

Eloff JN (1998a). Which extractant should be used for the screening and isolation of antimicrobial components from plants? J. Ethnopharmacol. 60:1-8.

Eloff JN (1998b). A sensitive and quick micro plate method to determine the minimum inhibitory concentration of plant extract for bacteria. Planta Med. 64:711-714.

Hamer M (2007). The beneficial effects of tea on immune function and inflammation: A review of evidence from in vitro, animal and human research. Nutr. Res. 27:373-379.

Hutchings A, Scot AH, Lewis G, Cunningham A (1996). Zulu Medicinal Plants University of KwaZulu-Natal Press.

Masoko P, Picard J, Eloff J N (2005). Antifungal activities of six South African Terminalia species (Combretaceae). J. Ethnopharmacol. 99:301-308.

Mulaudzi RB, Ndhlala A R, Finnie JF, Van Staden J (2009). Antimicrobial, anti-inflammatory and genotoxicity of Alepidea amatymbica and Alepidea natalensis (Apiaceae). S Afr.J. Bot. 75: 584-487.

Pfaller MA, Diekema DJ (2004). Rare and Emerging Opportunistic Fungal Pathogens: Concern for Resistance beyond Candida albicans and Aspergillus fumigatus. J. Clin. Microbiol. 42 (10):44419-431.

Rabe T, Van Staden J (1997). Antibacterial activity of South African plants used for medicinal purposes. J. Ethnopharmacol. 56 (1):81-87

Rustaiyan A, Sadjadi AS (1987). Kaurene drivatives from Alepidea amatymbica. Phytochemistry 26:2105-2107.

Van Wyk BE (2008). A broad review of commercially important southern African medicinal plants. J. Ethnopharmacol. 119:342-355.

Walsh JT, Anaissie JE, Denning WD, Herbrecht R, Kontoyiannis PD, Marr A K, Morrison A, Segal HB, Steinbach JW, Stevens DA, Van BurikWingard JR Patterson TF (2008). IDSA Guidelines for Aspergillosis Clin. Infect. Dis. 46:329

Watt JM, Breyer-Brandwijk MG (1962). Medicinal and Poisonous plants of Southern and Eastern Africa.2nd Ed E & S Livingstone, Edinburgh p 300.

Yff BTS, Lindsey KL, Taylor MB, Erasmus DG, Jager A. K (2002). The pharmacological screening of Pentanisia prunelloides and the isolation of antibacterial compound, palmitic acid. J. Ethnopharmacol. 79:101-107.

Palliative treatment of cancer in resource poor settings: Traditional medicine perspective

Florence Dushimemaria[1] and Davis R. Mumbengegwi[2]

[1]Science, Technology and Innovation Division, Multi-disciplinary Research center, University of Namibia, Private Bag 13301, 340 Mandume Ndemufayo Avenue, Pionier spark, Windhoek, Namibia.
[2]Science, Technology and Innovation Division, Multi-disciplinary Research center, University of Namibia, Private Bag 13301, 340 Mandume Ndemufayo Avenue, Pionier spark, Windhoek, Namibia.

This study aimed to determine the suitability of ethnomedicinal plants as a suitable option for palliative care of cancer in Namibia. To achieve this, key informant interviews were conducted in central and northern parts of Namibia on the use of ethnomedicinal plant products for palliation of cancer. Information from surveys on the medicinal use of plants in Oshikoto and Zambezi regions of Namibia for ailments such as tumors were used to select plants for phytochemical analysis. Plants were collected and extracts were prepared for analysis for phytochemical detection using thin layer chromatography, anti-protease, antioxidant and phytochemical quantification of *Colophospermum mopane* and *Shinziophyton rautanenii* plants. Findings from key informant interviews revealed pain management for cancer patients was the primary form of disease management at health care facilities in contrast to an established holistic palliative care system. As a result, patients looked towards alternative treatment from ethnomedicinal plant sources in their bid to palliate cancer and seek hope. Phytochemical analysis of indigenous plants collected, revealed the presence of class compounds such as flavonoids, alkaloids, triterpenes, coumarins and anthraquinones as well as biological activities such as anti-protease, antioxidant properties. In conclusion, phytochemical properties of the six plants were consistent with their ethnomedicinal use, making them a suitable option for treatment of cancer in resource poor settings such as Namibia. Further studies are required to evaluate safety and mode of action.

Key words: Palliative care, Namibia, medicinal plants, anti-cancer.

INTRODUCTION

Non-communicable diseases (NCD) such as cancer, diabetes, cardiovascular disease, as well as Human immunodeficiency virus infection and acquired immune deficiency syndrome (HIV/AIDS) and chronic respiratory disease were responsible for over 63% of the fifty seven million mortalities that occurred in 2008 (WHO, 2011). The World Health Organization (2011) report on NCD, shows that over 85% of premature deaths from NCD occurred in low-middle income countries. In Namibia, 19% of deaths were due to cardiovascular diseases while cancer, chronic respiratory disease and diabetes contributed 3% each respectively. The incidence of cancer

*Corresponding author. E-mail: dmumbengegwi@unam.na.

in Namibia is on the rise. Kaposi sarcoma and prostate cancers are the leading cancers among the male population while breasts and cervical cancer are more common in females (Namibian Cancer Registry, 2011). Between 2006 and 2009, the frequencies were 22.1 and 19.2%, respectively, while statistics (Namibian Cancer Registry, 2009) showed a lower proportion of 19.2 and 12%, for Kaposi sarcoma and prostate cancer in males respectively. During the period of 2006 to 2009 (Namibian Cancer Registry, 2011), the most prevalent cancers in women were breast cancer (27.6%) and cervical cancer (17.1%). During the previous reporting period (Namibian Cancer Registry, 2009), a total of 4,949 cancer cases were recorded in comparison to 6,464 total cases between the period of 2006 to 2009 (Namibian Cancer Registry, 2011). These numbers reflect that cancer is a public health concern in Namibia, and hence emphasize the necessity of care and support for individuals with life-limiting conditions (Webster et al., 2007; Thomson, 2012).

Despite the evolution of treatment options of cancer such as chemotherapy, radiotherapy, surgery, hormonal treatment or a combination of these, effective and affordable cancer treatment is still illusive for many individuals. Factors such as disease progression, type of cancer, cost of treatment, lack of cancer management professionals and resources all hamper effective cancer treatment and management. In Namibia, a patient has to go through a long period of referrals before accessing proper treatment. First report is at a local clinic, from which patient is sent to a district hospital, followed by regional district, where one can consult with an oncologist; a patient may need to be referred to the central hospital in Windhoek before effective treatment and monitoring is initiated. By the time an opportunity for effective treatment is available, prognosis is often very poor and treatment options are expensive and beyond the reach of 56% of the Namibian population who live in rural resource poor settings.

Palliative care is a multi-dimensional, multi-disciplinary approach to treatment, which focuses on alleviating symptoms and distress arising from treatment serious disease and its treatments (Powell et al., 2010), for both the patient and their relatives (WHO, 2011). The African Palliative Care Association (APCA) of Namibia, in conjunction with partners such as the Cancer Association of Namibia, the Ministry of health and social services, United States Agency for International Development (USAID), Catholic AIDS Action (CAA) and Hospices of Hope, strive to increase awareness for the need for palliative care as well as access. Despite these efforts, access to effective palliative care is still illusive in Namibia (Palliative care training ends in capital, 2014). The APCA further advocates to avail morphine in order to effectively manage suffering of patients. Options for addressing chronic pain in palliative care involve use of opioids such as morphine (Webster et al., 2007). In resource poor settings, poverty makes it hard to access effective palliative treatment (Harding, 2008). In addition to this, legislative policies are not in place, especially when it comes to inclusion of alternative therapy options such as traditional medicines, further hampering effective palliative care (Webster et al., 2007; Powell et al., 2011; Logie and Harding, 2005).

Traditionally, plants have been a vital resource of medicines for health care provision (Thomson, 2010; Maliwichi-Nyirenda and Maliwichi, 2010), yet there is a renewed interest in research towards the discovery and development of plant-derived medicines for mainstream usage as, many medicines in clinical use owe their origin to plants (Thomson, 2010). In addition, Sharma et al. (2011) observed increased reliance on traditional medicine evident in developing countries as a primary healthcare provision. Medicinal plants owe their chemotherapeutic properties to the presence of bioactive constituents such as alkaloids, terpenes and particularly polyphenols, which are known for antioxidant plus anti-inflammatory qualities (Farombi and Owoeye, 2011). For instance, Bernard and Alayinka (2010) reported pharmacological effects that cucurbitacins, a triterpenoid steroid conjugate possess analgesic, anti-inflammatory, antioxidant and antiproliferative activities. The antioxidant properties of plant derived medicines are capable of palliative, curative and preventative pharmacological effects for chronic disease such as cancer (Thomson, 2010). Traditional medicine has two goals: to cure disease and thereby prolong life or provide comfort and relief, therefore making disease easier to live with (Mudigonda and Mudigonda, 2010; Powell et al., 2011).

In this study, the potential usage of Namibian indigenous plants for palliative care in a resource poor setting, with emphasis on cancer and other non-communicable diseases, is discussed. Furthermore, key informant interviews were conducted. Chemical profiles of plants used as baseline data for characterization and validation of plants' usage in traditional settings.

MATERIALS AND METHODS

Key informant interviews

The Key informants (KI) interviews were conducted with practitioners in cancer treatment and care in the Khomas and Oshana regions of Namibia on the incidences of cancer in Namibia. Five key informants (referred to as KI1, KI2, KI3, KI4 and KI5) were interviewed on the use of alternative medicines in treatment of cancer within cancer patients in Namibia.

Plant species reviewed

Plants with an ethnomedicinal background were obtained using literature search (Watt and Breyer-Brandwijk, 1962; Palgrave, 1981; von Koenen, 2001; Cheihkyoussef et al., 2011a; Cheihkyoussef et al., 2011b), and based on responses obtained in a survey conducted in the Zambezi region of Namibia (Du Preez et al.,

2010). Further search revealed little or no evidence of proven medicinal evidence of plants. Plant material was sustainably harvested from the Zambezi region of Namibia, using guidelines from the National Botanical Research Institute (NBRI). Voucher specimen were prepared and sent for authentication at the NBRI as different ethnic names can refer to the same plant or different names to the same plant. Confirmation of scientific names can lead to proper identification of collected plants.

Preparation of bioactive extracts

Harvested plant material was cut into small pieces and dried at room temperature for two weeks before being ground to a fine powder. The ground plant material was then used to prepare organic plant extracts using methanol as solvent and sterilized distilled water to prepare aqueous extracts. After soaking ground plant for 7 days, mixture was filtered and solvent was evaporated. This was followed with dry freezing to totally remove solvent, resulting in dry crude extracts of various plant parts, such as leaf, root, twig and bark.

Chemical profile investigation

Plants were screened for known anti-cancer properties using chemical assays such as anti-protease activity, antioxidant activity and selected phytochemical compounds. Firstly, the antioxidant and anti-protease activity of the different plant extracts was investigated using 2,2'-azino-bis(3-ethylbenzothiazoline-6-sulphonic acid)(ABTS) and radiograph film with gelatin respectively. Methanolic portions of different plant parts were screened for various selected phytochemical compounds, such as flavonoids, alkaloids, triterpenoids, coumarins and anthraquinones, according to Harborne (1998). Table 1 shows the various solvent systems and chromogenic reagent used to detect the listed phytochemicals using thin layer chromatography.

Phytochemical quantification

Plant material from *Colophospermum mopane* and *Shinziophyton rautanenii* were analyzed for the total content of saponins, alkaloids and phenols. Total saponin and alkaloid was quantified using methods adapted from Edeoga et al. (2005) to determine percentage yield. Total phenolic content was analyzed using a method contained in Jing et al. (2010) with slight modifications, and gallic acid was used to develop a calibration curve in order to expresses phenolic content as gallic acid equivalents (GAE) µg/ml. Antioxidant activity was investigated using a method adopted from Jing et al. (2010) and Re et al. (1999). A standard graph developed from ascorbic acid was used to estimate the antioxidant activity. Each phytochemical was quantified in triplicate from each sample.

RESULTS

Collected plants were identified (Table 2) using local names within the community and their identity was validated scientifically by the NBRI. The validation of plant names, by scientific means affords universal comparison of the same plant, even if it's from different communities.

Chemical profiling of the plants revealed the presence of different phytochemicals. High anti-protease and anti-oxidant activity was detected in all plant parts, with the exemption of *Acanthosicyos naudinianus* shoots, which contained no detectable anti-protease activity. Different phytochemicals such ascoumarin, anthraquinone, alkaloids, flavonoids and triterpenoids were detected and were observed to be distributed in different tissues of the plants (Table 3). This development implies that the local community members may sustainably utilize plant material with the assurance that either plant parts contain potentially therapeutic phytochemicals.

Furthermore, based on literature review (Watt and Breyer-Brandwijk, 1962; Palgrave, 1981; von Koenen, 2001; Cheihkyoussef et al., 2011; Cheihkyoussef et al., 2011), responses on the use of medicinal traditional plants and phytochemical profiles of the six collected plants (Table 2), two plants; *S. rautanenii* and *C. mopane* root ant bark extracts were analyzed for the total content of alkaloids, saponins, phenols and antioxidant activity (Figure 1). Both the roots of *S. rautanenii_*(9.64±4.6% yield) and *C. mopane* (11.13±2.7% yield) displayed the highest alkaloid, content while the bark extract of *S. rautanenii* (2.08±0.5% yield) had the lowest alkaloid content. Meanwhile, the *C. mopane* root (205.4±9.3 GAE µg/ml) had the highest phenol content and the *C. mopane* bark (12.6±1.7 GAE µg/ml) extract had the lowest phenolic content. Saponin quantification revealed that the bark of *S. rautanenii* (13.6±10.4 %) was the highest saponin content while the root extract of *S. rautanenii* (1.8±0.7%) was the lowest saponin yield. The *S. rautanenii* root (945.6±231.1 AAE µg/ml) and bark (226.7±17.6 AAE µg/ml) extracts had the highest and lowest antioxidant activity, respectively.

DISCUSSION

Namibia has a wealth of traditional practices, which includes substantial ethnomedicine knowledge. This is passed on from a traditional knowledge holder to younger members of the community. Sadly, this does not happen in all instances, which leads to loss of traditional heritage. Namibia needs to take advantage of its current wealth of information, to properly document and validate Namibia's heritage. This will increase awareness of traditional based medicines in the country and potentially lead to inclusion of traditional plant based therapies in mainstream medicine.

In Namibia, some individuals suffer from cancer experience chronic pain, which is partly associated with the disease and also as a result of side effects from cancer treatments. Such pain makes living with cancer difficult and can be unbearable in advanced stages of cancer. In Namibia, since many patients present very late (KI1) progressive cases, at which time pain levels need to be managed to bearable levels, the availability of affordable pain relieving medications is vital. In Namibia, morphine is the medication of choice for individuals experiencing excruciating pain, in cancer patients or

Table 1. Solvent systems and chromogenic reagents for thin layer chromatography.

Phytochemical	Solvent system	Chromogenic solvent
Alkaloid	Ammonium hydroxide: Methanol. 3:200	Dragendorff reagent
Anthraquinone	Ethyl acetate: Methanol:Water, 100:17:13	10% KOH in methanol
Triterpenoid	Hexane:Ethyl acetate, 17:3	Liebermann burchard reagent
Coumarin	Chloroform	10% KOH in methanol
Flavonoid	Butanol:Aceticacid:Water, 4:1:5	1% Aluminium chloride in methanol

Table 2. Medicinal plants collected for the study, their reputed use, local names and voucher specimen numbers deposited with NBRI.

Scientific name	Local name	Family	Traditional use	Voucher specimen #
S. rautanenii	Mankettii	Euphorbiaceae	Sores on body surface	FD03
C. mopane	Omusati	Fabaceae	Swollen testis	FD02
Capparis tomentosa	Mudyangwe	Capparaceae	Poison, wound healing and anti-inflammatory	FD08
Lessertia benguellensis	Ndendeoma	Fabaceae	Syphilis, bloody urine and tonsils	FD06
Commiphora africana	Muwowo	Burseraceae	Abdominal cramps, anticancer and snake bite remedy	FD05
Acanthosicyos naudinianus	Muputwi	Curcubitaceae	Poison, wound healing, edible and antiinflammatory	FD04

those suffering from other NCD, according to KI5. The APCA and Namibia's Ministry of Health and Social Services are currently working on legislature which supports availability of morphine, even to the healthcare analyst I (MIA) levels in health care institutions (KI4).

However, the effectiveness of such a strategy relies hugely on the availability of such drugs. With lacking supporting legislation (Logie and Harding, 2005) coupled with lack of monetary funds in poor resource settings, palliative care is often unattainable. According to KI1, many cancer sufferers already seek assistance from traditional healers within the Namibian setting. KI2 and KI3 however presented a contradicting picture regarding the level to which individuals seek health care from elsewhere. According to KI1, mangosteen juice, Ativan (Lorazepam) and SOLAL are among natural products in use by cancer patients in Namibia. Mangosteen juice is derived from a fruit of *Garcinia mangostana*, a tropical tree, growing in Asian countries. Numerous studies have been conducted on the chemical properties of the "Queen of fruits". These studies reveal compounds such as many variations of xanthones (Towatana et al., 2010). Its physiological properties include, high antioxidant activity, antitumor, anti-inflammatory, antiviral, antibacterial, anti-allergy properties but are not exclusive, (Pedraza-Chaverri et al., 2008). Use of combination treatments such as lorazepam, diphenhydramine plus metoclopramide and dexamethasone, to control vomiting and nausea as side effects arising from anticancer treatments are also common (Kris et al., 1987).

A source, (Olowokudejo et al., 2008) concedes that traditional medicine is a reliable source of effective, affordable and easily accessible therapeutic entities. However, it's important to know that effective palliative care does not take the place of a prescribed treatment regimen. A look at these six Namibian plants (Table 2) revealed the presence of different bands of phytochemical compounds, using thin layer chromatography. Phytochemical compounds have been shown to confer anti-inflammatory (Bellik et al., 2013) and analgesic properties (Ojieh et al., 2013), which are all beneficial to combat NCDs. Thin layer chromatography (TLC) results suggests that different kinds of triterpenoids and anthraquinones are present, as evidenced by the numerous bands observed on TLC plates (Table 3). It follows that, observed antioxidant activity may be due to the presence of phytochemicals (Table 3). In another study conducted in Botswana (Motlhanka, 2008), *C. mopane* methanolic extracts displayed radical scavenging activity. Antioxidant activity is commonly attributed to phenolic compounds, however, spearson correlation analysis revealed a correlation=0.58 (n-12, p=0.048) between alkaloid content and antioxidant activity. Plants from the euphorbiaceae family, such as *S.*

Table 3. Phytochemical profile of medicinal plants collected from the Zambezi region, Namibia.

Plant sample	Anti-protease	anti-oxidant	Coumarin	Alkaloid	Flavonoid	Triterpene	Anthraquinone
S. rautanenii bark	+++	+++	++	+	+	+++	-
S. rautanenii root	+++	+++	+	+	+	++++	+++
C. mopane bark	+++	+++	++	+	+	+++	-
C. mopane root	+++	+++	++	+	+	+++	-
A. naudinianus shoot	-	+++	+	+	+	++	++
A. naudinianus tuber	+++	+	-	+	-	+	+
C. africana twigs	+++	+++	-	-	-	+	+
C. africana roots	+++	+++	+	+	+	+	++
L. benguellensis leaf	+++	++	+	+	+	++	++++
C. tomentosas hoot	+++	+++	+	+	-	++	++
C. tomentosa root	+++	+++	+	+	-	++	-

Key: ++++ = high, + = low, - = no detection.

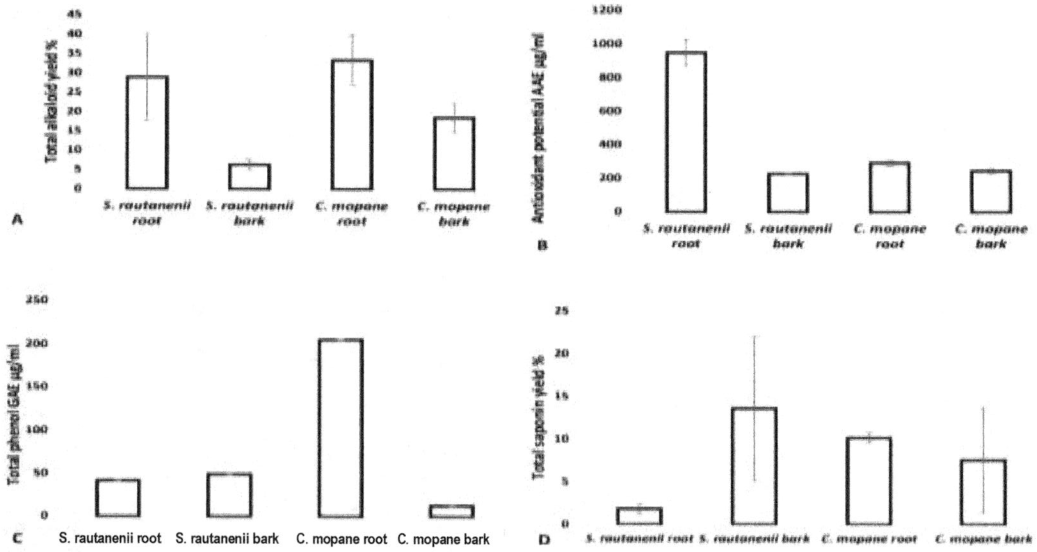

Figure 1. Quantification of phytochemicals in the root and bark of *C. mopane* and *S. rautanenii* depicted as depicted in A) Alkaloids, B) Antioxidant activity, C) Phenolic content and D) Saponin.

rautanenii have been found to confer antineoplastic activities (Soetan and Aiyelaagbe, 2009), antioxidant activity (Dasari et al., 2012) and this was attributed to the presence of phenolic acids. The phytochemical profile (Table 3) and quantification (Figure 1) suggests that the use of these plants in the traditional setting is rational and may be useful as an anticancer traditional alternative treatment (Wahab et al., 2010).

In the traditional setting, water is used as a solvent for preparation of medicinal treatments. However, organic solvents such as methanol, dichloromethane are used because they extract bioactive compounds more efficiently (Jo et al., 2011; Govindappa et al., 2011; Elkady, 2012). In addition to water, palm wine made from a tree, locally known as makalani palm (*Hyphaenepetersiana*) is used to prepare medicinal portions, even though this method is rare. Therefore, with the wealth of opportunities presented by Namibia's abundance of indigenous plants, there is a need for research into the safety and efficacy of plant derived extracts using *in vitro* assays to determine the anticancer effects of these plants. Further studies may also lead to standardization and dosage regimen of plant based supplements for use as alternative anticancer medicinal implements.

Conclusion

Cancer is an increasingly common cause of morbidity and mortality in Namibia. Providing healthcare to cancer patients in Namibia is a challenge not only because of the lack of treatment options, but also because of the lack of financial resources for treatment. This study shows the potential of medicinal plants to provide an option for palliative care of cancer patients. Further study of such medicinal plants may result in their becoming a mainstream as either a palliative treatment option or a potential cure for some early stage cancers in rural and even urban settings.

ACKNOWLEDGEMENTS

The authors of this study wishes to acknowledge the support of the Multidisciplinary research center and the Biological Sciences Department at the University of Namibia. The funds were provided by the University of Namibia Research and Publications Office and the German Academic Exchange Programme (DAAD). Rutgers State University of New York and the Global Institute of Bio-exploration (GIBEX) for the use of Screen-to-Nature Kits.

REFERENCES

Bellik Y, Boukraa L, Alzahrani HA, Bakhotmah BA, Abdellah FA, Hammoudi SM, Iguer-Ouada M (2013). Molecular mechanism underlying anti-inflammatory and anti-allergic activities of phytochemicals: An update. Molecules 18:322-353.

Bernard SA, Olayinka OA (2010). Search for a novel antioxidant, anti-inflammatory/analgesic or anti-proliferative drug: Cucurbitacins hold the ace. J. Med. Plants Res. 4(25):2821-2826.

Cheihkyoussef A, Shapi M, Matengu K, Mu Ashekele H (2011). Ethnobotanical study of indigenous knowledge on medicinal plant use by traditional healers in Oshikoto region, Namibia. J. Ethnobiol. Ethnomed. 7:10-21.

Cheikhyoussef A, Mapaure I, Shapi M (2011). The use of some indigenous plants for medicinal and other purposes by local communities in Namibia with emphasis on Oshikoto region: A review. Res. J. Med. Plants 5(4):406-419.

Dasari NP, Rao GB, Rao SE, Rao MT. Praneeth DVS (2012). Quantification of phytochemical constituents and In Vitro antioxidant activity of Synadiumgrantii. Free Radic. Antioxid. 2(2):68-72.

Du Preez I, Nepolo E, Siyengwa R, Shapi M, Cheikhyoussef A, Mumbengegwi D (2010). Study on indigenous medicinal knowledge in Caprivi region. Multidisciplinary resource center: Windhoek.

Edeoga HO, Okwu DE, Mbaebie BO (2005). Phytochemical constituents of some Nigerian medicinal plants. Afr. J. Biotechnol. 4(7):685-688.

Elkady A (2012). Crude extracts of Nigella sativa inhibits proliferation and induces apoptosis in human cervical carcinoma HeLa cells. Afr. J. Biotechnol. 11(64):12710-12720.

Farombi EO, Owoeye O (2011). Antioxidant and chemopreventative properties of *Vernonia amygdalina* and *Garcinia biflavonoid*. Int. J. Environ. Res. Public Health 8:2533-2555.

Govindappa M, Kumar ANV, Santoyo G (2011).*Crotalaria pallida* extracts as a putative HIV- protease inhibitors. J. Res. Biol. 1(4):285-291.

Harborne JB (1998). Phytochemical methods: A guide to modern techniques of plant analysis. 3ed. Chapman & hall: London p 302.

Harding R (2008). Palliative care in Resource-poor settings: Fallacies and misapprehensions. Commentary 36(5): 515-517.

Jing LJ, Mohamed M, Rahmat A, Bakar MFA (2010). Phytochemicals, antioxidant properties and anticancer investigations of the different parts of several ginger species (*Boesenbergia rotunda, Boesenbergia pulchellavar attenuate* and *Boesenbergia armeniaca*). J. Med. Plants Res. 4(1):27-32.

Jo KJ, Lee JM, Lee SC, Park HR (2011). Anticancer activity of persimmon (*Diospyros kaki* L.) calyx extracts on human cancer cells. J. Med. Plants Res. 5(12):2546-2550.

Kris MG, Gralla RJ, Clark R A, Tyson LB, Groshen S (1987). Antiemetic control and prevention of side effects of anti-cancer therapy with lorazepam or diphenhydraminewhen used in combination with metoclopramide plus dexamethasone. Cancer 60:2816-2822.

Logie DE, Harding R (2005). An evaluation of a morphine public health programme for cancer and AIDS pain relief in Sub-Saharan Africa. BMC Public Health 5:82-87.

Maliwichi-Nyirenda CP, Maliwichi LL (2010). Medicinal plants used to induce labour and traditional techniques used in determination of onset of labour in pregnant women in Malawi: A case study of Mulanje district. J. Med. Plants. Res. 4(24):2609-2614.

Motlhanka DM (2008). Free radical scavenging activity of selected medicinal plants of Eastern Bostwana. Abstract. Pak. J. Biol. Sci. 11(5):805-808.

Mudigonda T, Mudigonda P (2010). Palliative cancer care ethics: Principles and challenges in Indian setting. Indian J. Palliat. Care16(3):107-110.

Namibian Cancer Registry (2011). Cancer in Namibia 2006-2009. Cancer association of Namibia: Windhoek.

Ojieh AE, Adegor EC, Lawrence EO (2013). Preliminary phytochemical screening, analgesic and anti-inflammatory properties of *Celosia*

isertii. European J. Med. Plants 3(3):369-380.
Olowokudejo JD, Kadiri AB, Travih VA (2008). An ethnobotanical survey of herbal markets and medicinal plants in lagos state of Nigeria. Ethnobot. Leaf. 12:851-865.
Palgrave KC (1981). Trees of southern Africa. Palliative care training ends in capital. Struik publishers: Cape town.
Pedraza-Chaverri J, Cardenas-Rodriguez N, Orozco-Ibarra M, Perez-Rojas JM (2008). Medicinal properties of mangosteen (*Garciniamangostana*). Food Chem. Toxicol. 46:3227-3239.
Powell RA, Mwangi-Powell FN, Kiyange F, Radbruch L, Harding R (2011). Pallaitive care development in Africa: How can we provide enough quality care? BMJ Support Palliat. Care 1(2):113-114.
Re R, Pellegrini N, Proteggente A, Pannala A, Yang M, Rice-Evans C (1999). Antioxidant activity applying an improved ABTS radical cationdecolorization assay. Free Radic. Biol. Med. 26(9/10):1231-1237.
Sharma H, Parihar L, Parihar P (2011). Review on cancer and anticancer properties of some medicinal plants. J. Med. Plants Res. 5(10):1818-1835.
Soetan KO, Aiyelaagbe OO (2009). The need for bioactivity-safety evaluation and conservation of medicinal plants-A review. J. Med. Plants Res. 3(5):324-328.
Thomson GE (2010). Further consideration of Asian medicinal plants in treating common chronic diseases in the west. J. Med. Plants Res. 4(2):125-130.
Towatana NH, Reanmongkol W, Wattanapiromsakul C, Bunkrongcheap R (2010). Acute subchronic toxicity evaluation of the hydroethanolic extracts of mangosteen pericarp. J. Med. Plants Res. 4(10):969-974.
Von Koenen E (2001). Medicinal, poisonous and edible plants of Namibia. Klaus Hess Publishers/ Verlag: Windhoek.
Wahab OM, Ayodele AE, Moody JO (2010). TLC phytochemical screening of Nigerian Loranthaceae. J. Pharmacogn. Phytother.. 2(5):64-70.
Watt JM, Breyer-Brandwijk MG (1962). Medicinal and poisonous plants of southern and eastern Africa. Bernard W. Riley: Santa Barbara.
Webster R, Lacey J, Quine S (2007). Palliative care: A public health priority in developing countries. J. Public Health Policy 28:28-39.
WHO (2011). Non-communicable diseases: country profiles. Available at: http://www.who.int/nmh/countries/en/

5

Ethnobotanical survey of healing medicinal plants traditionally used in the main Moroccan cities

Messaoudi Moussi I.*, Filali, H., Tazi, A. and Hakkou, F.

Laboratory of Pharmacology and Toxicology, Faculty of Medicine and Pharmacy of Casablanca, University Hassan II. Morocco.

The present study is a survey conducted to indicate the healing medicinal plants, traditionally used by the Moroccan population, and especially to select the healing plants mainly used in the form of essential oils. This survey allowed an inventory of 59 species of healing plants belonging to 37 families. The results showed that the whole plant is the most commonly used part (31%), followed by the leaves (29%). Most plants are Moroccan and are used as a single powder and as essential oils. The most common frequency of use is 2 times per day and the treatment duration depends mainly, on the pathological field and the nature of the wound. Also, the results revealed that plants whose leaves are the most used as essential oils are: *Rosmarinus officinalis*, *Lavandula angustifolia* and *Artemisia tridentata.* This study showed that medicinal plants play an important role in healing practices. It's a very valuable source of information for the studied areas and for national medicinal flora. So, it could be a database for further research in the field of herbal medicine, pharmacology and in order to manufacture new drugs based on medicinal plants.

Key words: Medicinal plants, pharmacological properties, healing, traditionnal medicine, ethnobotanical survey, Morocco.

INTRODUCTION

Since ancient times, man has always used medicinal plants to treat himself; and for fifteen years, researches have increased worldwide and have sought to investigate the pharmacological activities of these plants. Indeed, it is estimated that 80% of the population of developing countries, use traditional medicine (Bousta and Ennabili, 2011). These countries include Morocco, whose knowledge of phytotherapy and traditional medicine is transmitted by the culture through generations. These knowledge are developed, and enriched, thanks to the strategic geographic position of the kingdom.

The geographical position of Morocco provides a remarkable range of bioclimates, a great biodiversity, a good wealth of medicinal and aromatic plants and a variety of traditional knowledge. Indeed, the Moroccan flora is composed of over 4200 species and subspecies belonging to a large botanical known family, with 130 families and 940 species represented by: *Ateraceae*, *Fabaceae*, *Poaceae*, *Brassicaceae*, *Caryophylaceae*, *Lamiaceae*, *Apiaceae*, *Scrophulariaceae* and other families (Bellakhdar, 1998). Medicinal plants are therefore a precious heritage for humanity and especially for Morocco.

Wounds have always had a considerable impact on

*Corresponding author. E-mail: messimane38@yahoo.fr.

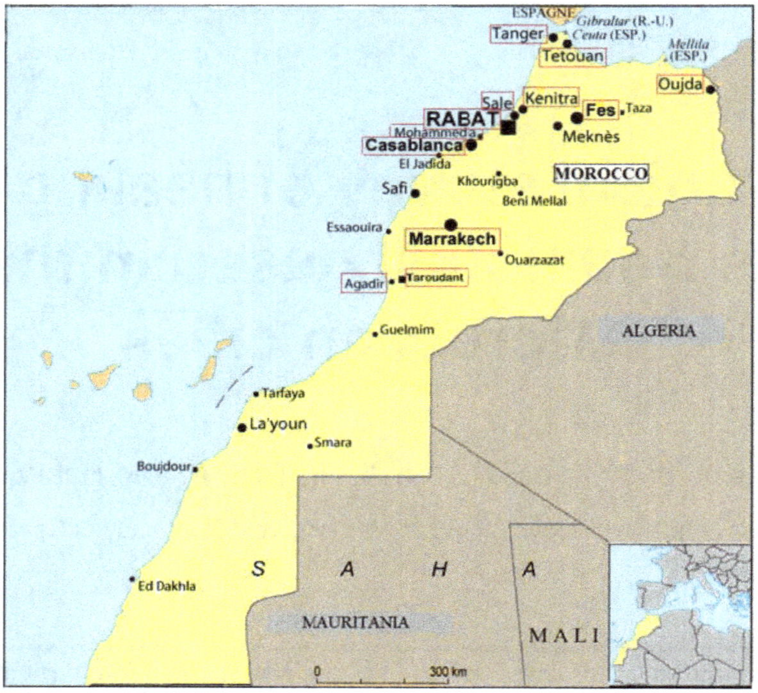

Figure 1. Map of Morocco showing the surveyed cities, Source: http://www.diplomatie.gouv.fr/fr/dossiers-pays/maroc/.

health especially those related to chronic skin wounds constitute a major health burden in developing countries (Agyarea et al., 2009). Subsequently, surgical wounds present in Morocco, a problem of drug therapy.Inflammation,swelling, pain and infection due to these wounds are closely related properties and involved in a big number of skin trauma.

To complete the partial and fragmentary studies conducted everywhere in Morocco, ethnobotanical surveys help to gather a very valuable source of information, ready to be scientifically exploited. In this context, the present study is part of the latter surveys. It aims to make a thorough inventory of medicinal plants with healing properties, traditionally used in Morocco and to choose the healing plants that are likely to be used in subsequent studies.

MATERIALS AND METHODS

Area of the study

Morocco is located at the north western tip of the African continent, separated from Spain by the 14 km of the Strait of Gibraltar. It is bathed in the west by the Atlantic Ocean and in the north by the Mediterranean Sea, both of which give it two coastlines spanning nearly 3500 km. Constituting a North-South passage area, Morocco has a surface of 710,850 km² and belongs to both the Mediterranean and the Sahara worlds (Bellakhdar, 1998). Due to its strategic location, Morocco has a rich flora. Changes in the climate and terrain are the major factors that can explain this floral wealth. Indeed, it has two coastlines and therefore receives rain streams from the Atlantic Ocean, which accumulate against the mountain barriers of the Atlas. This leads to heavy rainfalls in the cities of Rabat, Casablanca, Fez and the formation of snow in the high peaks of the Atlas, while the south and east stay arid.Moreover, the botanical interest of Morocco is intense and contains at least 2.5 million hectares of forest (about 15% of the total area) which contains cedars, palms, date palms, fig trees, olive trees, almond trees, acacias, fruit trees, cork oaks, pines, eucalyptus, and endemic plant that is the Argan tree, which is found nowhere else in the world, but in Morocco. (Bellakhdar, 1998).

Among the big and great cities in this country, we find Casablanca, Marrakech, Agadir, Fez, Tetouan, Tangier and Oujda, in addition to the towns of Mohammedia, Salé, Kenitra and Taroudant in the Agadir area. The study chose to carry out its investigation in these cities because they belong to the most populated regions of Morocco. They are not only best known for their richness on medicinal plants, climate and biodiversity, but also for their cultural diversity. They are a home from the numerous herbalists who live there. The surveyed cities (framed in red) are illustrated in Figure 1.

METHODOLOGY

This study was conducted to establish an inventory, as complete as possible, of medicinal plants traditionally used because of their healing properties by herbalists located in the main Moroccan cities to treat their patients. The study investigation lasted about five months (from 21 September, 2014 to 16 January, 2015). The total number of herbalists contacted is 202 whose distribution is represented in Table 1.

To have an overview of the local traditional uses and the pharmacopoeia's floristic diversity of these Moroccan cities, the ethnobotanical survey was conducted using series of direct and telephonic interviews with herbalists of the cities cited in Table 1. It was carried out using a predetermined questionnaire with specific questions about the healing plant: its local name, its origin (country,

Table 1. Number of herbalists contacted per city.

Surveyed cities	Number of herbalists	Surveyed cities	Number of herbalists
Casablanca	80	Marrakech	20
Fès	20	Tanger	18
Kenitra	8	Tétouan	5
Mohammedia	5	Agadir	10
Rabat	18	Taroudant	3
Salé	12	Oujda	3

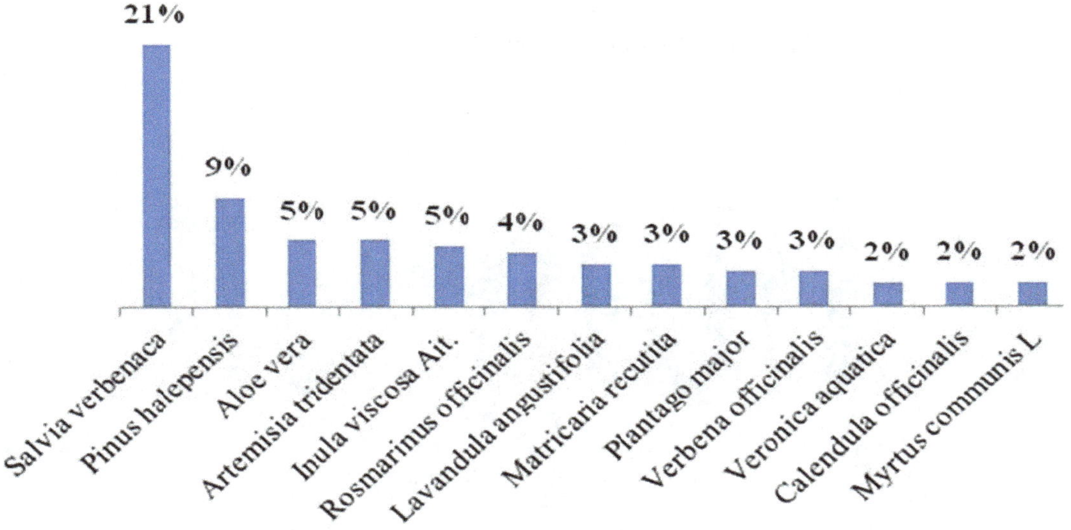

Figure 2. Distribution of collected healing plants.

region or city), its harvest season, its parts used, its form of preparation, the administration way of the plant, the frequency of use per day, the duration of the treatment, and if the plant is used alone or in combination with other plants.

Interviews were conducted in the dialect language of the country. The identification of the scientific names of the medicinal plants was carried out by a Professor Pharmacognosist at the High School of Technology (EST) in Casablanca, and with reference to the book of traditional medicinal plants (Bellakhdar, 1998). The study was able to collect 211 questionnaires in relation with the healing plants. Among the 202 herbalists contacted, 152 accepted to answer to the questions, while the others either refused to respond to our request, or were not specialized in medicinal plants or were unreachable.

The study was especially interested to find a relationship between the criteria of the plants that were collected during the investigation, in order to highlight information that will be used for the selection of healing plants for further experimental studies.

Statistical analysis

The counting of the results was carried out by an established mask on Statistical Package for the Social Sciences (SPSS) software, version 21. The relationship between the variables was evaluated by the test of independence Chi-square (χ^2) with a confidence level of 95% and by calculating the p-value. The results are considered significant when the p-value is less than 0.05.

RESULTS

Floristic screening

Scientific name of the listed plants

The survey allowed an inventory of 59 species of healing medicinal plants. So, the analysis identified several plants but the most represented are: *Salvia verbenaca* at a frequency of 21%, *Pinus halepensis* (9%), *Aloe vera* (5%), *Artemisia tridentata* (5%), *Inula viscosa ait.* (5%), *Rosmarinus officinalis* (4%) and *Lavandula angustifolia* of 3%. The classification of these species by their frequency is represented in Figure 2. All the indexed healing plants and their corresponding properties are listed in Table 6 and 7,

Families of healing plants

The recorded healing medicinal plants belong to 37 families four of which are predominant: *Lamiaceae* (34%), *Asteraceae* (18.7%), *Pinaceae* (8.9%) and

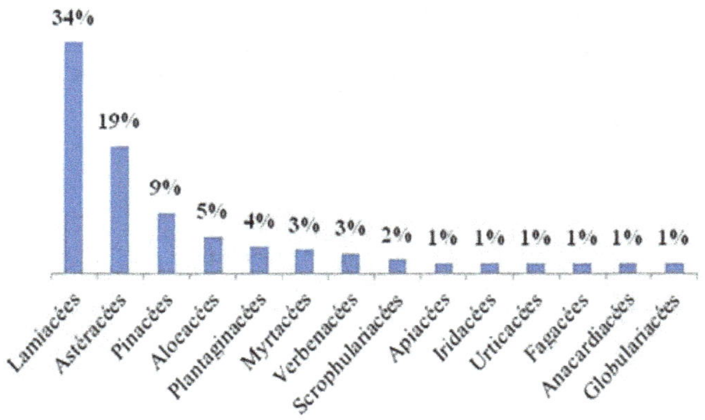

Figure 3. Distribution of healing plants families.

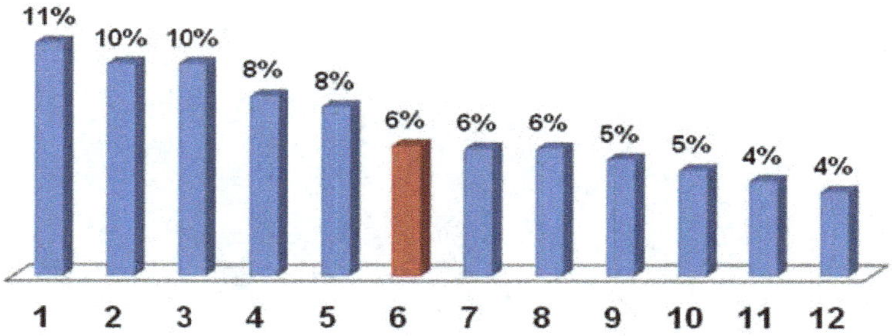

Figure 4. Distribution of healing plants based on Moroccan regions, (1) Souss-Massa-Draa, (2) Marrakech-Tensift-Al Haouz, (3) Gharb-Chrarda-BeniHssen, (4) Meknes-Tafilalet, (5) Tangier- Tetouan (6) No Moroccan, (7) Taza-Al Hoceima-Taounate, (8) Fez-Boulemane, (9) Tadla-Azilal, (10) Oriental, (11) Doukkala-Abda, (12) Rabat-Sale-Zemmour- Zaër.

Aloaceae (5.4%). The rest of results are shown in Figure 3.

Origin of plants

The plants were classified according to their original area and where they are most prevalent. Most of Moroccan healing plants are distributed in the region of Souss-Massa-Draa (11%), followed by the region of Marrakech-Tensift-Al Haouz and the region of Gharb-Chrarda-Beni Hssen with 10%, while 6% of the plants are not Moroccan Figure 4.

Plants season

The availability and distribution of plants depend on the season and climate. The study obtained information on the harvest season for each plant. Spring is the season with high percentage of plants (50%), followed by summer (14%), winter (9%) and autumn (5%). Figure 5 illustrates the obtained results.

Ethnobotanical and pharmacological screening

Used parts of plant

The used parts of plants were collected and classified according to their order of importance. The whole plant is the most commonly used form with a frequency of 31%, followed by leaves with 29%, flowers (12%), bark (7%) and seeds (7%). The term "Other" refers to other parts of the plant found, as mucilage for *Aloe vera* species and stigma for *Crocus sativum* species. Figure 6 includes all these results.

Form of use

To facilitate the use of medicinal plants, herbalists recommend several types of preparations: powder, decoction, infusion and cold water, use as essential oils and many others. The most widely used form is a single powder of 57%, followed by the form of essential oils of 22% and by other forms (11%), like the application of the plant directly on the wound, or formed into a wound

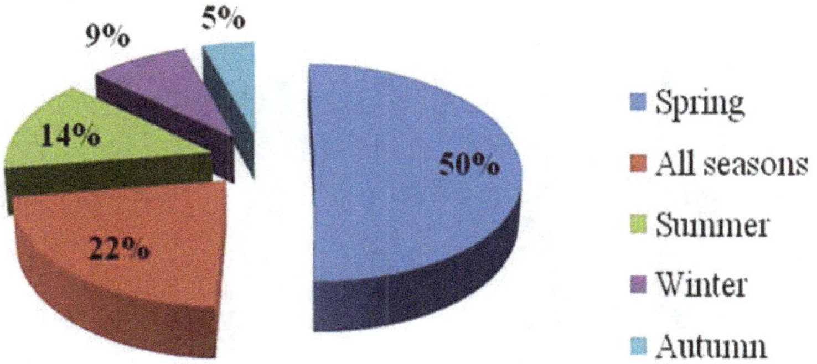

Figure 5. Distribution of healing plants by season.

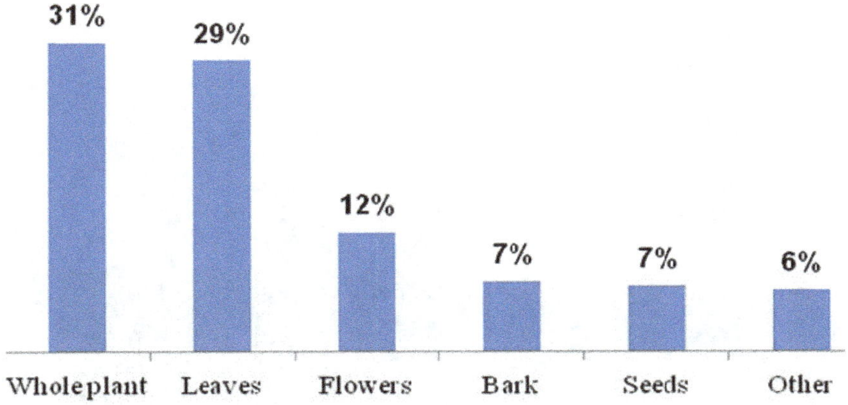

Figure 6. Distribution's frequency of used parts of healing plants.

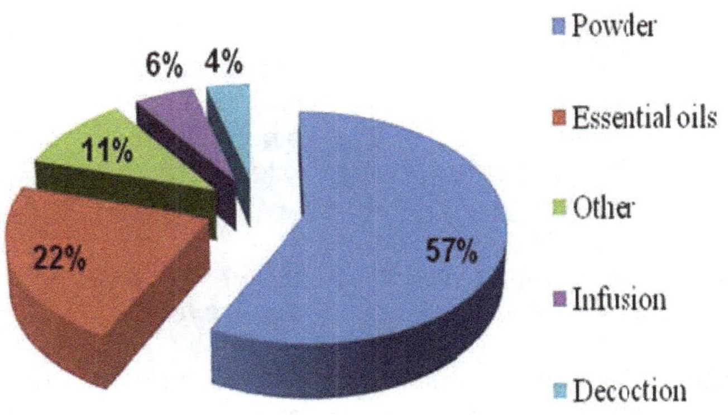

Figure 7. Dosage form of recorded healing plants.

dressing or applied as a cream Figure 7.

Way of administration

The most common ways of drugs administration are dermal and oral. In this study, the extreme majority staffs for dermal administration (90.5 %), 16% for a combination of dermal and oral administration and 2% for the oral way were found out.

Frequency and duration of use

According to each herbalist, medicinal plants are applied one to five times a day and the diagnosis may sometimes

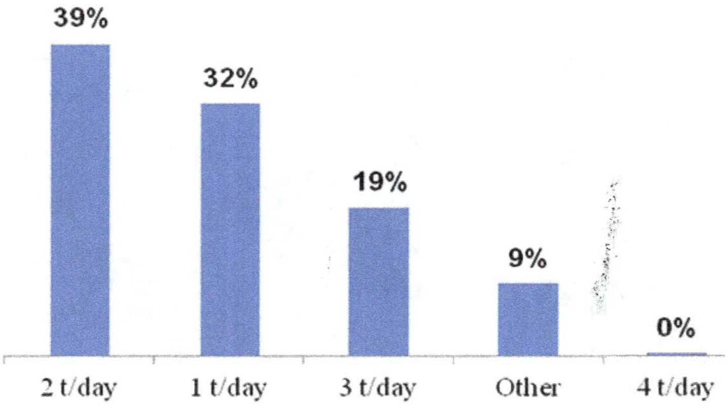

Figure 8. Frequencies of use of healing plants.

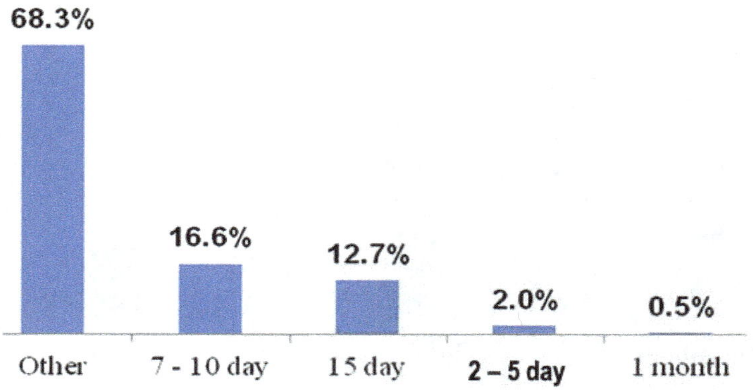

Figure 9. Distribution's frequency of the treatment's duration.

vary depending on the wound. The treatment period for its part, can extend to a month, but that depends on the pathological field (case of the patient) and on the depth of the wound. In this study, 39% for a frequency use of 2 times a day (morning and evening), 32% for 1 time a day (especially at night), 19% for 3 times a day, and 9% represents the frequency that depends on the wound and the treated patient's case were obtained (Figure 8). For the duration of treatment, the majority of herbalists were unable to inform us about the exact duration of therapy because it depends on the wound, the patient's healing duration, the response to the treatment and the effectiveness of this latter. The study got a major frequency of 68.3% for the criterion "Other" (depending to the wound, to the patient's case and the response of the latter to the treatment), 16.2% for a period of 1 week to10 days and 12.7% for a period of 2 weeks (Figure 9).

Plants association

According to herbalists, there are plants that can be associated with other species or mixed with vegetable or essential oils from other plants. The study investigation revealed that the predominant part (66.4 %) is for a single use of plants without any association with other species and the rest (33.6 %) is for the association of plants with others. Names and frequencies of associated plants are listed in Table 2.

Evaluation of the independence of variables with Chi-square test

Let X and Y be two qualitative variables with l and k modalities, respectively. The study test that X and Y are independent (H_0). The Chi-square variable is associated with a number of degrees of freedom (v) calculated including: $v = (k-1)\ (l-1)$ (Mountassir, 2014). The study also based on the calculation of p value to test the independence of two variables. The test is significant and H_0 is rejected when the p value is less than 0.05.

Crossing between used parts and form of use

Consider X as the qualitative variable that represents the part of the plant used and Y qualitative variable that

Table 2. List and frequencies of associated plants.

Healing plant	Associated medicinal plants
Aloe vera	*Myrtus communis L.*(1)
Amica L.	*Artemisia absinthium* (1)
Artemisia tridentata	*Lavandula angustifolia* (3), *Myrtus communis L.* (1), *Matricaria recutita* (1), *Thymus vulgaris* (1), *Artemisia absinthium* (1), *Quercus faginea lamk* (1), *Rhus albidum schousb.* (1), *Tea melaleuca* (1)
Calendula officinalis	*Lavandula angustifolia (1), Rosmarinus officinalis (1)*
Inula viscosa ait.	*Argania spinosa* (2), *Matricaria rectutita* (1)
Saponaria vaccaria L.	*Argania spinosa* (1)
Globularia alypum L.	*Salvia verbenaca* (1)
Lavandula angustifolia	*Argania spinosa* (1)
Marrubium vulgare	*Artemisia abstinthium* (1)
Rosmarinus officinalis	*Calendula officinalis* (1), *Thymus vulgaris* (1)
Salvia verbenaca	*Plantago major* (6), *Verbena officinalis* (9), *Pinus halepensis* (6), *Thymus vulgaris* (1), *Plantago psyllium* (1), *Inula viscosa ait.* (1), *Argania spinosa* (1), *Myrtus communis L* (1), *Artemisia tridentata* (1), *Marrubium vulgare* (2), *Lavandula angustifolia* (1)
Thymus vulgaris	*Rosmarinus officinalis* (1)
Laurus nobilis L.	*Argania spinosa* (1)
Smilax aspera L.	*Matricaria recutita* (1)
Pinus halepensis	*Salvia verbenaca* (2), *Verbena officinalis* (2), *Artemisia tridentata* (2), *Myrtus communis L.* (1), *Marrubium vulgare* (1), *Plantago major* (1)
Plantago major	Salvia verbenaca (1), Verbena officinalis (1)
Urtica dioica	Thymus vulgaris(1), Rosmarinus officnalis(1)
Verbena officinalis	Salvia verbenaca (1), Plantago major (1), Papaver rhoeas L. (1)
Curcuma longa.	Artemisia tridentata (1), Marrubium vulgare (1), Allium cepa (1)

(Frequency).

Table 3. Contingency table: Used parts*form of use.

Form of use/ Part	Leaf	Flower	Roots	Bark	Fruit	Seeds	Whole plant	Other	Total
Powder	2.98	0.21	0.00	2.86	0.06	0.14	4.96	0.64	11.85
Decoction	0.70	0.34	0.32	0.03	0.52	0.64	0.97	0.01	3.53
Infusion	4.70	0.51	0.19	0.94	0.59	0.07	2.71	0.47	10.18
Essential oils	1.65	1.85	0.79	1.73	0.33	0.01	1.76	0.51	8.64
Other	0.00	0.00	0.43	1.83	0.64	0.09	1.58	5.37	9.95
Total	10.05	2.91	1.74	7.40	2.14	0.95	11.97	6.99	44.15

represents the use form of the plant. The study want to test that X and Y are independent (H_0), for a significance level of 95% using a contingency table with double entry. Table 3 summarizes the results of this test. According to this table, $v = 28$, $\chi^2_{obs}=44.15$ and $\chi^2_{v;\alpha}=16.93$ so $\chi^2_{obs} > \chi^2_{v;\alpha}$. Therefore, H_0 is rejected.

Crossing between used parts and use form as essential oils

Let the qualitative variable X: Used parts, and Y: Use form as essential oils. According to the contingency Table 4, $v=7$, $\chi^2_{obs}=69.1$ and $\chi^2_{v;\alpha}=2.17$ so $\chi^2_{obs} > \chi^2_{v;\alpha}$. There-

Table 4. Contingency table: used parts*use as essential oils form.

Form of use	Leaves	Flower	Roots	Bark	Fruit	Seeds	Whole plant	Other	Total
Use as essential oils	47.81	1.36	5.88	5.88	2.91	0.98	1.36	2.91	69.10

fore H_0 is rejected.

In order to exactly know the part of the plant which is most often used in the form of essential oils, or in other words, the part of the plant which is most often used as essential oils form, the study has made the crossing between using form as essential oil and every part of the plant (leaf, flower, fruit, root, bark, seeds and whole plant) (Table 5). From Table 5, the *p* value of the Chi-square test of 0.003 (less than 0.05) made the study to conclude that the use in the form of essential oils depends on the leaves.

For the second crossing, the *p* value: 0.116 is higher than 0.05, the study doesn't reject H_0, and reached the conclusion that the use form of essential oils doesn't depend on the flowers. The *p* value of the third crossing (0.214) higher than 0.05 doesn't reject H_0 and conclude for an independence between the use form as essential oils and roots (at a confidence level of 95%). For the fourth crossing, the *p* value (0.06) is higher than 0.05; therefore study didn't reject H_0 and conclude that the use form as essential oils is independent of the barks. For the fifth crossing, the *p* value (0.663) is higher than 0.05, so the study didn't reject H_0 and conclude that the use form as essential oils doesn't depend on the fruit. Then, the *p* value (0.567) of the sixth crossing is higher than 0.05, so the study did not reject H_0 and conclude that the use form as essential oils does not depend on seeds. Finally, according to the Chi-square of the seventh crossing, the *p* value is less than 0.05. So the study rejects H_0 and concludes that the use in the form of essential oils depends on the whole plant.

Crossing between use form of essential oil and the healing plant

Here, the study wants to test if the use in the form of essential oils form depends on the plant species. According to Table 5, the *p* value is less than 0.05 (0.000). These results are significant and the H_0 hypothesis is rejected.

Crossing between use form of essential oil, leaf-part and healing plant

The study wants to show through this crossing that the use of the leaves in the form of essential oils depends on the healing plant species. Indeed, Table 5 gives a *p* value less than 0.05. Furthermore, plants whose leaves are more often used in the form of essential oils are: *R. officinalis*, *L. angustifolia*, *A. tridentata*, *M. communis L* and *T. vulgaris* (Figure 10)

DISCUSSION

The phytotherapy is frequently used by the Moroccan population. In fact, according to some study, 70 to 80% of Moroccan people use medicinal plants to heal: 60% of them are female, and more than 50% are illiterate (Zeggwagh et al., 2013). 55 to 90% of people use plants to treat chronic diseases of which 16.8% are for the dermatological affections and wounds in Fez (Zeggwagh et al., 2013). Moreover, in the region of Ksar Lakbir, 11.6% of plants are employed to treat skin diseases (Merzouki et al., 2000), 15% in the region of Essaouira (Mehdioui et al., 2007), 17% in Ifran (Rhafouri et al., 2014) and 12.5% in the region of Zaêr (Lahsissene et al., 2010). On the other hand, medicinal plants are used for dermatological affections by 27% in the region of El Hajeb (EL Amri el al., 2014), by 11.80% in the region of Agadir (El Hafian et al., 2014), by 10% in Kenitra (Salhi et al., 2010), by 12% in the region of Haut Atlas Oriental (Belamdini et al., 2014) and by 16% in the region of Meknes-Tafilalet (Fadil et al., 2014).

Indexed healing medicinal plants

A number of 59 species of healing medicinal plants has been inventoried in this study, of which majority are: *S. verbenaca*, *P. halepensis*, *A. vera*, *A. tridentata*, *I. viscosa* ait , *R. officnalis*, *L. angustifolia*. In parallel, the national literature review enabled us to screen 59 Moroccan healing plants including: *S. verbenaca*, *P. halepensis, I. viscosa ait.*, *A. tridentata* and *A. vera, in addition to 54 other healing plants* (Bellakhdar, 1998). Another national ethnobotanical study shows that *A. vera, L. officinalis, M. recutita, M.s communis, C. officinalis* and *T. vulgaris* have wound healing properties (Sijelmassi, 2011). This shows the proximity of the results of this study with those found in the literature.

On the other hand, an ethnobotanical survey confirmed that *S. verbenaca*is has been employed by the local population to facilitate the wound healing, in the region of Zaër (Lahsissene et al., 2009), Haut Atlas Oriental (Belamdini et al., 2014) and of Settat (Bammi et al., 2002). Moreover, it has been shown that *S. verbenaca* and *I. viscosa ait.* have a healing potential on wounds,

Table 5. Chi-square test: use as essential oils and used part of plants.

Parameter		Pearson Chi-square			Fisher's exact test		Interpretation
Crossing		Value	DOF	P value	Signification exacte (bilateral)	Exact significance (unilateral)	Significance
1	Use as essential oils form*Leaves	8.787	1	0.003	0.004	0.003	S
2	Use as essential oils form*Flowers	2.466	1	0.116	0.168	0.092	NS
3	Use as essential oils form*Roots	1.541	1	0.214	0.293	0.195	NS
4	Use as essential oils form*Bark	3.391	1	0.066	0.075	0.052	NS
5	Use as essential oils form*Fruit	0.190	1	0.663	0.705	0.457	NS
6	Use as essential oils form*Seeds	0.327	1	0.567	0.556	0.380	NS
7	Use as essential oils form*Whole plant.	7.204	1	0.007	0.008	0.005	S
8	Use as essential oils form*Name ofplant.	128.265	55	0.000	-	-	S
9	Use as essential oils form*Leaf-part*Name of plant.	8.787	1	0.003	0.004	.003	S

*DOF: Degree Of Freedom; NS: No Significant; S: Significant.

Table 6. Inventory of healing plants recorded in our ethnobotanical survey.

Family	Scientific name	Local name	% of plant	Used part	Usedform	Additive	Frequency of use	Treatment duration	Administration way	Content in EO	Properties	Plants association	Corresponding References
Aloeaceae	*Aloevera*	الصبار	5.7%	Mg (4), Pu (2), L (2), Fl (1), W (2), Ba (1)	Di (6), Cr (1), Po (1), Dr (1), EO (3)	Olive oil (2), Argan oil (2)	1t/d (4), 2t/d (6), 3t/d (2), Other (1)	2 We (4), Other (8)	Cu (10)	Yes (4), No (3)	**[1]**	Yes	Sijelmassi (2011), Bellakhdar (1998)
Amaryllidaceae	*Allium cepa*	البصلة	0.5%	F (1)	Dr (1)	Honey (1)	1t/d (1)	3 D (1)	Cu (1), Or (1)		**[2]**	No	El Hafian et al. (2014)
	Pistacialenticus L.	الضرو	0.5%	F (1)	Po (1), EO (1)	-	4 t/d (1)	Other (1)	Cu (1)	Yes (1)	**[3]**	No	Daoudi et al (2015)
Anacardiaceae	*Pistaciaterebinthus L.*	ايك البطم	0.5%	F (1)	Po (1)	-	3t/d (1)	2 We (1)	Cu (1)	No (1)	**[4]**	No	-
	Rhusalbidums chousb.	الزواية	0.5%	Ba (1)	Po (1) Dec (1)	-	2 t/d (1) 3t/d (1)	2 We (1)	Cu (1)	No (1)	**[5]**	No	-
	Carum carvi L.	الكروية	0.5%	S (1)	Po (1)	-	2t/d(1)	Other(1)	Cu (1) Or (1)	-	**[6]**	No	-
Apiaceae	*Centellaasiatica*	القسط الهندي	0.5%	Ba (1), R (1)	Po (2)		1 t/d (1), 2 t/d (1)	Other (2)	Cu (2)	No (1)	**[7]**	No	-
	Coriandrum sativum	القزبر	0.5%	L (1), R (1) S	Po (1)		3 t/d (1)	1 We (1), 2 We (1)	Cu (1), Or (1)	Yes (1)	**[8]**	No	-

Table 6. Contd.

Aristolochiaceae	*Aristolochia long.*	برزطم	0.5%	Ro (1), Bo (1)	Po (1)	Honey (1)	1t/d (1)	1 Mo (1), Other (1)	Cu (1)	No	**[9]**	No	Bellakhdar (1998)
	Arnica L.	الحلحال	0.9%	L (1), Fl (1) W (1)	Po (1), Dec (1), EO (2), Dr (1)	Salt (1)	2 t/d (1), 3 t/d (2)	Other (2)	Cu (2)	Yes (2)	**[10]**	**Yes**	-
	Artemisia tridentata	الشيح	5.2%	L (6), Fl (2), W (2), S (2), Ro (1), F (1)	Po (7), Dec (3), Inf (3), EO (5), with honey, Di (1)	Argan oil (2), Honey (2), Grease (1)	1 t/d (3), 2 t/d (7), 3 t/d (4), 4 t/day (1), Other (1)	1 We (2), 2 We (2), Other (7)	Cu (11), Or (1)	Yes (9)	**[11]**	**Yes**	Salhi et al. (2010), Fakchich and Elachouri (2014)
	Calendula officinalis	الجمرة	1.9%	Fl (4) L (1)	Po (1) Dec (1) Inf (1) EO (1) Oil (1) Mac (2)		1 t/d (2) 2 t/d (3) 3 t/d (2)	2 We (1) Other (3)	Cu (4) Or (2)	Yes (2) No (2)	**[12]**	**Yes**	Sijelmassi (2011), Bellakhdar (1998)
	Chamaemelu mnobile	البابونج	0.5%	L (1) R (1)	Po (1)	Oil (1)	1 t/d (1), 2 t/d (1)	Other (1)	Cu (1)	Yes (1)	**[13]**	No	Tahri et al. (2012)
Asteraceae	*Inulaviscosa ait.*	مكرمان الترهل	5.2%	L (12)	Po (11), Dec (1), Inf (1), EO (1), Di (2),	Water (1), Resin (1), Argan oil (2), Olive oil (3), Cider vinegar (1,) Propolis (1)	1 t/d (9), 2t/d (3), Other (2)	1 We (1), Other (10)	Cu (11), Or (1)	Yes (9), No (1)	[14]	Yes	Tahri et al. (2012), Salhi et al. (2010)
	Matricaria recutita	البابونج الألماني	3.3%	W (2), Fl (3), F (1), L (1), R (1),	Po (2), Inf (2), EO (5)	Vegetal oil (2)	1t/d (4), 2 t/d (4), 3 t/d (1)	2 We (1), Other (6)	Cu (7), Or (2)	Yes (7)	[15]	No	Sijelmassi (2011), Fakchich et al. (2014), Merzouki et al. (2000)
	Pulicaria arabica	العطازة	0.5%	F (1)	EO (1)	Jojoba oil (1)	1t/d (1)	Other (1)	Cu (1)	Yes (1)	[16]	No	-
	Saussurea coctus	القسط البحري	0.5%	R(1)	Po(1)		1t/d (1)	Other (1)	Cu (1)	No (1)	[17]	No	-
	Tanacetum parthenium	البابونج الكبير	0.5%	L (1) R (1)	Po (1)	Oil (1)	1 t/d (1), 2 t/d (1)	Other (1)	Cu (1)	Yes (1)	[18]	No	-

Table 6. Contd.

Cactaceae	*Opuntia ficus-indica*	الكرموص الهندي	0.5%	F (2) S	EO (1), Other (1)		1t/d (2)	1 We (1), Other (1)	Cu (2)	Yes (1)	[19]	No	Fakchich et al. (2014)
Caryophyllaceae	*Saponaria vaccaria L.*	الصابونية	0.5%	L (1)	Po (1), Mac (1)	Oilve oil (1), Argan oil(1)	1t/d (1)	Other (1)	Cu (1)		[20]	Yes	Bellakhdar (1998)
Cesalpiniaceae	*Cassia absus L.*	حبة البركة	0.5%	F (1)	Po(1) EO (1)		1t/d (1)	Other (1)	Cu (1)	Yes (1)	[21]	No	-
Chenopodiaceae	*Chenopodium L.*	المخينزة	0.5%	L (1)	Di (1), EO (1)		2t/d (1)	Other (1)	Cu (1)	Yes (1)	[22]	No	Bellakhdar (1998)
Fabaceae	*Vicia sativa L.*	عين الأرنب	0.5%	L (1)	Po (1)	Honey (1)	1t/d (1)	Other (1)	Cu (1)	Yes	[23]	No	-
Fagaceae	*Quercus faginea lamk.*	العفصة	1.4%	Nu (2), F (2)	Po (3)		2 t/d (3), 3 t/d (1)	1 We (1), 2 We (1), Other (1)	Cu (3)	No (1)	[24].	No	Fakchich et al. (2014), Merzouki et al. (2000)
Geraniaceae	*Geranium L.*	لمعطرشة	0.9%	W (1), Fl (1)	Po (1), EO (1)	Oil (1)	1 t/d (1), 2t/d(1)	Other (2)	Cu (2)	Yes (2)	[25]	No	Fadil et al. (2014)
Globulariaceae	*Globularia alypum L.*	تسلغا	1.4%	L (2), Fl (1)	Po (3), EO (1)	Almond oil (1), Olive oil (1)	1 t/d (1), 2t/d (3) 3 t/d (1)	1 We (1), 2 We (1), Other (1)	Cu (3)	Yes (2), No (1)	[26]	Yes	-
Hypericaceae	*Hypericum perforatum*	يوفارقون	0.9%	Fl (2), F (1)	Po (2), EO (2)	Honey (1)	1t/d (2), 2 t/d (1)	Other (2)	Cu (2)	Yes (2)	[27]	No	Bammi and Douira (2002)
Iridaceae	*Crocus sativum*	زعفران لحر	1.4%	Sg (2), L (1)	Po (2), Dr (1), Di (1)	Honey (1), Argan oil (1)	1t/d (3)	1 We (2), Other (1)	Cu (3)	No (3)	[28]	No	-
Lamiaceae	*Lavandula angustifolia*	الخزامة	3.3%	L (4), Fl (1), W (3)	Po (4), EO (6), Dec (1)	Honey (1), Vaselin (1), Butter (1), Argan oil (1), Vegetal oil (1), Cider vinegar (1), Lavender water (1)	1 t/d (3), 2t/d (3), 3t/d (2)	1 We (1), 1 Mo (1), Other (5)	Cu (7)	Yes (7)	[29]	Yes	Sijelmassi (2011), Tahri et al. (2012)

Table 6. Contd.

Marrubium vulgare	مريوت	1.4%	W (2) L (1)	Po (1), Di (1), Dr 1)	Salt (1), Olive oil (1)	1 t/d (1), 2 t/d (1), 3 t/d (1)	2 We (1), Other (2)	Cu (3)	Yes (2)	[30]	Yes	Fakchich et al. (2014), Lahsissene et al. (2009), Daoudi et al. (2015)
Mentha x piperita L.	النعناع	0.9%	L (2)	Inf(1), EO (1), Mac (1), Dr (1)	Vaselin (1), Oil (1),Alcohol (1)	1 t/d (2), 2 t/d (1)	Other (2)	Cu (2), Or (1)	Yes (2)	[31]	No	-
Ocimum basilicum	الحبق	0.9%	L (1), Fl (2)	Po (1), EO (2)	Honey (1)	2 t/d (1), Other (1)	1 Mo (1), Other (1)	Cu (2)	Yes (2)	[32]	No	-
Origanum vulgare	زعيترة	0.5%	L (1)	Inf Dec (1), EO (1)	Castor oil (1)	2 t/d (1)	2 We (1)	Cu (1)	Yes (1)	[33]	No	-
Rosmarinus officinalis	اليازير	4.3%	L (5), Fl (1) F (1), W (3)	Po (3), Inf (2), Dec (2), EO (7)	Honey (2), Vegetal oil (3)	1 t/d (2), 2 t/d (6), 3t/d (2)	Other (5), 1 We (3)	Cu (7), Or (2)	Yes (8)	[34]	Yes	Fakchich et al. (2014), El Amri et al. (2014),Lahsissene et al. (2009), Salhi et al. (2010), Bellakhdar (1998)

and are used by the population of Settat's province (Tahri et al., 2012). Indeed, *S. verbenaca, I. viscosa ait., A. tridentata* and *R. officinalis* are recorded as healing medicinal plants by a survey in the region of Gharb of Morocco (Mechraâ Bel Ksir) (Benkhnigue et al., 2011), whereas it was found that *A. tridentata*, *I. viscosa*, *R. officinalis* and *S. verbenaca* have healing properties against wounds, in Kenitra (Salhi et al., 2010).

Families of healing plants

The study has indexed 37 families of which*Lamiaceae*, *Asteraceae*, *Pinaceae* and *Aloaceae* are predominant. In fact, several studies have confirmed the dominant presence of these families. An ethnobotanical survey in Fez (Zeggwagh et al., 2013), at Kenitra (Salhi et al., 2010) and in the region of Haut Atlas Oriental (Belamdini et al., 2014) showed that *Lamiceae*, *Asteraceae* and *Apiaceae* are the most represented. Another one, has demonstrated that *Lamiaceae*, *Fabaceae* and *Apiaceae* are the dominant families at the region of Agadir (El Hafian et al., 2014), Whereas, two other research teams found that *Lamiaceae*, *Asteraceae* and *Liliaceae* are the major families used by the local population of Ifran (Rhafouri et al., 2014) and Essaouira (Mehdioui et al., 2007). Finally, the national study of medicinal plants found that *Asteraceae, Fabaceae* and *Poaceae* are the predominant families in Morocco, which explains this similar distribution through regions (Bellakhdar, 1998).

Origin of plants and season

The plants were found in most parts of Souss-Massa-Draa, followed by the region of Marrakech-Tensift-Al Haouz and the region of Gharb-Chrarda-Beni Hssen. This distribution can be explained by climate changes, soil and reliefs type from one region to another (Bellakhdar, 1998), and also by the cultural outcome of each region which has its own traditional use of medicinal plants. On the other hand, spring is the season of flowering aromatic plants and it's an ideal bioclimatic period for them, that is why the study

Table 6. Contd.

	Salvia verbenaca	الخياطة	21.3%	W (37), L (3), R (2), Fl (2), F (3), Ro (1)	Po (44), Inf (2), EO (1)	Olive oil (2), Honey (2), Butter (1), Cider vinegar (2), Alcohol (1), Water (1)	1t/d (19), 2 t/d(13), 3 t/d (8), 5t/d (1), Other (8)	1 We (9,) 2 We (5), Other (32)	Cu (43), Or (12)	Yes (6), No (2)	**[35]**	No	Fakchich et al. (2014), Lahsissene et al (2009), Merzouki et al. (2000), Daoudi et al. (2015), Belamdini et al. (2014), Bammi and Douira.(2002), Tahri et al. (2012), Salhi et al. (2010), Bellakhdar (1998)
	Thymus vulgaris	الزعتر	1.4%	L (1) W (1)	EO (2), Inf (1)	Vegetal oil (1)	2 t/d (2), 3 t/d (1)	1 We (1), Other (1)	Cu (2), Or (1)	Yes (2)	**[36]**	**Yes**	Sijelmassi (2011), Bellakhdar (1998)
Lauraceae	*Laurus nobilisL.*	ورق سيدنا موسى	0.5%	L (1)	Po (1), EO (1)	Argan oil (1)	1 t/d (1), 2 t/d(1)	Other (1)	Cu (1)	Yes (1)	**[37]**	**Yes**	-
Liliaceae	*Cinnamomumv erum*	القرفة	0.5%	Ba (1)	Po (1), EO (1)	Oil (1)	2t/d (1)	1 We (1)	Cu (1), Or (1)	Yes (1)	**[38]**	No	-
	Smilax aspera L.	ورق العليق	0.5%	L (1)	Po(1)	Cider vinegar(1) Propolis (1)	1t/d(1)	Other(1)	Cu (1)	Yes(1)	**[39]**	**Yes**	-
Lythraceae	*Lawsonia inermis*	لحنا	0.5%	L	Po (1), Dec(1), Inf(1)	Honey (1)	2t/d (1)	2 We (1)	Cu (1)	No (1)	**[40]**		Fakchich et al. (2014), Semwal et al. (2014), Hseini and Kahouadji (2007), ;Zeggwagh (2013), Lahsissene and Kahouadji (2010), Bellakhdar (1998)
Myristicaceae	*Myristica fragrans*	الوردالمسكي	0.5%	Fl (2), L (1)	EO(2), Po (1)	-	1t/d (2), 2t/d (1)	Other (2)	Cu (2)	Yes (2)	**[41]**	No	-

found the majority of aromatic plants in spring. Also, the season of harvesting can influence the composition of the plant on several essential metabolites.

Used parts of plant

The high frequency use of the whole plant can be explained by the facility of the manipulation of the plant. In fact, another study showed that people are more likely to pick the whole plant and to use it instead of choosing a specific desired part (Tahri et al., 2012). This can probably explain the high use of the whole plant in this study. The high use of the leaves can be explained by the fact that they are the seat of several reactions (photosynthesis for example) and they contain several metabolites that are primordial for the pharmacological properties of the plant (Salhi et al., 2011). Also, their performances are better compared to other parts of the plant. Indeed, other studies have shown that essential oils yield of leaves of some plants is higher compared to flowers (Bassole et al., 2001).

Table 6. Contd.

Myrtaceae	*Melaleucatea*	اتاي	1.4%	S (2)	Po (3)	Castor oil (1) Almond oil (1)	1t/d (2), 2t/d (2)	Other (3)	Cu (3)	Yes (1)	**[42]**	No	-
	Myrtus communis L.	الريحان لحلموس	1.9%	L (2), Fl (1), W (1)	Po (1), EO (3)	Vegetal oil (1), Almond oil (1), Castor oi l(1)	1 t/d (1), 2 t/d (2), 3t/d (1), Other (1)	Other (3), 2 We (1)	Cu (4)	Yes (4)	**[43]**	No	Sijelmassi (2011), Wahid (2013), Tahri et al. (2010), Bellakhdar (1998)
Papaveraceae	*Papaver rhoeas L.*	بلعمان	0.5%	Fl (1)	Po (1) Di (1)		1t/d (1)	Other (1)	Cu (1)	No (1)	**[44]**	No	Fakchich et al. (2014)
Pédaliaceae	*Sesamum indicum*	السمسم	0.5%	S (1)	EO (1)		1t/d (1)	Other (1)	Cu (1)	Yes (1)	**[45]**	No	Zeggwagh et al (2013)
Pinaceae	*Pinus halepensis*	التايدة	9.0%	W (7), R (2), Ba (4), Fl (1)	Po (14), Inf (1)	Olive oil (1), Rancid butter (1), Cider vinegar (1)	1t/d (7), 2 t/d (6), Other (3)	1 We (3), 2 We (1), Other (11)	Cu (14), Or (2)	Yes (1), No (4)	**[46]**	**Yes**	Bammi and Douira. (2002)
Plantaginaceae	*Plantago major*	المصاصة	2.8%	W (1), F (1), L (1), Fl (1)	Po (2), Di (1)	-	1 t/d (1), 2 t/d (1), 3 t/d (1)	Other (3)	Cu (3), Or (1)	Yes (1), No (1)	**[47]**	**Yes**	Sijelmassi (2011), ElAmri et al. (2014), Bellakhdar (1998)
	Plantago psyllium	زرقطونة	0.9%	W (1)	Po (1)	-	1t/d (1)	Other (1)	Cu (1)	-	**[48]**	No	Bellakhdar (1998)
Poaceae	*Avena sativa L.*	الخرطال	0.5%	S (1)	Po (1)	Lemon juice (1)	1t/d (1)	Other (1)	Cu (1)	No (1)	**[49]**	No	-
Rhamnaceae	*Rhamnus alaternus L.*	مليلس	0.5%	L (1)	Po (1), EO (1)		1t/d (1)	1 Mo (1)	Cu (1)	Yes (1)	**[50]**	No	-
Ranunculaceae	*Clematis cirrhosa L.*	ايكودي	0.5%	R (1)	Mac (1)	Milk juice (1)	1t/d (1)	Other (1)	Cu (1)	No (1)	**[51]**	No	-
Salicaceae	*PopulusL.*	أسفساف	0.5%	L (1)	Po (1)	-	2t/d (1)	2 We (1)	Cu (1)	Yes (1)	**[52]**	No	-
Sapotaceae	*Argania spinosa*	أركان	0.9%	F (3)	EO (1), Other (2)	-	1t/d (2), Other (1)	1 We (1), Other (2)	Cu (3)	-	**[53]**	No	Zeggwagh et al. (2013)
Solanaceae	*Capsicum annuum*	التحميرة	0.9%	W(2)	Po (2)	-	1t/d(2)	Other (2)	Cu (2)		**[54]**	No	

Table 6. Contd.

Scrophulariaceae	*Veronica aquatica*	الحريكةالملسة	1.9%	W (2) L (1)	Po (2), Inf (3), EO (1), Dr (1)	-	2 t/d(2), 3 t/d (2)	1 We (1), Other (2)	Cu (3), Or (3)	Yes (2), No (1)	**[55]**	No	-
Urticaceae	*Urtica dioica*	الحريكة	1.4%	W (2), L (2), R (1), Bo (1)	Po (3), Inf (3), Dec (1), EO (1), Mac (1)	Alcohol (1), Cider vinegar (1)	1 t/d (1), 2 t/d (2), 3t/d (2)	1 We (1), Other (3)	Cu (4), Or (3)	Yes (4)	**[56]**	**Yes**	-
Verbenaceae	*Verbena officinalis*	بايموت	2.8%	W (3) Ro (1)	Po (4)	-	1 t/d (1), 2 t/d (1), 3 t/d (2), Other (1)	1 We (1), Other (3)	Cu (4)	-	**[57]**	**Yes**	Bellakhdar (1998)
Zingiberaceae	*Curcuma longa*	الخرقوم	0.5%	W (1)	Po (1)	Honey (1), Butter (1)	Other (1)	Other (1)	Cu (1)	-	**[58]**	**Yes**	-
Zygophyllaceae	*Peganum harmala L.*	الحرمل	0.5%	S (1)	Po (1)	-	2t/d (1)	1 We (1)	Cu (1)	Yes (1)	**[59]**	No	Fakchich et al. (2014), Bellakhdar (1998)

(Frequency) ; Ba: Barks; Bo: Boughts; Bu: Bulb; Cu: Cutaneous; Cr: Cream; Dec: Decoction; Di: Direct application; Dr: Dressing; D: Day; EO: Essential oils; F: Fruit; Fl: Flowers; Inf: Infusion; L: Leaves; Mac: maceration; Mo:Month; Mu: Mucilage; Nu: Nuts; Po: Powder; Pu: Pulp; Ro: Rods; R: Roots; S: Seeds; W: Whole plant; We: Week. t/d: time/day.
*Other: Depending the pathological field and to the wound.

Form of use

The high use of the plant as a powder form, according to herbalists, can be explained by the facility and the rapidity of the operation, the nature of the herbalist's profession and his experience. But it can also be explained by the effectiveness of this method on the healing of skin wounds. This was confirmed by other regional studies which found that the use of plant in powder form is frequently used by the local population of Essaouira (25%) (Mehdioui et al., 2007), Ifran (22%) (Rhafouri et al., 2014), Kenitra (25.9%) (Salhi et al., 2010), in the region of Zaêr (11.5%), Atlas Oriental (27.92%) (Belamdini and Douira, 2002) (Lahsissene et al., 2010), and in the region of Haut.

The important use of essential oils can be explained by the fact that they contain several essential compounds, and active ingredients responsible for the plant's activities and its effectiveness.

Way of administration

The important frequency of use of dermal way can be explained by the nature of the disease, which is the skin healing, and also because the effectiveness of treatment is direct and more important by dermal way.

Frequency and duration of use

The frequency and the duration of use changes from one herbalist to another because everyone has its personal diagnosis of the pathological field and of the patient's case. However, majority of herbalists recommend using the plant 2 twice a day in the morning and at the night, but they were not able to adjudicate about the treatment duration. They estimate that they have to examine thepatient before giving a diagnosis decision.

Plants association

These plant associations are explained by the fact that the efficiency of the plant increases when it associated with one or more other plants and that the wound healing time decreases. For example, consider *S. verbenaca* which is the main inventoried species. The herbalists interviewed

Table 7. Inventoried properties list of recorded healing plants.

Plant	Properties
Aloe vera	Healing, antidiabetic, anticancer, against burns, against redness, for hair and face care, against kidney problems, against stretch marks and varicose veins
Allium cepa	Healing, against cold
Pistacia lenticus L	Healing, against skin abscesses
Pistacia terebinthus L.	Healing, against abscesses, hair care
Rhusalbidumschousb.	Healing, anti diarrhea and abscesses
Carum carvi L.	Healing
Centella asiatica	Healing
Coriandrum sativum	Healing, antidiuretic, antiseptic, antispasmodic, anti diarrhea, carminative
Aristolochia long.	Healing, against pimples
Arnica L.	Healing, antiseptic, antidiabetic, antiinflammatory
Artemisia tridentata	Healing, hemostatic, anticancer, antiseptic, antidiabetic, antibiotic, draining, wormer, against sinusitis, against cold, digestive, against stomach problems, acne, eczema
Calendula officinalis	Healing, anti-hepatitis, anticancer, antifungal, assists delivery
Chamaemelum nobile	Healing
Inula viscosa ait.	Healing, against stomach ulcers, against burns, against anal fissures
Matricaria recutita	Healing, antipyretic, anti-inflammatory, antispasmodic, antiallergic, soothing, softening, black marks
Pulicaria arabica	Healing
Saussurea coctus	Healing
Tanacetumparthenium	Healing, antispasmodic, antiseptic, antiviral, for breathing and digestive apparatus, calming
Opuntia ficus-indica	Healing, against stretch marks, anti wrinkles
Saponaria vaccaria L.	Healing, against constipation
Cassia absus L.	Healing
Chenopodium L.	Healing, antipyretic, antirheumatic
Vicia sativa L.	Healing. against stomach problems
Quercus faginea lamk.	Healing, anti-haemorrhagic, anti diarrhea, blackening
Geranium L.	Healing
Globularia alypum L.	Healing, antidiabetic, against burns
Hypericum perforatum	Healing
Crocus sativum	Healing, antiseptic, against herpes, against eyes problems
Lavandula angustifolia	Healing, toning, strengthens immunity, antiseptic
Marrubium vulgare	Healing, antirheumatic, against pimples and abscesses
Mentha x piperita L.	Healing, against burns, against stomach problems, against cold, against headaches
Ocimum basilicum	Healing, antiseptic, calming
Origanum vulgare	Healing
Rosmarinus officinalis	Healing, hypertensive, antioxidant, antiseptic, anti-hepatitis, antifungal, Antibiotic, detoxifying, energizing, antioxidant, enhances memory
Salvia verbenaca	Healing, antidiabetic, antispasmodic, against pimples, against stomach problems, against bad cold, against bloating, anti acne
Thymus vulgaris	Healing, antibiotic, antiseptic, strengthens immunity, digestive, hair care
Laurus nobilisL.	Healing, against facial tasks
Cinnamomum verum	Healing, antiseptic, antirheumatic, constipating, against gases
Smilax aspera L.	Healing
Lawsonia inermis	Healing, antimycosic, antidiarrhea, against abscess, hair care
Myristica fragrans	Healing, face care
Melaleuca tea	Healing
Myrtus communis L.	Healing, antispasmodic, antiseptic, hair care

Table 7. Cont'd.

Papaver rhoeas L.	Healing.
Sesamum indicum	Healing, anti tasks, against sunlight
Pinushalepensis	Healing, antiseptic, analgesic, against burns, against digestive problems
Plantago major	Healing, antiinflammatory, analgesic, against urinary and digestive problems
Plantago psyllium	Healing, antiseptic.
Avena sativa L.	Healing
Rhamnus alaternus L.	Healing, against black tasks
Clematis cirrhosa L.	Healing, against black tasks
PopulusL.	Healing
Argania spinosa	Healing, against sunburn, face care, anti wrinkles, anti tasks, anti eczema
Capsicum annuum	Healing, antiseptic
Veronica aquatica	Healing, antihemorrhagic, against pimples, anticancer, kidney problems, anemia, diarrhea, remineralizing, against anemia
Urtica dioica	Healing, anti-haemorrhagic, antirheumatic, antidiuretic, against hair loss, against hemorrhoids
Verbena officinalis	Healing, antiinflammatory, activates immune system
Curcuma longa	Healing
Peganum harmala L.	Healing

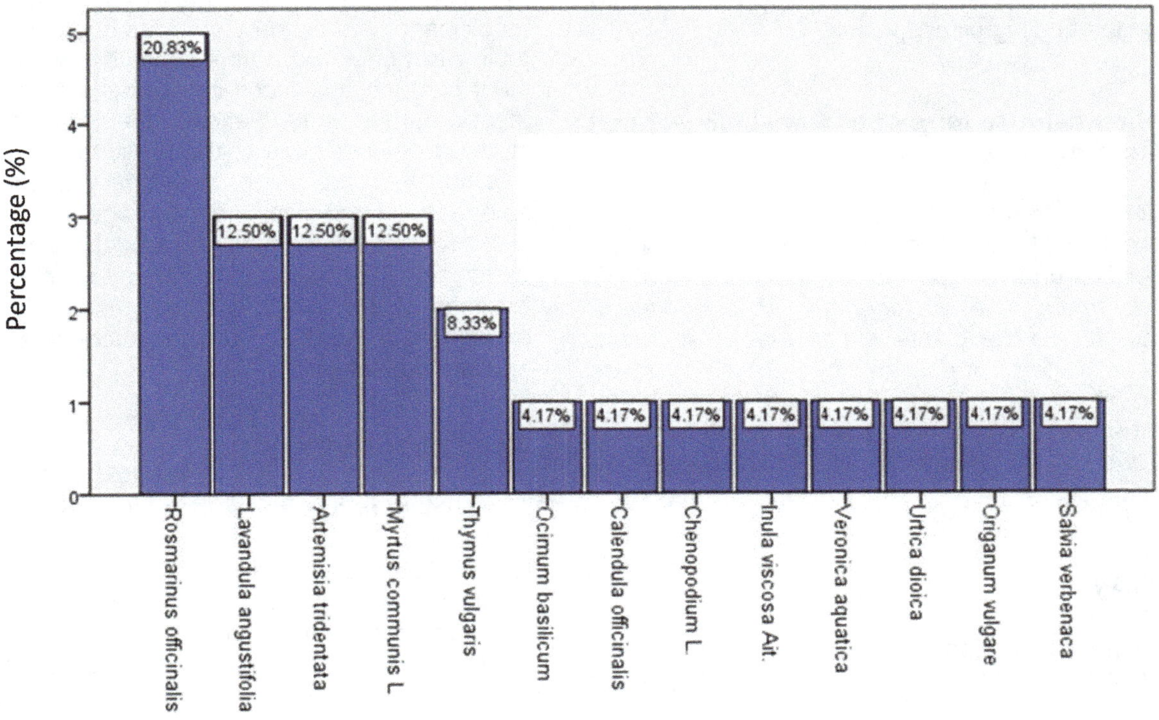

Figure 10. Workforce of healing plants whose leaves are used as essential oils.

said that *S. verbenaca* is used most often when it is associated with other plants, and its efficiency increases exceeding 80% if it is associated with *P. halepensis* or *V. officinalis*. Indeed, this result was confirmed by another ethnobotanical study, which showed that *S. verbenaca* is often associated with these plants (Bellakhdar, 1998).

Crossing between used parts and form of use

From this crossing, the study obtained that $\chi^2_{obs} > \chi^2_{v;\ \alpha}$. Therefore, H_0 is rejected. The study concluded that the used form of the plant depends on the used parts.

Crossing between used parts and use as essential oils

The study found out, through this crossing, the use in the form of essential oils depends on the leaves and on the whole plant but it is independent of the other parts like: flowers, roots, barks, fruit and seeds. The dependence of the use in essential oils to the whole plant confirms the results of the Chi-square test of Table 4. So, the study can conclude from the results, that the use of essential oils depends on part of the plant which is used and more specifically on the leaves. This can be explained by the fact that leaves contain all the essential plant metabolites including essential oils.

Crossing between use form of essential oil with healing plant

The statistical results of the crossing (Table 5) allowed us to conclude that the use of essential oils form actually depends on the healing plant species.

Crossing between use form of essential oil, leaf-part and healing plant

This crossing enabled us to conclude that the use of the leaves as essential oils depends on the nature of the healing plant. Furthermore, the study found that *R. officinalis*, *L. angustifolia*, *A. tridentata*, *M. communis L* and *T. vulgaris* are the plants whose leaves are more often used in the form of essential oils. Based on these results, the study has chosen to use these plants in subsequent experimental studies, as part of of the study research work, to develop and manufacture a phytomedicine.

CONCLUSION

The use of medicinal plants has been in existence for decades; it has been and remains until today requested by the Moroccan population. Furthermore, phytotherapy is a discipline that is changing these days, and people are more likely to go to the natural products to heal and for treatments of wounds.

Indeed, this study was conducted in order to make the most complete inventory of the healing medicinal plants used in Morocco and to gather all the necessary information about the therapeutic uses of these plants and their specific properties. Thus, the ethnobotanical survey allowed us to reveal a large number of information. It allowed the identification of 59 species of healing plants belonging to 37 families, whose *S. verbenaca* is the major species. It is presented in this study that among these families, *Lamiaceae* is the most represented family in the surveyed citie

On the pharmacological side, the whole plant is the most used part; powder is the most common used form. There is a relationship between the form of use and the used part of the plant; especially for essential oils use form. It was also discovered that the leaves which are the most commonly used part as essential oils, and that, of course, depends on the nature of the plant. The indexed plants are distributed specifically in the Souss-Massa-Draa region and their distribution varies from one region to another. Plants are more available in spring, they are used most often 2 times per day and the duration of the use varies depending to the wound and the pathological field.

This study is the result of a series of ethnobotanical surveys made with herbalists and traditional healers in the cities of Casablanca, Mohammedia, Rabat, Salé, Kenitra, Fez, Marrakech, Agadir, Taroudant, Tangier, Tetouan and Oujda. Using direct and telephonic interviews, the survey was carried out over a period of five months, and allowed the study to know the healing medicinal plants used by the Moroccan population of the main cities of Morocco. It revealed the wealth of floral and plant heritage and much other relevant information. It is therefore, necessary to expand the field/population of this study to other regions of the Kingdom, to include all the healing medicinal plants traditionally used, and also to safeguard this precious plant heritage.

These conclusive results allowed the study to justify (as preliminary information gathered in the field) the choice of healing plants that will be used in subsequent experimental studies, to manufacture a new wound healing product.

AKNOWLEDGMENTS

The authors of this article thank the University Hassan II for financing the publication costs. We are very grateful to AIT FARAJI S., from the Direction of Studies and Financial Forecasts, of Ministry of Economy and Finance in Rabat, for his help in the statistical analysis of the results. They are also grateful to Messaoudi Moussi A., from the Moroccan-Libyan Chamber for his assistance in interviews with herbalists, and to traditional herbalists of surveyed cities for their availability and their assistance.

REFERENCES

Agyarea C, Asase A, Lechtenberg M, Niehues M, Deters A, Hensel A (2009). An ethnopharmacological survey and in vitro confirmation of ethnopharmacological use of medicinal plants used for wound healing in Bosomtwi-Atwima-Kwanwoma area, Ghana. J. Ethnopharmacol, 125:393-403.

Bammi J, Douira A (2002). Les plantes médicinales dans la forêt de l'Achach (Plateau central, Maroc). Acta Botanica Malacitana. 27:131-145.

Bassole IHN, Ouattara AS, Nebie R, Ouattara CAT, Kabore ZI, Traore SA (2001). Composition chimique et activités antibactériennes des huiles essentielles des feuilles et des fleurs de *Cymbopogon proximus* (stapf.) et d'*Ocimum canum* (sims). Pharm. Med. Trad. Afr. 11 : 37-51.

Belamdini N, El Hafian M, Rochdi A, Zidane L (2014). Etude floristique et ethnobotanique de la flore médicinale du Haut Atlas oriental (Haute Moulouya). J. Appl. Biosci. 78:6771-6787.

Bellakhdar J (1998). La Pharmacopée marocaine traditionnelle : Médecine arabe ancienne et savoirs populaires. Mazars Guy Revue d'histoire de la pharmacie 30:86-84.

Benkhnigue O, Zidane L, Fadli M, Elyacoubi H, Rochdi A, Douira A (2010). Etude ethnobotanique des plantes médicinales dans la région de Mechraâ Bel Ksiri (Région du Gharb du Maroc). Acta Botanica Barcinonensia *53*:191-216.

Bousta D, Ennabili A (2011). L'Institut national des plantes médicinales et aromatiques au service du développement de la phytothérapie au Maroc. Phytothérapie 9:297-303.

Daoudi A, Bammou M, Zarkani S, Slimani I, Ibijbijen J, Nassiri L (2015). Etude ethnobotanique de la flore medicinal de la commune rurale d'Aguelmouss province de Khénifra. Phytothérapie 1-9.

El Amri J, El Badaoui K, Zair T, Bouharb H, Chakir S, Alaoui TEM (2014). Ethnobotanical study of medicinal plants in the region El Hajeb (Central Morocco). J. Res. Biol. 4(8):1568-1580.

El Hafian M, Benlamdini N, El Yacoubi H, Zidane L, Rochdi A (2014). Etude floristique et ethnobotanique des plantes médicinales utilisées au niveau de la préfecture d'Agadir-Ida-Outanane (Maroc). J. Appl. Biosci. 81:7198-7213.

Fadil M, Farah A, Haloui T, Rachiq S. (2014). Diagnosis of the aromatic and medicinal plant sector in Morocco: Case of the cooperatives and associations of the Meknès-Tafilalt area. Lazaroa (35):155-166.

Fakchich J, Elachouri M (2004). Ethnobotanical survey of medicinal plants used by people in Oriental Morocco to manage various ailments. J. Ethnopharmacol. 154:76-87.

Hseini S, Kahouadji A (2007). Etude ethnobotanique de la flore médicinale dans la région de Rabat (Maroc occidental). Lazaroa 28:79-93.

Lahsissene H, Kahouadji A, Tijane M, Hseini S (2009). Catalogue des plantes médicinales utilisées dans la region de Zaër (Maroc occidental). Lejeunia 186-192.

Lahsissene H, Kahouadji A (2010). Usages traditionnels des plantes médicinales dans le Maroc occidental : cas de la région de Zaër. Phytothérapie 8(4):210-217.

Mehdioui R, Kahouadji A (2007). Etude ethnobotanique auprès de la population riveraine de la forêt d'Amsittène: cas de la Commune d'Imi n'Tlit (Province d'Essaouira). Bulletin de l'Institut scientifique, Rabat, section Sciences de la vie. 29 :11-20.

Merzouki A, Derfoufi FEd, Mesa M (2000). Contribution of the knowledge of Rifian traditional mediane: II: Folk medicine in Ksar Lakbir district (NW Morocco). Fitoterap 71:278-307.

Mountassir M (2014). Probabilités et statistique : Cours, Exercices, Etudes de cas et Modules technologiques. Afr. Orient. pp. 357-360.

Rhafouri R, Aafi A, Zair T, Strani B, El Omari M, Ghanmi M, Bentayeb A (2014). Ethnobotanical study of medicinal plants in Ifran's National Park (Morocco). J. Mater. Environ. Sci. 6 (3):619-630.

Salhi S, Fadli M, Zidane L, Douira A (2010). Etudes floristique et ethnobotanique des plantes médicinales de la ville de Kénitra (Maroc). Lazaroa 31:133-143.

Semwal RB, Semwal DK, Combrinck S, Cartwright-Jones C, Viljoen A (2014). *Lawsonia inermis L.* (henna): Ethnobotanical, phytochemical and pharmacological aspects. J. Ethnopharmacol. 155(1):80-103.

Sijelmassi A (2011). Les plantes médicinales au Maroc. Editions le Fennec. Casablanca, Morocco. p 285.

Tahri N, El Basti A, Zidane L, Rochdi A, Douira A (2012). Etude Ethnobotanique Des Plantes Medicinales Dans La Province De Settat (Maroc). Kastamonu Üniversitesi Orman Fakültesi Dergisi. 12(2):192-208.

Wahid N (2013). Perspectives de la valorisation de l'usage et de la culture du Myrtus communis L. au Maroc. Phytothérap 11:237-243.

Zeggwagh AA, Lahlou Y, Bousliman Y (2013). Enquête sur les aspects toxicologiques de la phytothérapie utilisée par un herboriste à Fès, Maroc. Pan Afr. Med. J. 14:125

Biochemical analysis of *Origanum vulgare* seeds by fourier-transform infrared (FT-IR) spectroscopy and gas chromatography-mass spectrometry (GC-MS)

Huda Jasim Al-Tameme, Imad Hadi Hameed*, Salah Ali Idan and Mohammed Yahya Hadi

Department of Biology, Babylon University, Hilla City, Iraq.

Medicinal plants are potential sources of natural compounds with biological activities, and therefore attract the attention of researchers worldwide. The objective of this research is to determine the chemical composition of methanolic seed extract. The phytochemical compound screened by spectroscopy and gas chromatography-mass spectrometry (GC-MS) method. Sixteen bioactive phytochemical compounds were identified in the methanolic extract of *Origanum vulgare*. The identification of phytochemical compounds is based on the peak area, retention time molecular weight, molecular formula, MS Fragment- ions and pharmacological actions. GC-MS analysis of *O. vulgare* revealed the existence of the 1,7-Dioxaspiro[5,5]undec-2-ene, 2,4-Dihydroxy-2,5-dimethyl-39(2H)-furan-3-one, 2,4-Difurobenzene, 1-benzyloxy, α-D-Glucopyranoside, O-α- Glucopyranosyl, 4-Hexenal, 6-hydroxy-4-methyl,dimethyl acetal, acetate, 4H-pyran-4-one,2,3,-dihydro-3,5-dihydroxy-6-methyl, Benzofuran, 4-Amino-1,5-pentandioic acid, 2-Methoxy-4-vinylphenol, d-Mannose, 7-Isopropyl-10-methyl-1-oxo-1,5-dithia-spiro[5,5]undecane-2-carboxy, Phytol, Cis-Vaccenic acid, N-Methyl-Nbenzyltetradecanamine, 3,8,8-Trimethoxy-3-piperidyl-2,2-binaphthalene-1,1,4,4-tetrone, and 17-(1,5-Dimethylhexyl)10,13-dimethyl. The FTIR analysis of *O. vulgare* seeds proved the presence of alkenes, aliphatic fluoro compounds, alcohols, ethers, carboxlic acids, esters and hydrogen bonded alcohols, phenols.

Key words: GC/MS, bioactive compounds, FT-IR, *O. vulgare*.

INTRODUCTION

Origanum vulgare L. is a perennial aromatic herb belonging to the family *Lamiaceae* (Skoula and Harborne, 2002) used for thousands of years as spices and as local medicines in traditional medicine (Altameme et al., 2015). *O. vulgare* L. is the most wide spread among all the species within the genus. It is distributed all over Europe, West and Central Asia up to Taiwan (Ietswaart, 1980; Hameed et al., 2015).

Aerial flowering parts of *O. vulgare* subsp. *viride* are used in Iranian traditional medicine as diuretic, stomachic, antineuralgic, antitussive and expectorant (Afsharypuor et al. 1997). *O. vulgare* plays a primary role

*Corresponding author. E-mail: imad_dna@yahoo.com.

among culinary herbs in world trade (Oliver, 1997). Taxonomic studies on the basis of morphological characters have led to the discrimination of several subspecies. Ietswaart (1980), distinguished six subspecies of *O. vulgare*, that is, *hirtum*, *vulgare*, *virens*, *viride*, *gracile* and *glandulosum*. Only *O. vulgare* L. subspecies *hirtum* has the leaf anatomy which corresponds to that of commercially marketed European oregano (Skoula and Harborne, 2002).

Oregano is used worldwide both as spice and crude drug, which is mainly provided by species of *Origanum* genus (Franz and Novak, 2002). Oregano was found to be strong antimicrobial agent and had a significant spasmolytic effect on smooth muscle (Hameed et al., 2015). The fumigant toxicity and insecticidal effect of oregano essential oils for storeroom insects has also been proved (Marn et al., 1999; Imad et al., 2015). Many herbs are commonly used in home-type cure therapies, complementary medicine and modern medicine because of their perceived antioxidant, antimicrobial, anticancer, etc. properties. Origanum species are counted among these herbs, since they show high activities according to their assessment for the above biological properties (Mechergui et al., 2010; Hussein et al., 2015). A remarkable phytochemical polymorphism with several chemotypes is also reported by several studies on this species that shows marked spatial segregation in nature (D'antuono et al., 2000; Radušiene et al., 2005; Hameed et al., 2015c).

Furthermore, *O. vulgare* has an antioxidant property and is applied in human health. Cervato et al. (2000), prove that the antioxidant activities of extracts of oregano's leaves (both aqueous and methanolic extracts) can inhibit all phases of lipid peroxidative process (Sahin et al., 2004; Singh, 2007; Hussein et al., 2015). The biological activity of essential oils and herb extracts cause a high pharmaceutical and industrial interest in *O. vulgare*, since antimicrobial, antifungal, insecticidal and antioxidative effects have been reported (Kulisic et al. 2004; Bakkali et al. 2008; et al., 2015). *Origanum* tea is a treatment for indigestion, coughs, and to stimulate menstruation. The oil of *Origanum* is used for toothache, and in some cosmetics. Its leaves and flowering stems are natural antiseptics because of high thymol content (Bhat et al., 2002; Singh, 2003; Dalpe, 2004; Bilalis et al., 2011).

The study, aim to study the analysis of chemical compounds of *Origanum vulgare* seeds by fourier-transform infrared (FT-IR) spectroscopy and gas chromatography-mass spectrometry (GC-MS).

MATERIALS AND METHODS

Collection and preparation of plant material

The seeds were dried at room temperature for two weeks, and when properly dried then powdered using clean pestle and mortar, and the powdered plant was size reduced with a sieve. The fine powder was then packed in airtight container to avoid the effect of humidity and then stored at room temperature. About thirteen grams of the plant sample powdered were soaked in 100 ml methanol individually. It was left for 96 h so that alkaloids, flavonoids and other constituents if present will get dissolved. The methanol extract was filtered using Whatman No.1 filter paper and the residue was removed (Jasim et al., 2015).

Gas chromatography – mass spectrum analysis

The GC-MS analysis of the plant extract was made in a (Agilent 7890 A) instrument under computer control at 70 eV. About 1μL of the methanol extract was injected into the GC-MS using a micro syringe and the scanning was done for 45 min (Imad et al., 2014a). As the compounds were separated, they eluted from the column and entered a detector which was capable of creating an electronic signal whenever a compound was detected. The greater the concentration in the sample, bigger was the signal obtained which was then processed by a computer. The time from when the injection was made (Initial time) to when elution occurred is referred to as the Retention time (RT). While the instrument was run, the computer generated a graph from the signal called Chromatogram. Each of the peaks in the chromatogram represented the signal created when a compound eluted from the Gas chromatography column into the detector. The X-axis showed the RT and the Y-axis measured the intensity of the signal to quantify the component in the sample injected. As individual compounds eluted from the gas chromatographic column, they entered the electron ionization (mass spectroscopy) detector, where they were bombarded with a stream of electrons causing them to break apart into fragments (Mohammed and Imad, 2013; Imad et al 2014b; Kareem et al., 2015).

The fragments obtained were actually charged ions with a certain mass .The M/Z (Mass / Charge) ratio obtained was calibrated from the graph obtained, which was called as the Mass spectrum graph which is the fingerprint of a molecule. Before analyzing the extract using gas chromatography and mass spectroscopy, the temperature of the oven, the flow rate of the gas used and the electron gun were programmed initially. The temperature of the oven was maintained at 100°C. Helium gas was used as a carrier as well as an eluent. The flow rate of helium was set to 1 ml per min. The electron gun of mass detector liberated electrons having energy of about 70eV. The column employed here for the separation of components was Elite 1(100% dimethyl poly siloxane). The identity of the components in the extracts was assigned by the comparison of their retention indices and mass spectra fragmentation patterns with those stored on the computer library and also with published literatures. Compounds were identified by comparing their spectra to those of the Wiley and NIST/EPA/NIH mass spectral libraries (Imad et al., 2014c; Muhanned et al., 2015).

RESULTS AND DISCUSSION

Gas chromatography and mass spectroscopy analysis of compounds was carried out in methanolic seeds extract of *O. vulgare*, shown in Table 1. The GC-MS chromatogram of the 16 peaks of the compounds detected was shown in Figure 1. Chromatogram GC-MS analysis of the methanol extract of *O. vulgare* showed the presence of sixteen major peaks and the components corresponding to the peaks were determined as follows. The First set up peak were determined to be 1,7-Dioxaspiro[5,5]undec-2-ene Figure 2. The second peak

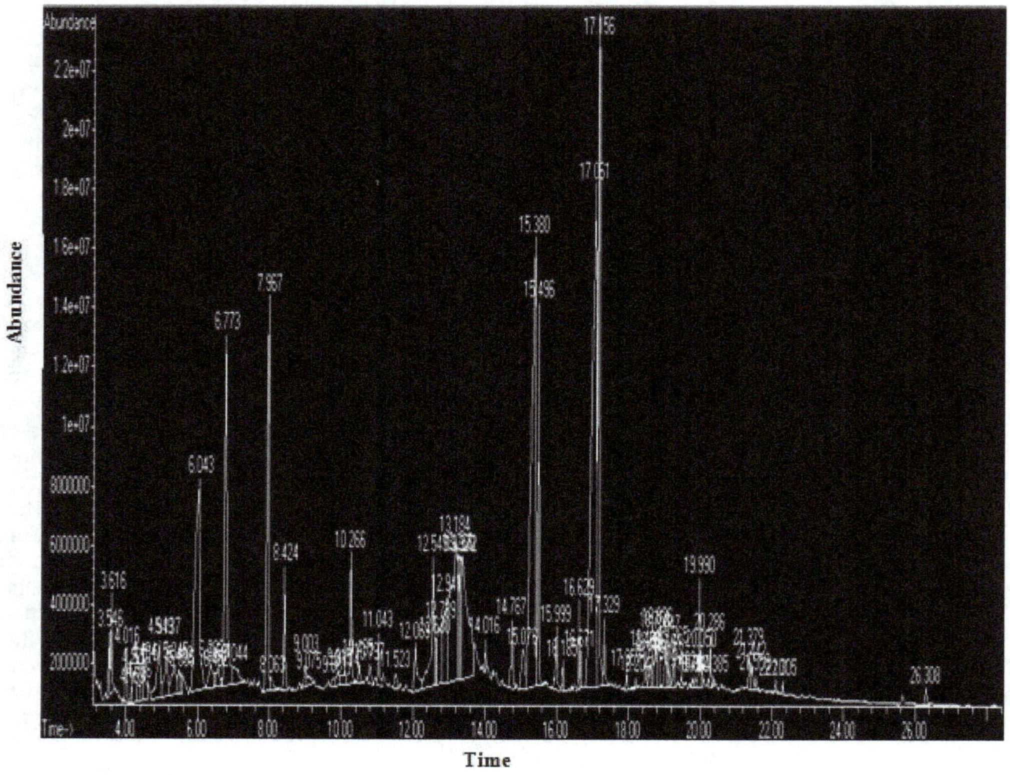

Figure 1. GC-MS chromatogram of methanolic extract of *O. vulgare*.

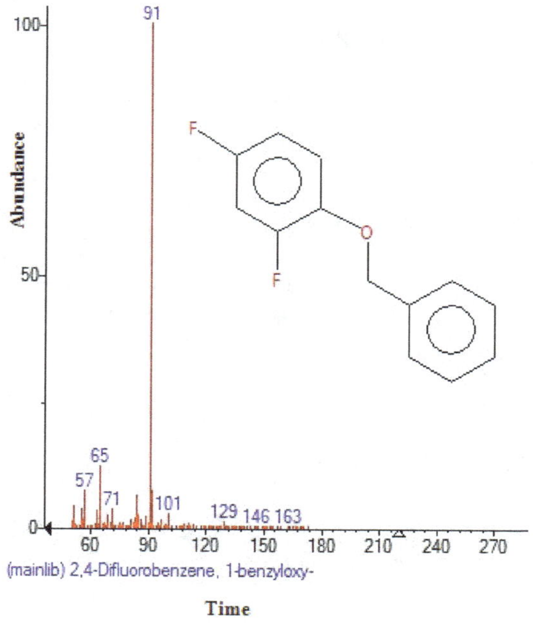

Figure 2. Mass spectrum of 2,4-Difurobenzene, 1-benzyloxy with Retention Time (RT)= 4.460.

indicated to be 2,4-Dihydroxy-2,5-dimethyl-39(2H)-furan-3-one Figure 3. The next peaks considered to be 2,4-Difurobenzene, 1-benzyloxy, α-D-Glucopyranoside, O-α-Glucopyranosyl, 4-Hexenal, 6-hydroxy-4-methyl,dimethyl acetal, acetate, 4H-pyran-4-one,2,3,-dihydro-3,5-dihydroxy-6-methyl, Benzofuran, 4-Amino1, 5-pentandiotic

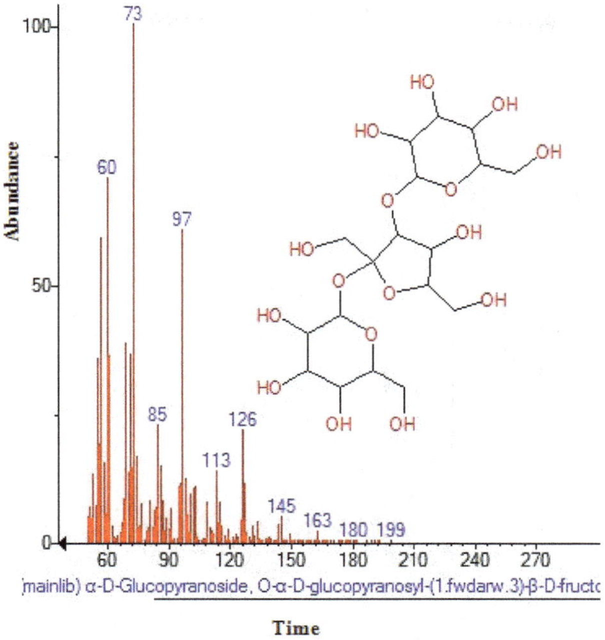

Figure 3. Mass spectrum of α-D-Glucopyranoside, O-α-Glucopyranosyl with Retention Time (RT)= 4.975.

Figure 5. Mass spectrum of 2,4-Dihydroxy-2,5-dimethyl-39(2H)-furan-3-one with Retention Time (RT)= 4.020.

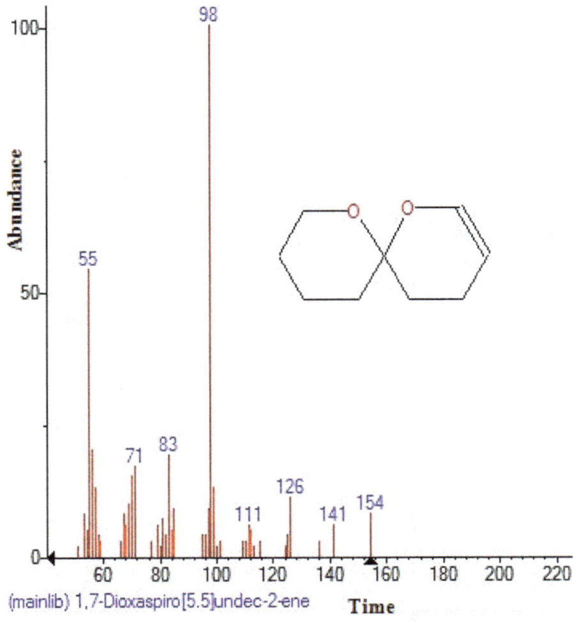

Figure 4. Mass spectrum of 1,7-Dioxaspiro[5,5]undec-2-ene with Retention Time (RT)= 3.585.

pentandioic acid, 2-Methoxy-4-vinylphenol, d-Mannose, 7-Isopropyl-10-methyl-1-oxo-1,5-dithia spiro[5,5]undecane-2-carboxy, Phytol, Cis-Vaccenic acid, N-Methyl-Nbenzyltetradecanamine, 3,8,8-Trimethoxy-3-piperidyl-2,2-binaphthalene-1,1,4,4-tetrone, and 17-(1,5-Dimethylhexyl)10, 13-dimethyl (Figure 4 to 17). The FTIR

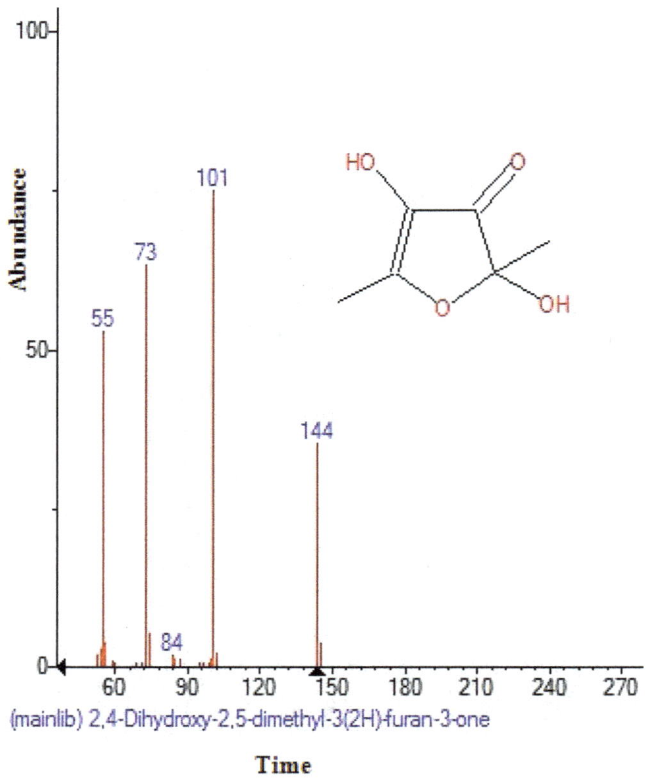

Figure 5. Mass spectrum of 2,4-Dihydroxy-2,5-dimethyl-39(2H)-furan-3-one with Retention Time (RT)= 4.020.

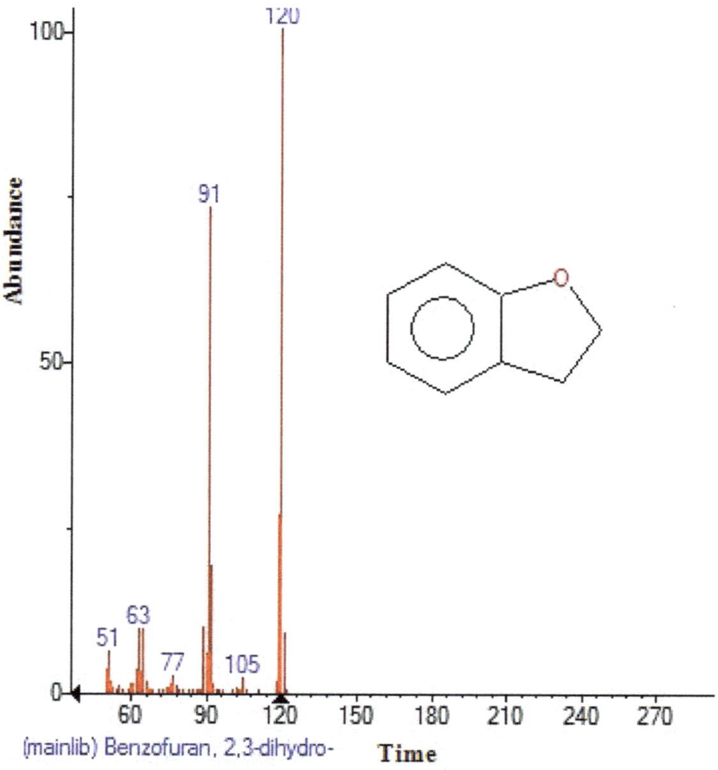

Figure 6. Mass spectrum of Benzofuran with Retention Time (RT)= 6.760.

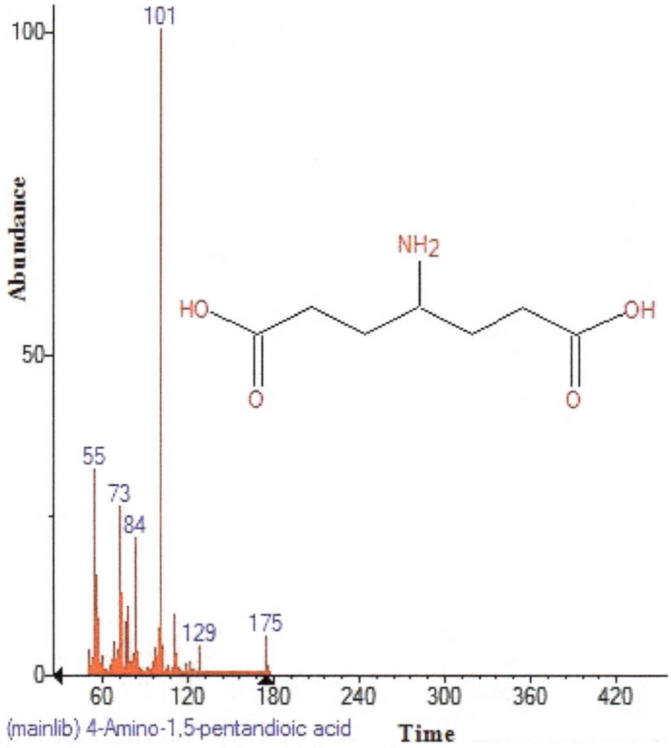

Figure 7. Mass spectrum of 4-Amino-1,5-pentandioic acid with Retention Time (RT)= 6.320.

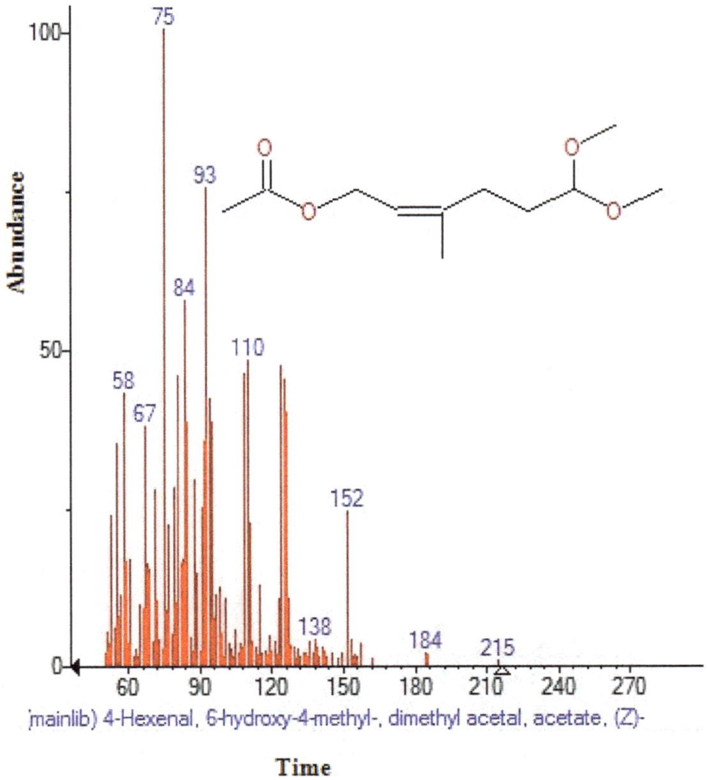

Figure 8. Mass spectrum of 4-Hexenal, 6-hydroxy-4-methyl,dimethyl acetal, acetate with Retention Time (RT)= 5.158.

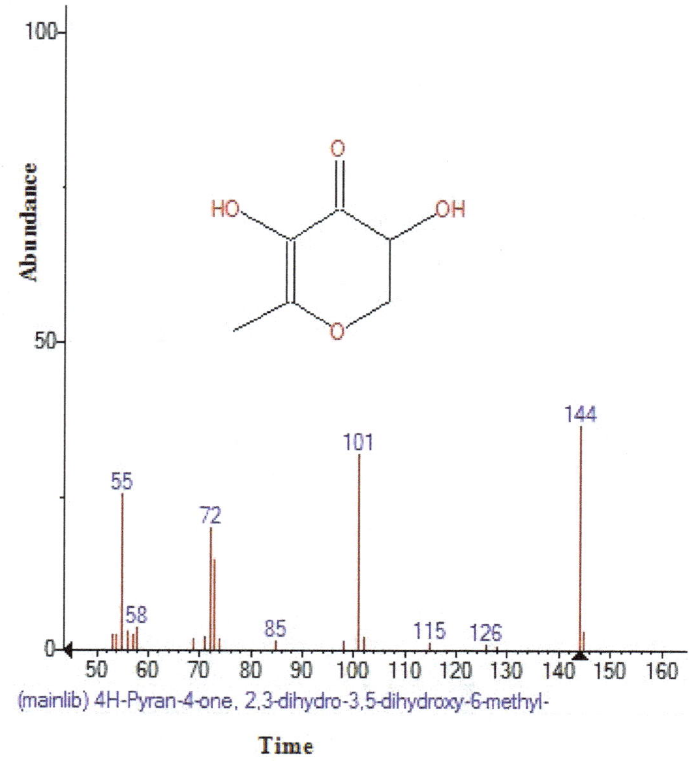

Figure 9. Mass spectrum of 4H-pyran-4-one,2,3,-dihydro-3,5-dihydroxy-6-methyl with Retention Time (RT)= 6.011.

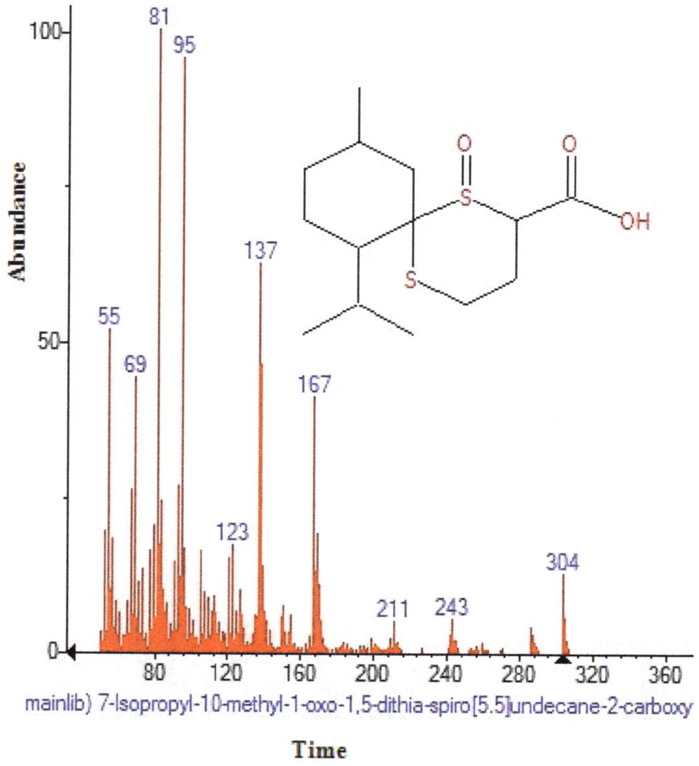

Figure 10. Mass spectrum of 7-Isopropyl-10-methyl-1-oxo-1,5-dithia-spiro[5,5]undecane-2-carboxy with Retention Time (RT)= 14.743.

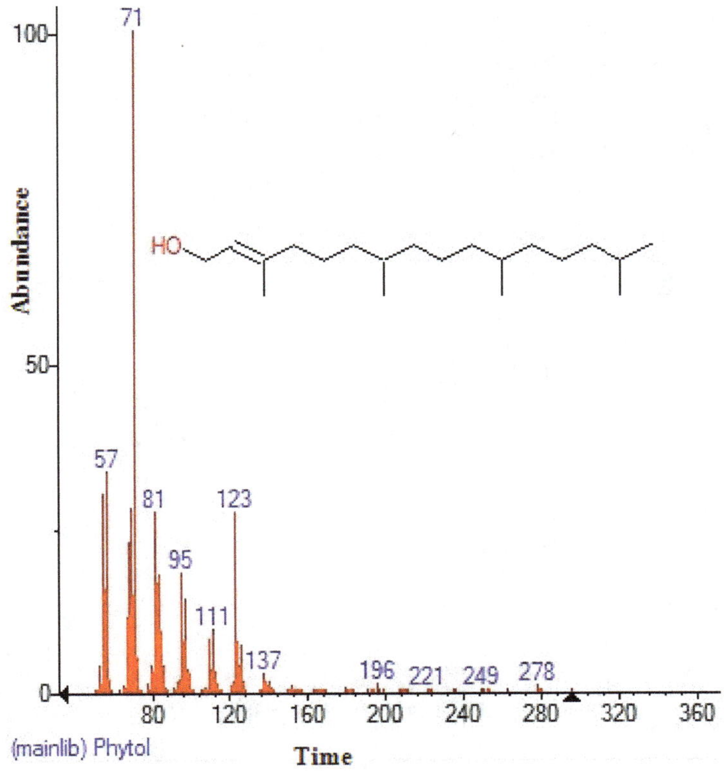

Figure 11. Mass spectrum of Phytol with Retention Time (RT)= 16.625.

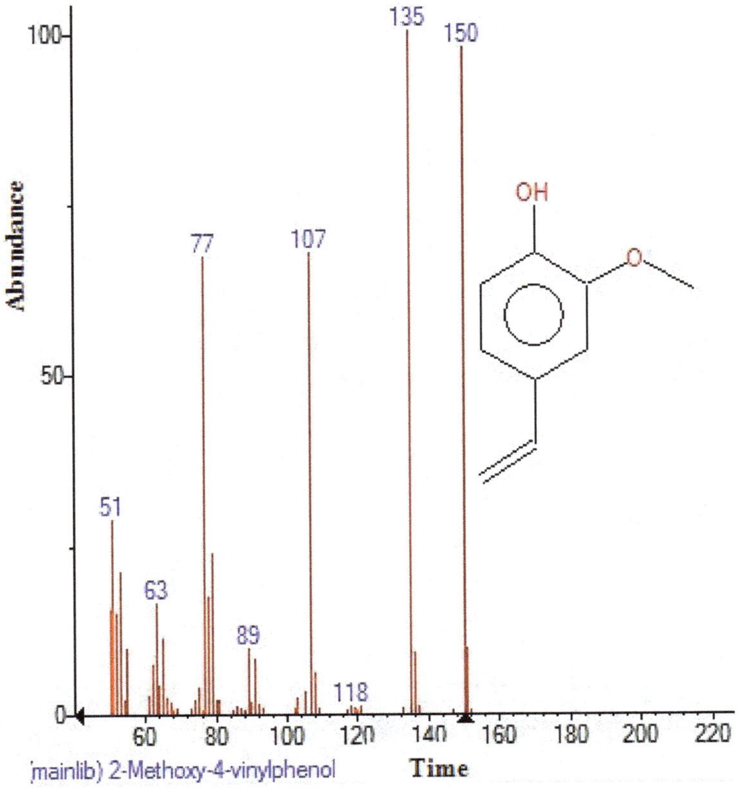

Figure 12. Mass spectrum of 2-Methoxy-4-vinylphenol with Retention Time (RT)= 7.974

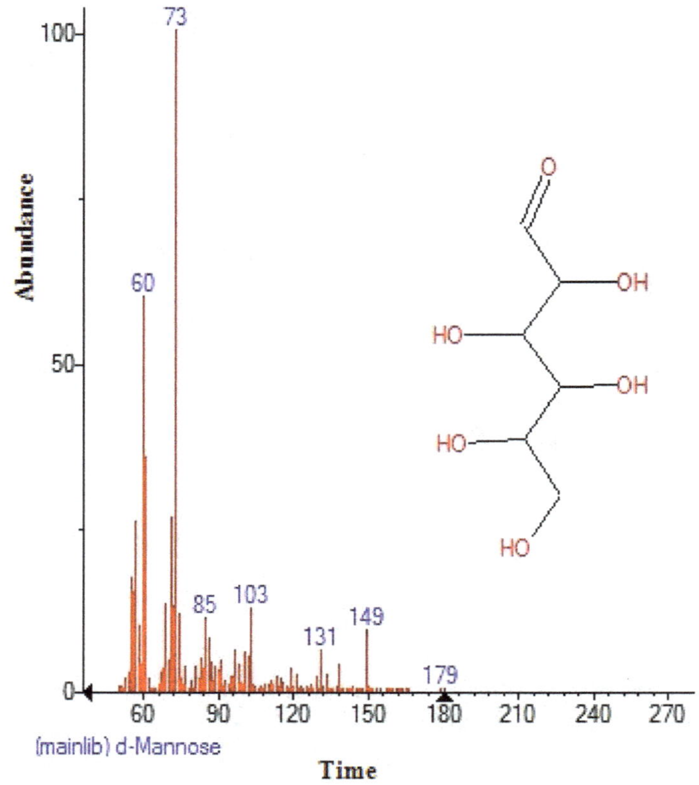

Figure 13. Mass spectrum of d-Mannose with retention time (RT)= 13.215.

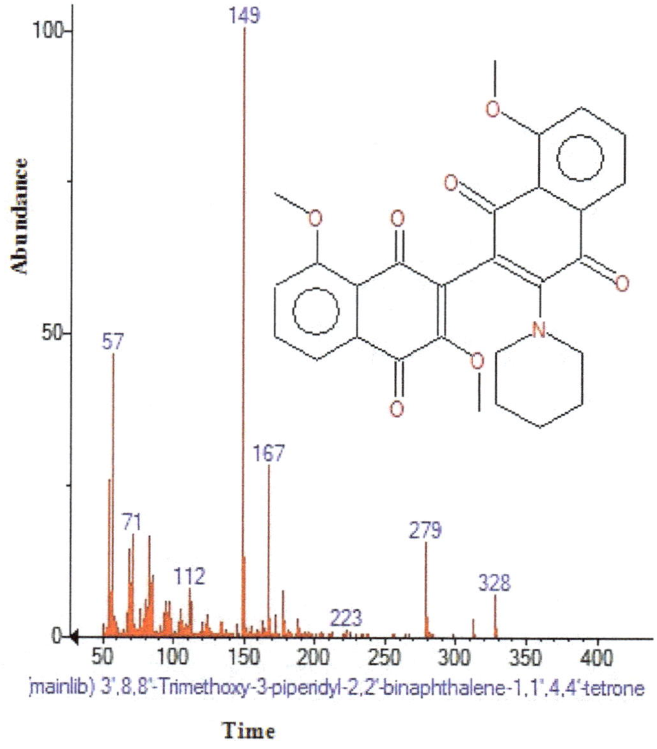

Figure 14. Mass spectrum of 3,8,8-Trimethoxy-3-piperidyl-2,2-binaphthalene-1,1,4,4-tetrone with retention time (RT)= 20.293.

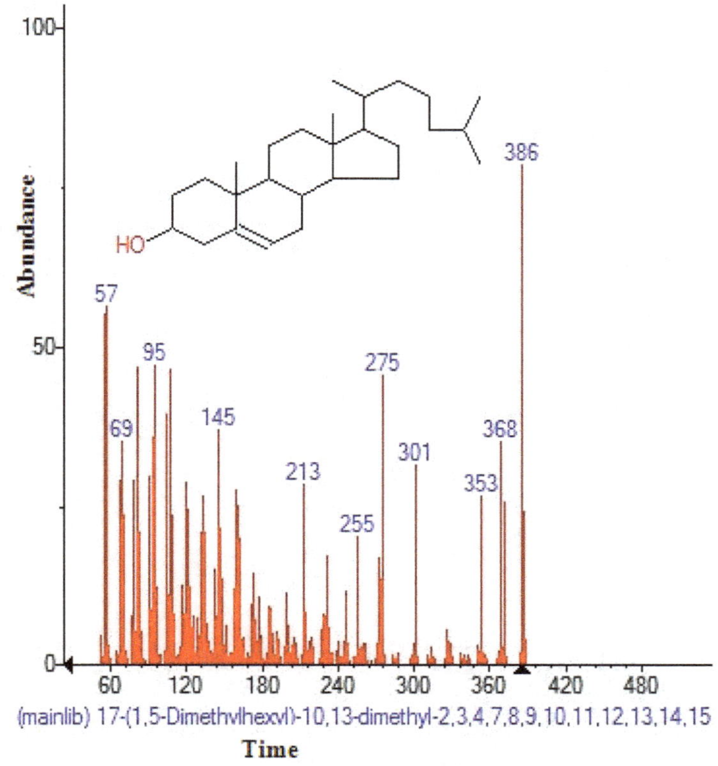

Figure 15. Mass spectrum of 17-(1,5-Dimethylhexyl)10,13-dimethyl with Retention Time (RT)= 26.284.

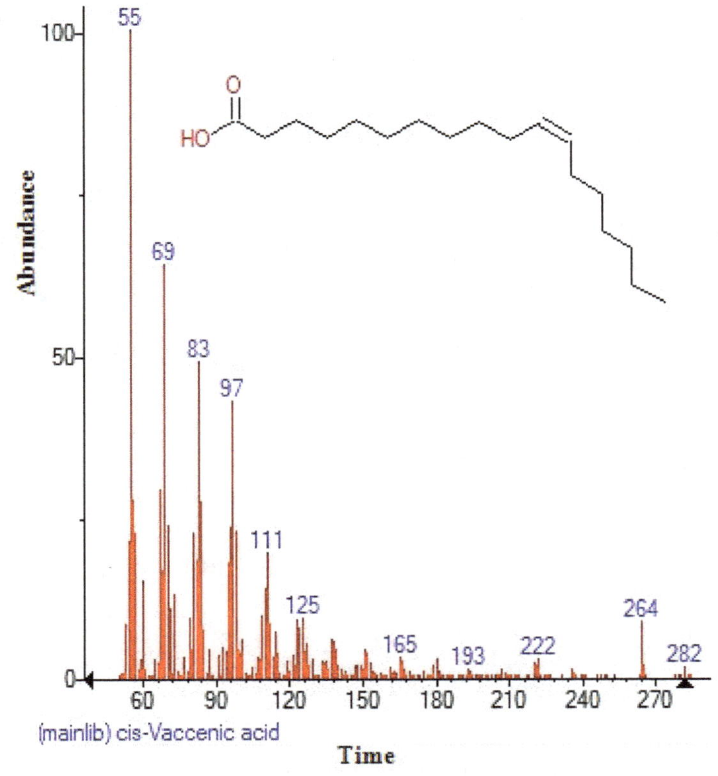

Figure 16. Mass spectrum of Cis-Vaccenic acid with retention time (RT)= 17.014

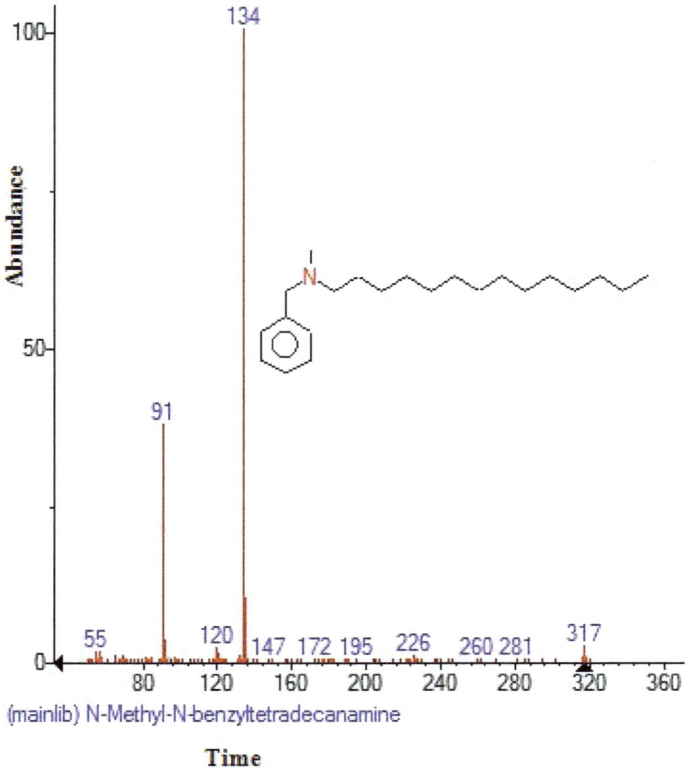

Figure 17. Mass spectrum of N-Methyl-Nbenzyltetradecanamine with Retention Time (RT)= 18.485.

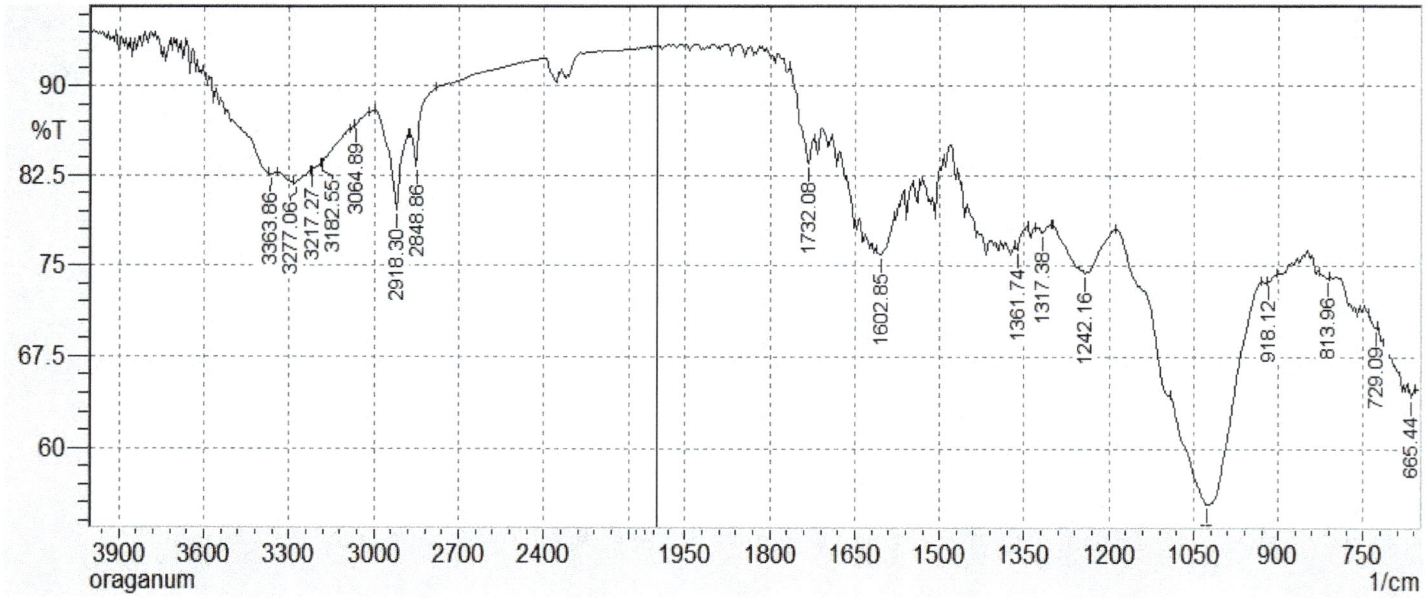

Figure 18. FT-IR peak values of *O. vulgare*

analysis of *O. vulgare* seeds proved the presence of alkenes, aliphatic fluoro compounds, alcohols, ethers, carboxlic acids, esters and hydrogen bonded alcohols, phenols which shows major peaks at 729.09, 1026.13, 1242.16, 1317.38, 2918.30, 3064.89 and 3363.86 (Table 2 and Figure 18).

Table 1. Major phytochemical compounds identified in methanolic extract of *O. vulgare*.

S/N	Phytochemical compound	RT(min)	Formula	Molecular weight	Exact mass	Chemical structure	MS Fragmentations	Pharmacological actions
1.	1,7-Dioxaspiro[5,5]undec-2-ene	3.585	$C_9H_{14}O_2$	154	154.09938	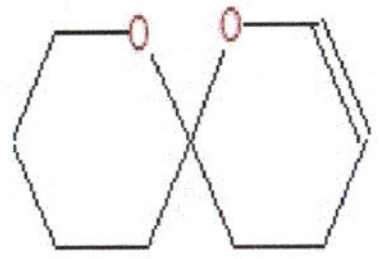	55,71,83,98,111, 126,141,154	Anti-inflammatory activity and anti-oxidative effects
2.	2,4-Dihydroxy-2,5-dimethyl-39(2H)-furan-3-one	4.020	$C_6H_8O_4$	144	144.042258	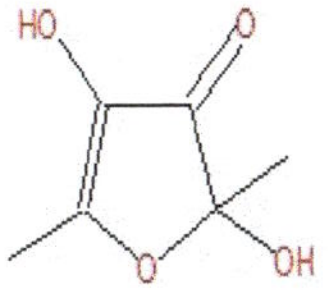	55,73,84,101,14 4	New chemical compound
3.	2,4-Difurobenzene, 1-benzyloxy	4.460	$C_{13}H_{10}F_2O$	220	220.069971	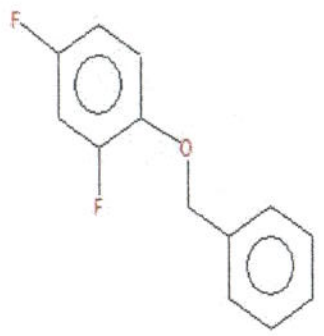	57,65,71,91,101, 129,146,163	Antihistamic and antibacterial
4.	α-D-Glucopyranoside, O-α- Glucopyranosyl	4.975	$C_{18}H_{32}O_{16}$	504	504.169035	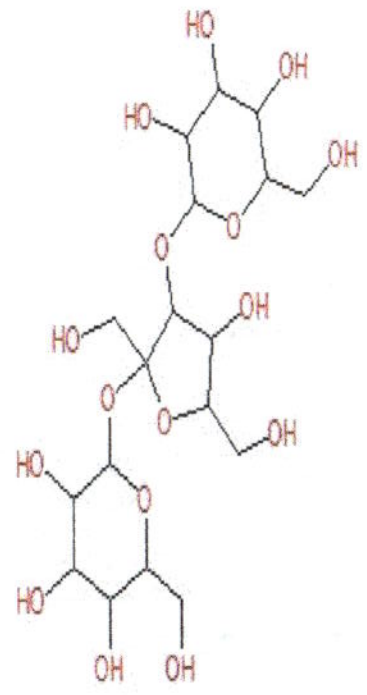	60,73,85,97,113, 126,145,163,180 ,199	Antidiabetic and anti-osteoporotic

Table 1. Cont'd.

5.	4-Hexenal, 6-hydroxy-4-methyl,dimethyl acetal, acetate	5.158	$C_{11}H_{20}O_4$	216	216.136159	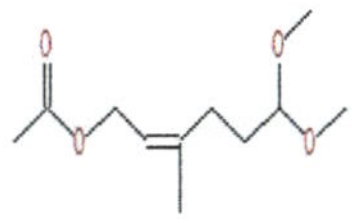	58,67,75,84,93,110,138,152,184, 215	Anagestic, anticoagulant and antipyretic
6.	4H-pyran-4-one,2,3,-dihydro-3,5-dihydroxy-6-methyl	6.011	$C_6H_8O_4$	144	144.042258	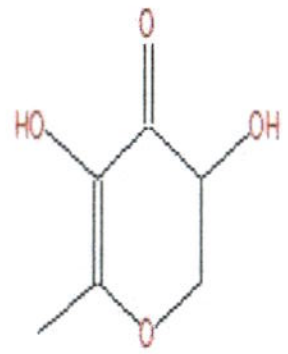	55,58,72,85,101, 115,126,144	Anti-tussive, antibacterial activities and antioxidant
7.	Benzofuran	6.760	$C_8H_8O_4$	120	120.0575147	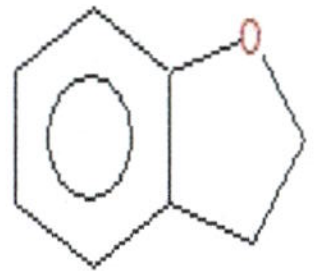	51,63,77,91,105, 120	Antimicrobial and anti-inflammatory activities.
8.	4-Amino-1,5-pentandioic acid	6.320	$C_7H_{13}NO_4$	175	175.084458	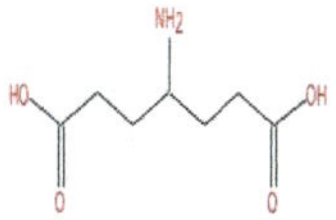	55,73,84,101,129,175	Anti-cancer agents
9.	2-Methoxy-4-vinylphenol	7.974	$C_9H_{10}O_2$		150.06808	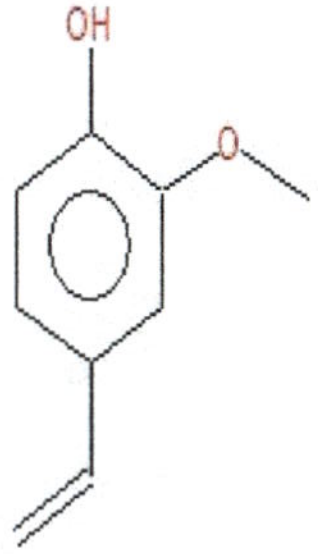	51,63,77,89,107, 118,135,150	Anti-inflammatory effect

Table 1. Cont'd.

10	d-Mannose	13.215	$C_6H_{12}O_6$	180	180.063388	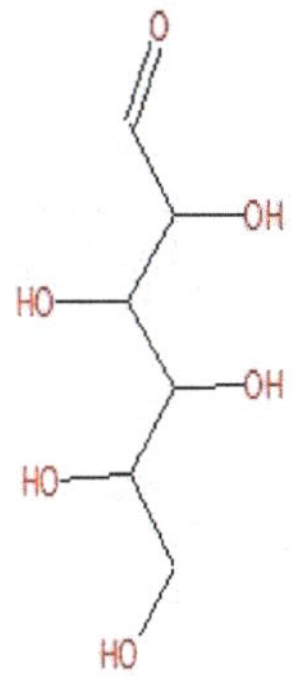	60,73,85,103,13 1,149,179	Anti-allergic and anti-bacterial
11.	7-Isopropyl-10-methyl-1-oxo-1,5-dithia-spiro[5,5]undecane-2-carboxy	14.743	$4H_{24}O_3S_2$	304	304.116686	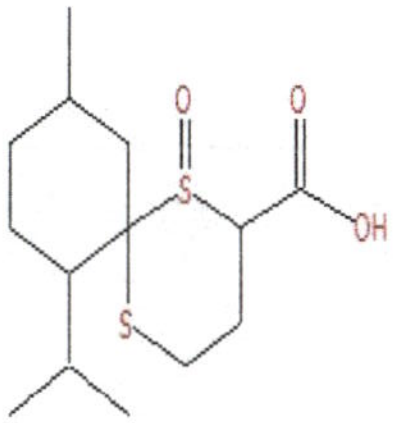	55,69,81,95,123, 137,167,211,243 ,304	New chemical compound
12.	Phytol	16.625	$C_{20}H_{40}O$	296	296.307917	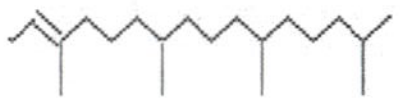	57,71,81,95,111, 123,137,196,221 ,249,278	Anti-inflammatory and antinociceptive activities
13.	Cis-Vaccenic acid,	17.014	$C_{18}H_{24}O_2$	282	282.25588	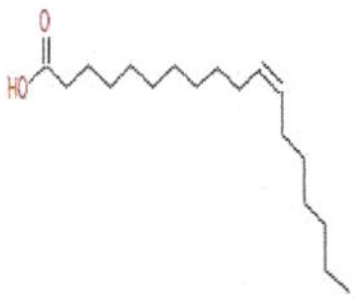	55,69,83,97,111, 125,165,193,222 ,264,282	Anti-carcinogenic effect
14.	N-Methyl-Nbenzyltetradecanami ne	18.485	$C_{22}H_{39}N$	317	317.30825	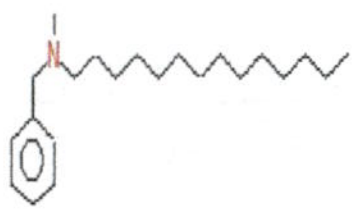	55,91,120,134,1 47,172,195,226, 260,281,317	Anti ulcer agents

Table 1. Cont'd.

15.	3,8,8-Trimethoxy-3-piperidyl-2,2-binaphthalene-1,1,4,4-tetrone,	20.293	$C_{23}H_{28}NO_7$	487	487.163101	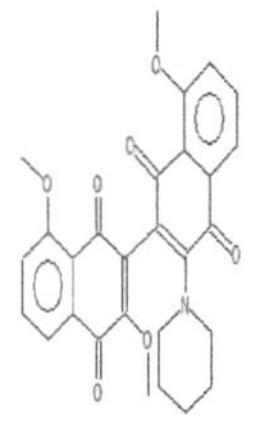	57,71,112,14916 7,223,279,328	Anticancer, antiarthritic and anti-inflammatory
16.	17-(1,5-Dimethylhexyl)10,13-dimethyl	26.284	$H_{69}NO_6Si_3$	386	386.354866	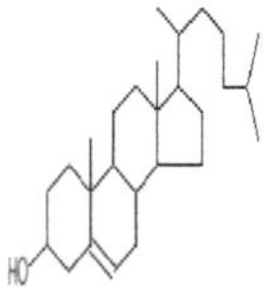	57,69,95,145,21 3,255,275,301,	Anti-HIV Agents

Table 2. FT-IR peak values of methanolic extract of *O. vulgare*

No.	Peak (Wave number cm^{-1})	Intensity	Bond	Functional group assignment	Group frequency
1.	665.44	64.274	-	Unknown	-
2.	729.09	69.940	C-H	Alkenes	675-995
3.	813.96	74.033	C-H	Alkenes	675-995
4.	918.12	73.759	C-H	Alkenes	675-995
5.	1026.13	55.406	C-F stretch	Aliphatic fluoro compounds	1000-10150
6.	1242.16	74.424	C-O	Alcohols, Ethers, Carboxlic acids, Esters	1050-1300
7.	1317.38	77.763	NO2	Nitro Compounds	1300-1370
8.	1361.74	76.351	NO2	Nitro Compounds	1300-1370
9.	1602.85	75.990	-	Unknown	-
10.	1732.08	83.527	-	Unknown	-
11.	2848.86	83.173	-	Unknown	-
12.	2918.30	79.612	C-H	Alkanes	2850-2970

Table 2. Cont'd.

13.	3064.89	86.700	H-O	H-bonded H-X group	2500-3500
14.	3182.55	83.546	H-O	H-bonded H-X group	2500-3500
15.	3217.27	82.889	O-H	Hydrogen bonded Alcohols, Phenols	3200-3600
16.	3277.06	81.843	O-H	Hydrogen bonded Alcohols, Phenols	3200-3600
17.	3363.86	82.552	O-H	Hydrogen bonded Alcohols, Phenols	3200-3600

CONCLUSION

O. vulgare is native plant of Iraq. It contain chemical constitutions which may be useful for various herbal formulation as anti-inflammatory, analgesic, antipyretic, cardiac tonic and antiasthamatic.

ACKNOWLGMENTS

The authors wish to express their deepest gratitude to Prof. Dr. Adul-Kareem for his valuable contributions and support throughout this study. They would also like to express their gratitude to Dr. Ali Al-Marzuki for his valuable suggestions and comments.

REFERENCES

Afsharypuor S, Sajjadi SE, Manesh ME (1997). Volatile constituents of Origanum vulgare ssp. viride (syn.: O. heracleoticum) from Iran. Planta Med. 63:179-180.

Altameme HJ, Hameed IH, Kareem MA (2015). Analysis of alkaloid phytochemical compounds in the ethanolic extract of Datura stramonium and evaluation of antimicrobial activity. Afr. J. Biotechnol.14 (19):1668-1674.

Bakkali F, Averbeck S, Averbeck D, Idaomar M (2008). Biological effects of essential oils-a review. Food Chem. Toxicol. 46:446-475.

Bhat S, Maheshwari P, Kumar S, Kumar A (2002). Mentha species: *In vitro* regeneration and genetic transformation. Mol. Biol. 3:11-23.

Bilalis D, Karkanis A, Konstantas A, Patsiali S, Triantafyllidis V (2011). Arbuscular mycorrhizal fungi: A blessing or a curse for weed Management in organic olive crops? Aust. J. Crop Sci. 5:858-864

Cervato G, Carabelli M, Gervasio S, Cittera A, Cazzola R, Cestaro B (2000). Antioxidant properties of oregano (Origanum vulgare) leaf extracts. J. Food Biochem. 24:453-465.

D'antuono LF, Galleti GC, Bocchini P (2000). Variability of Essential Oil Content and Composition of Origanum vulgare L. Populations from a North Mediterranean Area (Liguria Region, Northern Italy). Ann. Bot.86:471-478.

Franz C, Novak J (2002). Breeding of Oregano. In: Kintzios SE (ed.) Oregano: The Genera Origanum and Lippia. Medicinal and Aromatic Plants, Industrial Profiles 25. Taylor & Francis/CRC Press, USA pp.163-175.

Hameed IH, Hussein HJ, Kareem MA, Hamad NS (2015a). Identification of five newly described bioactive chemical compounds in methanolic extract of *Mentha viridis* by using gas chromatography-mass spectrometry (GC-MS). J. Pharmacogn. Phytother. 7(7):107-125.

Hameed IH, Ibraheam IA, Kadhim HJ (2015b). Gas chromatography mass spectrum and fourier-transform infrared spectroscopy analysis of methanolic extract of *Rosmarinus oficinalis* leaves. J. Pharmacogn. Phytother. 7(6):90-106.

Hameed IH, Jasim H, Kareem MA, Hussein AO (2015c). Alkaloid constitution of *Nerium oleander* using gas chromatography-mass spectroscopy (GC-MS). J. Med. Plants Res. 9(9):326-334.

Hussein AO, Hameed IH, Jasim H, Kareem MA (2015). Determination of alkaloid compounds of *Ricinus communis* by using gas chromatography-mass spectroscopy (GC-MS). J. Med. Plant. Res. 9 (10):349-359.

Ietswaart JH (1980). A taxonomic revision of the genus Origanum (Labiatae), Leiden botanical series, vol 4. Leiden University Press, The Hague, Leiden.

Imad H, Mohammed A, Aamera J (2014a). Genetic variation and DNA markers in forensic analysis. African J. Biotechnol. 13(31):3122-3136.

Imad H, Mohammed A, Cheah Y, Aamera J (2014b). Genetic variation of twenty autosomal STR loci and evaluate the importance of these loci for forensic genetic purposes. Afr. J. Biotech. 13: 1-9.

Imad H, Muhanned A, Aamera J, Cheah Y (2014c). Analysis of eleven Y-chromosomal STR markers in middle and south of Iraq. Afr. J. Biotech. 13(38):3860-3871.

Jasim H, Hussein AO, Hameed IH, Kareem MA (2015). Characterization of alkaloid constitution and evaluation of antimicrobial activity of *Solanum nigrum* using gas chromatography mass spectrometry (GC-MS). J. Pharmacogn. Phytother. 7(4):56-72.

Kareem MA, Hussein AO, Hameed IH (2015). Y-chromosome short tandem repeat, typing technology, locus information and allele frequency in different population: A review. Afr. J. Biotechnol. 14(27):2175-2178.

Kulisic T, Radoni A, Katalinic V, Milos M (2004). Use of different methods for testing antioxidative activity of oregano essential oil. Food Chem. 85:633-640.

Marn M, Novak J, Franz Ch (1999). Evaluierung von Nachkommenschaften von *Origanum vulgare*. Zeitschrift für Arznei- und Gewürz Pflanzen. 4:171-176.

Mechergui K, Coelho JA, Serra MC, Lamine SB, Boukhchina S, Khouja ML (2010). Essential oils of *Origanum vulgare* L. subsp. *Glandulosum* (Desf.) Ietswaart fromTunisia: chemical composition and antioxidant activity. J. Sci. Food Agric. 90:1745-1749.

Mohammed A, Imad H (2013). Autosomal STR: From locus information to next generation sequencing technology. Res.

J. Biotechnol. 8(10):92-105.

Muhanned AK, Ameer IA, Imad HH, Mohammed AJ (2015). A New Polymorphic Positions Discovered in Mitochondrial DNA Hypervariable Region HVIII From Central and North-Central of Iraq. Mitochondrial DNA. pp. 1-5.

Oliver GW (1997). The world market of oregano. Oregano. Proc. IPGRI Intl. Workshop on Oregano, Bari, Italy pp. 142-146.

Radušiene J, Stankevičiene D, Venskutonis R (2005). Morphological and chemical variation of *Origanum vulgare* L. from Lithuania. Acta Horticu. 675:197-203.

Sahin F, Güllüce M, Daferera D, Sökmen A, Sökmen M, Polissiou M, Agar G, Özer H (2004). Biological activities of the essential oils and methanol extract of *Origanum vulgare* ssp. vulgare in the Eastern Anatolia region of Turkey. Food Control 15:549-557

Singh S (2007). Effect of sources and levels of sulphur on yield, quality and nutrient uptake by linseed *(Linum usitatissimum)* Indian J. Agron. 52:158-159.

Skoula M, Harborne JB (2002). Taxonomy and chemistry. In: Kintzios SE (ed.) Oregano: The Genera Origanum and Lippia. Medicinal and Aromatic Plants - Industrial Profiles, Volume 25, Taylor & Francis CRC Press, USA pp. 67-108.

Analgesic and anti-inflammatory effects of the ethanol extract of *Elytraria marginata* Vahl (whole plant) in Wistar rats

J.S. Ashidi[1*], O.J. Ojetola[1], P.I. Aziba[2] and E.O. Ajaiyeoba[3]

[1]Department of Plant Science and Applied Zoology, Olabisi Onabanjo University, Ago-Iwoye. Ogun State, Nigeria.
[2]Department of Pharmacology, Obafemi Awolowo College of Health Sciences, Olabisi Onabanjo University, Sagamu, Ogun State, Nigeria.
[3]Department of Pharmacognosy, University of Ibadan, Ibadan, Nigeria.

The analgesic and anti-inflammatory effects of the ethanol extract of *Elytraria marginata* were studied using hot plate, thermal-induced pain and carrageenan-induced acute inflammation models in adult Wister rats. The preliminary phytochemical constituents of the extract were also ascertained. Inflammation was induced by injecting 0.1 ml of 1% carrageenan into the sub-planter surface of the right hind paw of the rats. Ethanol extract of *E. marginata* with doses of 50, 100 and 150 mg/kg and diclofenac 10 mg/kg were administered orally to separate groups of rats. Control group received 10 ml/kg of distilled water. The results showed that the extract (50, 100 and 150 mg/kg) significantly ($p<0.05$) reduced the carrageenan-induced rat paw oedema in a dose-dependent manner. The oedema reductions at a dose of 150 mg/kg at the 4th h were comparable to that obtained for diclofenac, the standard anti-inflammatory drug at the 3rd hour. The extract also showed a very good analgesic response against hot plate-induced analgesia (thermal stimuli) in the rats. Administration of the extract doses (50, 100 and 150 mg/kg) and ibuprofen 100 mg/kg produced a significant ($p<0.05$) reduction in the pain induced by the hot plate (thermal stimuli) in all the experimental groups when compared with the control. Preliminary phytochemical analysis showed the presence of alkaloids, flavonoids, tannins and saponins. These findings indicate that the ethanol extract of *E. marginata* has both analgesic and anti-inflammatory effects and could be beneficial in alleviating painful inflammatory conditions.

Key words: *Elytraria marginata* plant, inflammation, analgesia, diclofenac sodium, ibuprofen.

INTRODUCTION

Inflammation is a pathophysiological reaction of living organisms to injuries that leads to the local accumulation of plasma fluids and blood cells. Though a defense mechanism, the complex events and mediators involved in the inflammatory reaction can induce, maintain, or intensify numerous diseases (Carey et al., 2009).

In recent times, attention to medicinal plants has increased globally, and a number of evidences have shown the immense potential of medicinal plants traditionally used in various parts of the world (Anosike et

*Corresponding author. E-mail: joseph.ashidi@kcl.ac.uk: ashidisenu@yahoo.com.

al., 2009). Medicinal plants are considered to be an important source of new chemical substances with potential therapeutic effects (Goji et al., 2010). However, studies on inflammatory diseases are gaining much responsiveness, and the side effects of the currently available anti-inflammatory drugs pose a major problem during their clinical use (Kayaalp, 1998). Hence, the development of newer and more powerful anti-inflammatory drugs with less significant side effects is imperative.

The study of plants which are used traditionally in treating inflammatory conditions should be useful in the search for new drugs with anti-inflammatory and analgesic potentials. In Nigeria, many plant products are employed for their analgesic and anti-inflammatory effects and their efficiency is traditionally acclaimed. One of such plant is *Elytraria.marginata* Vahl. (Acanthaceae).

E. marginata is locally known as "*ewe eso*" in Yoruba in Nigeria. It is an annual or short-lived perennial herb, the stem is up to 9 inches high, with small white or bluish flowers and it is widely found in Tropical Africa. The plant has been reported for its use in the treatment of measles in traditional practices in Nigeria (Sonibare et al., 2009), and has been reported as one of the plants used locally in the treatment of sterility in women in Ivory Coast (Assi, 1980). Djah and Nueba (2011) also reported that *E. marginata* is used traditionally by Anyi-Ndenye women during pregnancy to ensure good development of pregnancy and to facilitate labour. *Elytrariaacaulis*, another species of *Elytraria* has been reported to be an anti-hyperglycemic agent on the alloxan-induced diabetes in rats (Kumudhavalli and Jayakar, 2011).

Though the plant has been used in traditional medicine in treating inflammatory condition, there is no scientific evidence for such activities available in literature. The objective of the present study is therefore to investigate the analgesic and anti-inflammatory effects of the ethanol extract of *E. marginata* on carageenan-induced oedema and hot plate-induced analgesia in experimental models in order to validate its traditional use and determine the probable phytochemical constituents present in the ethanol extract of *E. marginata* as the basis for its pharmacological actions.

MATERIALS AND METHODS

Plant collection and identification

The fresh plant of *E. Marginata* was purchased from Ago-Iwoye local market in August, 2012 and was identified by Mr. Shosanya, O.S. of the Forestry Herbarium at the Forestry Research Institute of Nigeria (FRIN), Ibadan, Oyo State, Nigeria. The voucher number allocated to the herbarium specimen is FHI 109760.

Experimental animals

A total number of 30 adult Wistar rats of both sexes were purchased from the Department of Physiology, College of Veterinary Medicine of the Federal University of Agriculture, Abeokuta, Ogun State, Nigeria. The animals weighed between 150 to 200 g. The animals were put under a well-ventilated condition and were housed in a cage of three animals each. They were allowed to acclimatize with the new environment before theexperiment commenced, and were adequately fed with pelletized feed and water *ad libitum*.

Chemical reagents and drugs

Absolute Ethanol, carrageenan, diclofenac sodium (reference drug), ibuprofen (reference drug), hydrochloric acid (HCl), distilled water, ammonia solution, dragendroff reagents, chloroform, lead acetate solution, concentrated sulphuric acid (H_2SO_4), glacial acetic acid, ferric chloride solution ($FeCl_3$), absolute ethanol (BDH) and Frankfurt or Diclofenac sodium (SWIPHA, London) were used in the study

Preparation of the extract

The dried plant of *E. marginata* was ground with an electric blender. The ground plant, 0.45 kg was macerated in 3 L ethanol for a period of one week. The resulting solution was filtered and the filtrate was concentrated to dryness using a water bath at 50°C. After determination of percentage yield, the extract was stored in the refrigerator (4°C) until needed for analysis.

Preliminary phytochemical screening

Phytochemical screening was carried out on *E. marginata* to test for alkaloids, anthraquinones glycosides, cardiac glycosides, flavonoids, saponins, tannins and cardenolides using standard protocols according to Sofowora (1993) and Ajaiyeoba (2002).

Test for alkaloid

To 0.2 g of the crude extract of *E. marginata,* 10 ml of 10%, HCl was added and placed on a water bath for 5 mins. The extract was then filtered and allowed to cool. The pH was then adjusted to about 6 to 7 by adding 10% ammonia and using litmus paper. Then 5 ml of the filtrate was taken into separate test tubes and small quantity of Wagner's, Mayer's and Dragendorff's reagents were added and observed. The presence of turbidity or precipitation indicates the presence of alkaloid (Sofowora, 1993).

Test for anthraquinone glycoside

To 0.2 g of the crude extract of *E. marginata,* 2 ml of 10% HCl was added and placed on a water bath for 5 mins and filtered while still hot, then allowed to cool. The filtrate was partitioned with equal volume of chloroform and shaken gently. The chloroform layer (lower layer) was transferred to a clean test tube and equal volume of the ammonia solution was added and then shaken gently. The presence of delicate rose-pink layer on the test solution indicated the presence of anthraquinones (Sofowora, 1993).

Test for cardiac glycoside

To 0.2 g of the crude extract was added water and 2 to 3 drops of lead acetate solution then was shaken gently and filtered. To the filtrate, 2 ml of chloroform was added and then 1 ml concentrated

H_2SO_4 was carefully added to form a lower layer. A reddish brown colour at interface was observed for cardiac glycoside (Sofowora, 1993).

Test for flavonoid

To 0.2 g of the crude extract of *E. marginata,* 10 ml of ethanol was added and 3 drops of Ferric chloride ($FeCl_3$) was added. A dark green colour indicated the presence of flavonoid (Ajaiyeoba, 2002).

Test for saponin

Crude extract of *E. marginata* (0.2 g) was placed in a test tube containing 10 ml of distilled water, and then boiled for f5 mins and then filtered. The filtrate was shaken vigorously and observed. The presence of froths indicated the presence of saponin (Sofowora, 1993).

Test for tannin

Crude extract of *E. marginata* (0.2 g) was decocted with 20 ml of distilled water by boiling for 10 mins and filtered while hot and allowed to cool. Ferric chloride reagent (0.1%) was added to the filtrate. A blue-black, green or blue green indicated the presence of tannins (Sofowora, 1993).

Test for cardenolides

Crude extract of *E. marginata* (0.2 g) was added 2 ml of glacial acetic acid containing a drop of $FeCl_3$ solution. Then 1 ml of concentrated H_2SO_4 was gently added to form under layer. A brown ring indicated the presence of cardenolides (Sofowora, 1993).

Anti-inflammatory response

The carrageenan-induced acute inflammation model was employed (Winter et al., 1962). A total number of fifteen rats were fasted for 6 h and divided into 5 groups of 3 rats per group. Deprivation of water was to ensure uniform hydration and to minimize variability in oedematous response (Winter et al., 1963). Various doses of the extract (50, 100 and 150 mg/kg) were administered orally to groups 1 to 3, respectively. Group 4 received oral administration of distilled water (10 ml/kg) as negative control while group 5 received oral administration of diclofenac sodium (10 mg/kg) as positive control. After 1 h, 0.1 ml of freshly prepared 1% carrageenan suspended in distilled water was injected into the subcutaneous region of the right hind paw of the rats. The measurement of the paw was taken before (initial paw volume) and after the injection of the carrageenan at 0.5, 1, 2, 3, 4 and 5 h using a Vernier caliper. The mean paw circumference and percentage inhibition of oedema was determined using the methods of Okpo et al. (2001) and Akah (2009). The percentage inhibition was calculated using the modified formula used by Ahmad et al. (1992) below:

Percentage inhibition = $(A–B)/A \times 100$

Where A is mean paw size of the control group and B is the mean paw size of the treated group.

Analgesic response (thermal stimuli)

Hot plate-induced analgesia was employed according to Ilodigwe and Akah (2009). Fifteen rats were fasted for 6 h and divided into 5 groups of 3 rats per group. The extract (50, 100 and 150 mg/kg) was administered orally to groups 1 to 3, respectively. Group 4 received oral administration of distilled water (10 ml/kg) as negative control while group 5 received oral administration of Ibuprofen (100 mg/kg) as positive control. After 1 h, each rat was gently placed on the hot plate maintained at 55±0.5°C and the time required by the rat to lick the paw or jump was taken as the response. The cut-off time or latency response was 15 seconds to avoid tissue damage. The percentage inhibition was calculated using the modified formula below:

Percentage inhibition = $(A–B)/A \times 100$

Where A is mean increase in latency of the treated group and B is the mean increase in latency of the control group.

Statistical analysis

The results of the experiment were expressed as Mean ± Standard error mean (SEM). Numerical data were analysed for homogeneity of variance using Bartlett's test. The data were then analysed using one-way ANOVA to determine whether results in a particular group is significantly different from those in the corresponding control groups. The analysis of variance was followed by Tukey post hoc for intergroup comparisons. $P<0.05$ were considered as significant.

RESULTS

The preliminary phytochemical screening of the ethanol extract of *E. marginata* (Table 1) showed the presence of alkaloids, cardiac glycoside, flavonoids, saponins and tannins. Other constituents like anthraquinones and cardenolides were absent.

Carrageenan-induced oedema

The effect of *E. marginata* ethanol extract on carrageenan-induced oedema is shown in Table 2. The extract produced a dose-dependent inhibition of oedema induced by carrageenan. The percentage inhibition produced by the extract EM (150 mg/kg) was comparable to that produced by diclofenac sodium, 10 mg/kg (standard drug) at the 3rd h post-carrageenan injection. Highest percentage of the inhibitory effect of the extract (39.56%) was observed at a dose of 150 mg/kg body weight at the 5th h. This inhibitory effect was comparableto that exhibited by diclofenac sodium (40.91%) at 10 mg/kg body weight at the 4th h.

Effect on hot plate analgesia

A significant ($p<0.05$) and dose-dependent elevation of the treatment reaction time to thermal pain was evident in the extract-treated animals. The effect of the extract (150 mg/kg) was comparable to that produced by 100 mg/kg of ibuprofen (standard drug) as displayed in Table 3.

Table 1. Result of phytochemical screening of the *E. marginata* ethanol extract.

Plant constituent	Occurrence
Alkaloid	+
Anthraquinone glycoside	-
Cardiac glycoside	+
Flavonoid	++
Saponin	++
Tannins	+
Cardenolides	-

Key: + Present in moderate concentration; ++ Present in abundance;Absent.

Highest percentage of the inhibitory effect of the extract (72.46%) was observed at a dose of 150 mg/kg. The inhibitory effect was greater compared to that of Ibuprofen at a dose of 100 mg/kg (67.15%).

DISCUSSION AND CONCLUSION

The present study showed some of the pharmacological basis for the ethnomedicinal use of *E. marginata* in the treatment of inflammation. Carrageenan-induced inflammation is one of the most employed models reported for screening of clinically effective anti-inflammatory agents. Oedema formation due to carrageenan in rat is a biphasic event. The initial phase of oedema is attributed to the release of histamine and serotonin, and the second phase of oedema is due to the release of prostaglandins, protease and lysosomal enzymes. However, it has been reported that the second phase is sensitive to the most clinically effective anti-inflammatory agents (Thakare et al., 2009).

The ethanol extract of *E. marginata* showed a good anti-inflammatory activity against acute inflammation induced by carrageenan in a dose-related manner at 3rd and 5th h. Oedema results from the action of inflammatory mediators such as histamine, serotonin and bradykinin at the site of a local inflammatory insult (Harriot et al., 2004). The early phase of oedema, beginning from 1 h after the administration of the irritant (carrageenan), is due to the release of histamine and serotonin, while the later phase, occurring from 3 to 5 h after the administration of the irritant (carrageenan) is induced by bradykinin, protease, prostaglandin and lysosome (Wallace, 2002; Harriot et al., 2004). The reduction in oedema exhibited by ethanol extract of the study plant showed that it contains active constituents which block the release of histamine and serotonin from mast cells and inhibit the activity of other inflammatory mediators.

From this study, *E. marginata* ethanol extract demonstrated significant (*$p<0.05$) and dose dependent anti-inflammatory activity against carrageenan-induced paw oedema. The effect of the extracts was most pronounced, 3 h after the induction of oedema, an action which was similar to that of diclofenac sodium, showing its usefulness in the management of acute inflammation. *E. marginata* (150 mg/kg) caused 39.56% inhibition of carrageenan-induced paw oedema compared to that of the standard drug (diclofenac sodium, 10 mg/kg) which was 40.91% at the 4th h.

Thermal painful stimuli are selective for the evaluation of centrally, but not peripherally acting analgesic drugs (Chau, 1989). *E. marginata* (150 mg/kg) produced 72.46% pain inhibition compared to that of the standard drug (Ibuprofen, 100 mg/kg) which produced 67.15% pain inhibition. These results suggest that the extract possesses non-steroidal anti-inflammatory drugs-like analgesic activities, mediated through both the peripheral and central mechanisms. However, the result of the thermal stimuli (hot plate) experiment showed that the extract is more effective in alleviating central pain. Since pain is an integral part of inflammation, the analgesic activity shall certainly be a beneficial factor during inflammatory condition.

The phytochemical screening of the plant showed that it contains alkaloids, flavonoids, saponins, tannins and phenols. To the best this study knowledge and within the scope of available literature, this is the first report of phytochemical screening on *E. marginata*. In a study on related species, *Elytrariaacaulis*, twopyrazole alkaloids were isolated and characterized to be with asomnine and 4'-hydroxywithasomnine (Ravikanth et al., 2001). In another study, asomnine was shown to have inhibitleukotriene metabolis mLTB4, and well had double inhibitory effect on COX-1 and COX-2 enzymes (Wube et al., 2008). Meanwhile, naturally occurring alkaloids, flavonoids and saponins have been found to elicit analgesic and anti-inflammatory properties (Fernanda et al., 2002; Anaga and Onehi, 2010). According to Manthey (2000), prostaglandins, a group of powerful pro-

Table 2. Effect of ethanol extract of *E. marginata* on the carrageenan-induced rat paw oedema.

Parameters	Mean paw size in centimeter ± standard error mean (SEM)						
	Paw sizes at different time intervals						
Treatment dose	0 min	30 min	60 min	120 min	180 min	240 min	300 min
EM (50 mg/kg)	0.46±0.02	0.71±0.03^{ns}(-4.41)	0.78±0.04^{ns}(-6.85)	0.82±0.03^{ns}(-3.80)	0.75±0.08^{ns}(9.64)	0.70±0.07* (20.45)	0.67±0.06* (26.37)
EM (100 mg/kg)	0.43±0.01	0.67±0.02^{ns}(1.47)	0.62±0.04* (15.07)	0.61±0.03* (22.78)	0.57±0.03* (31.33)	0.58±0.02* (34.09)	0.57±0.02* (37.36)
EM (150 mg/kg)	0.47±0.01	0.62±0.03^{ns}(8.82)	0.62±0.04* (15.07)	0.59±0.03* (33.90)	0.56±0.03* (32.53)	0.57±0.03* (35.23)	0.55±0.01*(39.56)
Distilled water (10 ml/kg)	0.46±0.01	0.68±0.03	0.73±0.03	0.79±0.02	0.83±0.01	0.88±0.02	0.91±0.02
Diclofenac sodium (10 mg/kg)	0.47±0.01	0.58±0.08* (14.71)	0.58±0.03* (20.55)	0.58±0.03*(26.58)	0.53±0.01* (36.14)	0.52±0.01*(40.91)	0.51±0.01* (43.96)

Percentage inhibition is shown in parenthesis, n=3, reduction in oedema of the treated groups (*p<0.05) was significant compared with the control groups. Values with (ns) are not significant when compared with the control groups. All values are expressed as mean paw size in centimetre (cm) ± standard error mean (SEM). The extract showed a dose-dependent inhibition of oedema induced by carrageenan. Percentage inhibition by the extract EM (150 mg/kg) can be compared with that produced by diclofenac (10 mg/kg), standard drug used after the 3rd h. EM= *Elytrariamarginata* ethanol extract. n= number of parameters (rats) in each group.

Table 3. Effect of *E. marginata* on the thermal pain induced by hot plate in rats.

Parameters	Mean increase in latency or time spent on the hot plate in seconds ± Standard error mean (SEM)		
Extract/Drug dose	Before treatment (sec)	After treatment (sec)	Percentage inhibition (%)
EM (50 mg/kg)	1.38±0.20	2.32±0.14*	40.52
EM (100 mg/kg)	1.69±0.20	3.68±0.60*	54.08
EM (150 mg/kg)	1.90±0.32	4.72±0.03*	72.46
Distilled water (10 ml/kg)	1.37±0.21	1.37±0.21^{ns}	-
Ibuprofen (100 mg/kg)	1.38±0.12	4.11±0.10*	67.15

The percentage inhibition for all the treated groups were significant (*p<0.05) compared with that of the control groups. Values with (ns) are not significant, n=3. EM (150 mg/kg) showed highest inhibitory effect and all values are expressed as Mean latency or time spent on the hot plate in seconds (sec) ± Standard error mean (SEM). The extract showed a dose-dependent inhibition of thermal pain by the hot plate.

inflammatory signaling molecules have been shown to be effectively inhibited by flavonoids. Therefore, the analgesic and anti-inflammatory activities of *E. marginata* may be due to the presence of alkaloids, flavonoids and other polyphenols.The ethanol extract of *E. marginata* showed significant analgesic effect, which justified its use in managing pain brought by high body temperature (heat) and pain during labour in pregnant women in traditional practices, the reason why it is called "*ewe eso*" meaning easy leaf". It also showed moderate and acute anti-inflammatory effect, which may be responsible for its use in treating measles and other skin sores. Using both the pharmacological and biochemical parameters in different animal models showed that the study plant, *E. marginata,* is a promising anti-inflammatory and analgesic agent and may be useful for the treatment of inflammatory conditions.

ACKNOWLEDGEMENT

The authors are grateful to Mr Olumide Adesanya for technical support.

REFERENCES

Ahmad F, Khan R, Rasheed S (1992). Studyof analgesic and anti-inflammatory activity from plant extracts of *Lactucascariola* and *Artemisia absinthium*. J. Islam. Acad. Sci.5:111-114.

Ajaiyeoba EO (2002). Phytochemical and antibacterial properties of *Parkiabiglobosa* and *Parkia bicolor* leaf extracts. Afr. J. Biomed. Res. 5:125-128.

Anaga AO, Onehi EV (2010). Antinociceptive and anti-inflammatory effects of the methanol seed extract of *Carica papaya* in mice and rats. Afr. J. Pharmacol. 4:140-144.

Anosike CA, Obidoa O, Ezeanyika LVS, Meshach MN (2009). Anti-inflammatory and anti-ulcerogenic activity of the ethanol extract of ginger (*Zingiber officinale*). Afr. J. Biochem. Res.3:379-384.

Assi LA (1980). Plants and the treatment of sterility in women in Ivory Coast. MPLW 19:13-22.

Carey WM, Dasi JMB, Rao NVGoltumukkala MK (2009). Anti inflammatory activity of methanol extract of *Bambusa vulgaris* leaves. Int. J. Green Pharm. 3:234-238.

Chau T (1989). Pharmacological methods in the control of inflammation. In: Modern methods in Pharmacology. R. Alan (Ed.). Liss Inc. New York. pp. 195-212

Djah FM, Nueba DFR (2011). Traditional practices and medicinal plants use during pregnancy by Anyi-Ndeye women (Eastern Cote d'Ivoire). Afr. J. Reprod. Health.15:85-93.

Fernanda LB, Victor AK, Amelia, TH,Elisabetsky E(2002). Analgesic properties of Umbellatine from *Psychotria umbellate*. Pharm. Biol. 44:54-56.

Goji ADT, Mohammed A, Tanko Y, Ezekiel I, Okpanchi AO,Dikko AVV (2010). A study of the anti-inflammatory and anagelsic activities of aqueous extract of *Nauclealatifolia* leaves in Rodents. Asian J. Med. Sci. 2:244-247.

Harriot M, Marion E, Martha A, Wellford S, Williams A (2004). Inflammation induced by histamine, serotonine, bradykinin and compound 48/480 in the rat. Antagonists and mechanisms of action. J. Pharmacol. Exp. Ther. 191:300-302.

Ilodigwe EE, Akah PA (2009). *Spathodeacampanulata*: An experimental evaluation of the analgesic and anti-inflammatory properties of a traditional remedy. Asian J. Med. Sci. 1:35-38.

Kayaalp SO (1998). Medical pharmacology in terms of rational treatment.3rd ed. Hacettepe-Tas Publication, New York pp. 946-948.

Kumudhavalli MV, Jayakar B (2011). Phytochemical and pharmalogical evaluation of the dried leaves of *Elytrariaacaulis* (I.F). Lindau. J. Pharm. Res. 4:3219-3221.

Manthey JA (2000). Biological properties of flavonoid pertaining to inflammation. Microcirculation 7:29-34.

Okpo SO, Fatokun F, Adeyemi OO (2001). Analgesic and anti-inflammatory activity of *Crinum glaunum* aqueous extract. J. Ethnopharmacol. 78:207-211.

Ravikanth V, Ramesh P, DiwanPV, VenkateswarluY (2001). Pyrazole alkaloids from*Elytrariaacaulis.* Biochem. Syst. Ecol. 29:753-754.

Sofowora A (1993). Medicinal plant and Traditional medicine in Africa. Spectrum Book Ltd, Ibadan, Nigeria p 289.

Sonibare MA, Moody JO, Adesanya EO (2009). Use of medicinal plants for the treatment of measles in Nigeria. J. Ethnopharmacol.122:268-272.

Thakare VN, Anupama AS, Avinash DD, Naik SR (2010). Stem bark extraction of *Ficusbengalensis* Linn for anti-inflammatory and analgesic activity in animal models. Indian J. Exp. Biol. 48:39-45.

Wallace JM (2002). Nutritional and botanical modulation of the inflammatory cascade: eicosanoids, cyclooxygenase and lipooxygenase as an adjunct in cancer therapy. Integr. Cancer Ther. 1:7-37.

Winter EA, Risley EA, Nuss GV (1962). Carrageenan induced oedema in hind paw of the rat as an assay for anti-inflammatory drugs. Proc. Soc. Exp. Biol. Med. 111:544-547.

Winter EA, Risley EA, Nuss GV (1963). Anti-inflammatory and antipyretic activities of indomethacin. J. Pharmacol. Exp. Ther. 141:369-376.

Wube AA, Wenzig EM, Gibbsons S, Asres K, Bauer R, Bucar F (2008). Constituentsof the stem bark of *Discopodiumpenninervium* and their LTB4 and COX-1 and -2 inhibitory activities. Phytochemistry 69:982-987.

8

Herbal medicines use among diabetic patients in Oriental Morocco

Zayneb Alami[1]*, Hayat Aynaou[2], Bouchra Alami[3], Youssef Hdidou[2] and Hanane Latrech[2]

[1]Department of Pharmacy and Clinical Pharmacology, Mohammed VI University Hospital, Medical and Pharmacy School, Mohammed First University, Oujda, Morocco.
[2]Department of Endocrinology and Metabolism, Mohammed VI University Hospital, Medical and Pharmacy School, Mohammed First University, Oujda, Morocco.
[3]Department of Ophtalmology, Mohammed VI University Hospital, Medical and Pharmacy School, Mohammed First University, Oujda, Morocco.

The aim of this study was to determine the prevalence of herbal medicines (HM) use among diabetic patients in Oriental Morocco, in order to establish an updated inventory of HM consumption and determine the predictive factors of their use in our patients. We conducted a cross-sectional study during three months from March, 2013 to May, 2013 including all diabetic patients consulting at the Department of Endocrinology and Metabolism of Mohammed VI University Hospital in Oujda. The study included 279 diabetics (200 women and 79 men). The prevalence of HM use was 54.8%. Females were 3.25 times more likely to use HM. All patients did not inform spontaneously their physicians about HM use. More than fifty species belonging to 29 families were used by our population. The five most common HM used were *Salvia officinalis* (Labiaceae), *Trigonella feoenum graecum* (Leguminosae), *Olea europea* (Oleaceae), *Artemisia herba-alba* (Asteraceae) and *Origanum vulgare* (Lamiaceae). Besides, education level (p = 0.027), menopause (p = 0.027), type 2 diabetes (p = 0.05) and taking both oral hypoglycaemic agents and insulin injection (p = 0.043) are significant factors associated with HM use. HM is very common among diabetic patients. There is an urgent need for health education regarding the use of herbs in conjunction with conventional medicines. Clinical and randomized trials may be needed in the future to assess the efficacy and the safety of the reported herbs.

Key words: Herbal medicines, medicinal plants, phytotherapy, diabetes, Morocco, complementary and alternative medicine.

INTRODUCTION

Diabetes mellitus is one of the major public health concerns. Data from the International Diabetes Federation (IDF) indicate that there are 382 million diabetics all over the world and in the next 20 years, diabetes may affect about five times more people than it does now. Moreover, diabetes caused 5.1 million deaths in 2013. Epidemiological data show that 80% of people with diabetes live in low- and middle-income countries. In

*Corresponding author. E-mail: zayneb.alami@gmail.com.

Africa, there are more than 19 million patients with diabetes (International Diabetes Federation, IDF, 2012).

Since ancient time, patients with particularly chronic diseases such as diabetes mellitus use traditional medicine and often without consulting or even informing their physicians. According to the World Health Organization, traditional medicine, referred to complementary and alternative medicine (CAM) in some countries, covers a wide variety of therapies and practices including the use of herbal medicines (HM). Even if traditional medicine is mostly used by developing countries where a large number of people have poor access to modern health care systems, it is recognized now that the use of CAM is increasing and is observed in both developed and developing countries (WHO, 2014). Population-based studies in many developed countries such as Australia (MacLennan et al., 1996), United Kingdom (Emslie et al., 1996), Taiwan (Lew-Ting, 2003), Singapore (Lim et al., 2005), Canada (McFarland et al., 2002) and the United States of America (Tindle et al., 2005) report that one-half to two-thirds of adults use CAM.

Morocco is characterized by a large diversity of biotopes allowing a rich flora with about 4,200 species of which more than 600 are described in the Moroccan pharmacopeia (Bellakhdar et al., 1991). Many ethno-pharmacological surveys were conducted in various regions of Morocco (center, south and oriental) so as to identify species of HM used by patients or counseled by the herbalists in chronic diseases such as diabetes, hypertension, cardiac diseases (Ziyyat et al., 1997; Jouad et al., 2001; Eddouks et al., 2002) and cancer (Kabbaj et al., 2012). However, none of them determined the related factors to the use of HM in diabetic patients. The objectives of the current study were to determine the prevalence of HM use among diabetic patients in Oujda, the largest city of Oriental Morocco, to establish an updated inventory of the used plants and to identify the factors predicting HM use.

MATERIALS AND METHODS

Study design

We carried out a cross-sectional study during three months from March, 2013 to May, 2013 at Mohammed VI University Hospital in Oujda. Each diabetic patient who consulted at the Department of Endocrinology and Metabolism was asked to participate in the study. All patients were informed of the aims of the study and gave their consent.

Data collection

A face-to-face interview was conducted using a semi-structured questionnaire to obtain data including:

1. Data on patient: age, sex, weight, province region (rural or urban), medical insurance, education level (no education, primary, secondary or higher), diabetes type, its duration and treatment.
2. Information on HM use, use duration, the vernacular name, the used part, preparation method, use frequency, use resources, the reason of its use and side effects related to its use. The following references were used to identify the vernacular name and then to match it to the scientific name and the family to which they belong: (Hmamouchi, 2001; Bellakhdar et al., 1991)

Statistical analysis

Statistical analysis of data was performed using the IBM SPSS Statistics Standard version 21.0. Descriptive data were expressed using means, medians, standard deviations and percentages. Categorical data were compared using chi-square test χ^2. Statistical significance was defined as $p < 0.05$.

RESULTS

Socio-demographic and clinical characteristics

The study included 279 diabetic patients (200 women and 79 men) with a mean age of 50 ± 17 years and a mean weight of 67 ± 12 kg. Most of them came from urban regions (93.7%), had no education (43.8%) or studied at a primary level (27.5%) and had no medical insurance (74.3%). Type 2 diabetes was more common in our population than type 1 (72.4% vs. 27.6%) with a median duration of 7 years [4 – 12]. Sixty five percent of patients had at least one cardiovascular risk factor. The main risk factors in our population were menopause followed by hypertension. Table 1 shows socio-demographic and clinical characteristics of our patients.

Prevalence and resources on HM use

The prevalence of HM use was 54.8%. Females used HM 3.25 times more likely than males. None of our patients disclosed HM use spontaneously to their physician. More than ninety percent of HM users (93.8%) reported HM usage for more than a month. The frequency of consumption of HM was everyday for 51.2% and once a week for 28.1%. Most patients learned about HM use primarily from friends, neighbors and families (84.8%), followed by media (radio in 9% and television in 5.5%). The majority of patients (80%) got HM from the herbalists and 17% of them directly from nature. Few patients (8%) reported gastro-intestinal effects while 91.7% had no side effects.

Patterns, attitudes, beliefs, and perceptions toward HM

Most HM users (81.1%) believed that HM can potentiate the effect of the drug medicines and can help them achieve better control in diabetes while only 7% of them used HM because they think that medicines are not

Table 1. Socio demographic and clinical characteristics of the population (n=279).

Characteristic	Variable*
Age [Min-Max]	50 ± 17 [11 – 87]
Weight (kg)	67 ± 12
Gender	
Female	200 (71.7)
Male	79 (28.3)
Origin	
Urban	254 (93.7)
Rural	17 (6.3)
Education level	
Illiterate	116 (43.8)
Primary	73 (27.5)
Secondary	53 (20)
Tertiary	23 (8.7)
Medical insurance	
Yes	69 (25.7)
No	199 (74.3)
Cardiovascular risk factors	175 (65.5)
Smoking	21 (11.9)
Hypertension	100 (56.8)
Dyslipidemia	46 (26.1)
Menopause	109 (61.9)
History of familial cardiovascular diseases	19 (10.8)
Diabetes type	
Type 1	74 (27.6)
Type 2	194 (72.4)
Duration of diabetes (years)	7 (4 – 12)
Treatment	
Insulin	97 (35.1)
Oral hypoglycaemic agents	122 (44.2)
Both	50 (18.1)

effective as they must be. Some use HM (4.9%) because they do not have any confidence in medicines (Table 2). Table 3 provides a comparison of characteristics between HM users (HM+) and no users (HM-). Patients with cardiovascular risk factors use HM more than patients who do not (p = 0.035). Menopause seems to be a significant risk factor associated to HM use (p = 0.027). We observed that patients with type 2 diabetes used HM (59.3%) more than patients with type 1 diabetes (45.9%), although this is not statistically significant (p = 0.05). Duration of diabetes did not differ between HM+ and HM- (p=0.48). Most HM users were treated by the combination of hypoglycaemic agents and insulin injection (p = 0.043). We also observed that the majority of patients treated only by insulin did not use HM (51.1%).

Inventory of plant species used by diabetic patients

In 60% of cases, a mixture of plants was used. More than

Table 2. Attitudes, beliefs and perceptions toward HM.

Attitudes, beliefs and perceptions toward HM	N (%)
Believe that HM potentiate the effect of drug medicines	117 (81.8)
No confidence on drugs medicines	7 (4.9)
Lack of effectiveness of medicines	10 (7)
Other (Cannot afford medicines)	9 (6.3)

Table 3. Association of characteristics between patients concerning the use of HM.

Characteristic	No HM use (HM-) n=126 (%)	HM use (HM+) n=153 (%)	P - value
Age			
< 40 years	35 (50.7)	34 (49.3)	0.334
≥ 40 years	88 (44)	112 (56)	
Gender			
Male	43 (54.4)	36 (45.6)	0.051
Female	83 (41.5)	117 (58.5)	
Education level			
No education	41 (35.3)	75 (64.7)	
Primary and secondary school	66 (52.4)	60 (47.6)	0.027
Above	11 (47.8)	12 (52.2)	
Medical insurance	32 (46.4)	37 (53.6)	0.756
Risk factors	71 (40.3)	105 (59.7)	0.035
Smoking	11 (52.4)	10 (47.6)	0.231
Hypertension	41 (41)	59 (59)	0.838
Dyslipidemia	19 (41.3)	27 (58.7)	0.877
Menopause	37 (33.9)	72 (66.1)	0.027
Familial history of cardiovascular disease	5 (26.3)	14 (73.7)	0.187
Diabetes type			
Type 1	40 (54.1)	34 (45.9)	0.05
Type 2	79 (40.7)	115 (59.3)	
Treatment			
Insulin	50 (51.5)	47 (48.5)	
Oral hypoglycaemic agents	50 (41)	72 (59)	0.043
Both	19 (38)	31 (62)	
Duration of diabetes	7 (4-12)	8 (4-12)	0.488

P-value was determined by Chi-square $\chi 2$.

fifty plant species belonging to 29 families were used by our population, of which the five most used were: *Salvia officinalis* (62 citations), *Trigonella feoenum-graecum* (36 citations), *Olea europea* (34 citations), *Artemisia herba alba* (32 citations) *and Origanum vulgare* (28 citations). An inventory of the 49 plants identified and used is given in Table 4 with the vernacular name, family name, part used, mode of use and number of citations.

Table 4. Medicinal plants used by patients with diabetes in Oujda.

Scientific name	Vernacular name	Family	Part of plant	No of citations	Mode of use
Ajuja iva	Chendgora	Lamiaceae	-	1	-
Allium cepa	Bessel	Liliaceae	Bulb	1	Directly, with honey
Aloe vera	Sabra	Liliaceae	-	2	-
Ammi visnaga	Bechnikha	Apiaceae	-	1	-
Anthemis nobilis	Babounj	Asteraceae	Oil, Leaves	1	Decoction
Argania spinosa	Argan	Saotaceae	Seeds	3	Decoction
Aristolochia longa	Berztem	Aristolocheae	Seeds	1	Decoction
Artemisia herba-alba	Acchih	Asteraceae	Leaves, seeds	32	Infusion, decoction
Astragalus sp.	Grayen Al Kabch	Fabaceae	-	1	-
Beta vulgaris	Selq	Chenopodiaceae	-	-	-
Centaurium spicalum	Merraret Al Hench	Gentianaceae	-	1	-
Cicer arientirum	Hemmous	Fabaceae	-	1	-
Cinnamonum cassia	Kerfa	Lauraceae	Bark	1	Decoction
Citrus aurantiifolia Swingle	Liymoun	Rutaceae	Leaves	1	Infusion
Coriandrum sativum	Kozbor	Apiaceae	seeds	1	Directly
Cynara cardumculus	Kherchouf	Asteraceae	Leaves	4	Decoction
Echinops spinousus	Taskra	Asteraceae	Seeds	2	Infusion
Eriobotyra japonica	Mzah	Rosaceae	Leaves	1	Infusion, decoction
Eucalyptus globulus	Calyptus	Myrtaceae	Leaves	1	-
Ficus carica	Kermouss	Moraceae	Fruit	1	-
Globularia alypum	Aîn Al Arnab	Globulariaceae	Leaves	1	Decoction
Linum susitatissimum	Kettan	Linaceae	Seeds	3	Directly
Marrubium vulgare	Merriwa	Lamiaceae	Leaves	2	Decoction
Mentha pulegium	Fliyou	Lamiaceae	Leaves	4	Infusion
Nerium oleander	Defla	Apocynaceae	Leaves	3	Decoction
Nigella sativa	Sanouj	Renonculaceae	Seed	6	Infusion, decoction
Olea europaea	Zitoun	Oleaceae	Leaves	34	Decoction
Opuntia ficus-indica	Al Hendiya	Cactaceae	-	1	-
Origanum compactum	Zâater	Lamiaceae	All, Leaves	28	Decoction, infusion
Peganum harmala	Al Harmel	Zigophylaceae	Seeds	2	Infusion
Pimpinella anisum	Hebbat Helawa	Apiaceae	Seeds	3	Decoction, with water
Prunus amygdalus	Allouz Al Harr	Rosaceae	Seeds	4	Decoction

Table 4. cont'd

Punica granatum	Remman	Rosaceae	-	1	-
Rosmarinus officinalis	Azir	Lamiaceae	Leaves	14	Decoction, with tea
Rubia tinctorum	Al foua	Rubiaceae	-	1	-
Ruta graveolens	Fejel	Rutaceae	Leaves	1	Directly, decoction
Salvia officinalis	Salmiya	Lamiaceae	Leaves	62	Decoction, infusion, with tea
Satureja calamintha	Nebta	Labiaceae	Leaves	1	Infusion
Sonchus arvensis	Kettann Al Hench	Asteraceae	Leaves	1	Infusion
Sorghum vulgare	Bechna	Gramieae	Seeds	2	Infusion, decoction
Tetraclinis articulate	Arâar	Cupressaceae	Leaves	1	-
The sinensis	Atay	Ternstroemiaceae	Seeds	1	-
Thymelea hirsuta	Methnane	Thymeliaceae	Seeds	1	Infusion
Trigonella-foenum graecum	Al Helba	Fabaceae	Seeds	36	Infusion, directly, with pickle and sparkling water, with water
Urtica dioica	Herriga	Urticaceae	Leaves	2	Decoction
Verbena officinalis	Allouiza	Verbenaceae	Leaves	4	Infusion, decoction
Viscum album	Lenjbar	Loranthaceae	Seeds	1	Infusion, mix with oil
Zingiber officinalis	Skinjebir	Zingiberaceae	Rhizome	1	-
Ziziphus lotus	Sedra	Rhamnaceae	Root	1	Infusion

DISCUSSION

The prevalence of HM use among diabetic patients in this study population was high (54.8%). The use of medicinal plants for diabetes treatment is reported worldwide. It is also a national widespread practice. However, this result is lower when compared to that of other national previous studies undertaken by Ziyyat et al. (1997) in the same region (67.5%) and in other regions of Morocco such as Fez-bouleman (76%) (Jouad et al., 2001) and Tafilalet (80%) (Eddouks et al., 2002). A large access to medicines and progressive awareness of population over the years may explain this finding. Another possible reason for the differences in the rate of HM use between these studies may be attributed to differences in the research methodology used. This prevalence remains higher in comparison to other Arabic countries such as Palestine, Jordan, Saudi Arabia, and Kuwait (Ali-Shtayeh et al., 2012; Otoom et al., 2006; Wazaify et al., 2011; Al-Rowais, 2002; Awad et al., 2008) where the following prevalence's were recorded: 51.9, 31, 16.6 to 17.4 and 13%. In Turkey, 41% of diabetic patients used at least one of CAM practices (Ceylan et al., 2009).

Females used HM more likely than males (58.5% vs. 45.6%), though not significant ($p = 0.05$). This is consistent with findings in other studies (Ziyyat et al., 1997; Jouad et al., 2001; Eddouks et al., 2002) and could be explained by the attachment of women in our country to traditional medicine. It may be also linked to the fact and that they stay more often at home as most of them are housewives.

Education level influences HM use ($p = 0.027$) whereas holding a medical insurance did not ($p = 0.57$). In fact, most HM+ were illiterate (64.7%) in comparison to HM- (35.3%). This is in contrast with the results of an Indian survey where higher levels of education and socio-economic status were significant positive correlates of CAM use (Kumar D et al., 2006). All patients practicing CAM used HM alongside allopathic treatment with a significant result with patients treated by both oral hypoglycaemic agents and insulin injection ($p = 0.043$). One possible reason for our findings is that patients with diabetes had poor blood-sugar control, as the conventional treatment requires them to be disciplined with respect to diet, lifestyle and behavior. So patients use HM to potentiate the anti-diabetic activity of the allopathic treatment and thus contribute to the management of their disease. In addition, 51% of patients with insulin therapy do not use HM. To explain this, patients at the stage of insulin therapy received improved diabetes education counseling. An alarming result is that none of our patients (100%) did inform us spontaneously about HM use. Similar studies conducted among Jordanian (Wazaify et al., 2011), Sudanian (Al-Rowais, 2002) and Palestinian patients (Ali-Shtayeh et al., 2012) have showed that respectively 84.3, 70 and 68% of patients did not tell their physicians or pharmacists about HM use. This result indicates that patients are not aware of the dangers that may occur when herbs are used in conjunction with medicines. The combination of herbal remedies and medical prescriptions may lead to ineffective diabetic management and adverse effects (Chavez et al., 2006). It is therefore important that patients disclose HM use to their health care professionals and physicians. This information about CAM usage should be incorporated into clinical practice and sought after by clinicians.

The most common sources of HM information were recommendation from friends, neighbors and families, followed by media. This finding highlights the importance of the patients close environment (friends, neighbors, family) in decision-making processes and health behaviors. So, health professionals should be aware of the impact of their beliefs and attitudes on the beliefs and attitudes of their patients. The present study indicates that we must involve patients' families during diabetes education counseling regarding the efficacy and potential side-effects of plants. In addition, health authorities should monitor advertising on radio and television by choosing qualified experts in the field to make advice to the population. The majority of plants used by patients was purchased locally. This highlights that plants are easy to access, available and cheap. In most cases (60%), patients did not use one plant but a mixture of plants. The reported number of herbs used by patients with diabetes in this work was about fifty species. This is slightly higher than the same study that was done earlier by Ziyyat et al. (Ziyyat et al., 1997) in Oriental Morocco (41 species) but considerably higher than that reported in Jordan (Wazaify et al., 2011) (12 species) and lower than a Palestinian study which reports 100 species (Ali-Shtayeh et al., 2012).

The most commonly used herbs by our population included *S. officinalis* (Labiaceae), *T. feoenum-graecum (Leguminosae), O. europea (Oleaceae), A. herba-alba (Asteraceae)* and *O. vulgare (Labiaceae).* Anti-diabetic activity has been demonstrated on diabetic animal models for *T. foenum-graecum* (Xue et al., 2007) and *O. europea* (Kaeidi et al., 2011). Many researchers have studied the hypoglycaemic effect of hydro-alcoholic extracts of *A. herba-alba* and confirmed the possibility of its use in the treatment of type 2 diabetes (Hamza et al., 2011) as well as in prevention (Hamza et al., 2010). Furthermore, some studies have suggested that the methanolic and the water ethanolic extracts of *S. officinalis* leaves have hypoglycaemic effects in Streptozotocin- and alloxan-induced diabetic animals without changes in insulin level (Eidi et al., 2005; Alarcon-Aguilar et al., 2002). In addition, the essential oil of sage has been tested and has proved its hypoglycaemic effect in normal and in alloxan-induced diabetic rats (Moradabadi et al., 2013) but not in streptozotocin-induced diabetic rats (Awad et al., 2008). (Lima et al., 2006) observed a metformin-like effect of infusion of *S. officinalis* on rat hepatocytes that may be useful as a food supplement in the prevention of type 2 diabetes by lowering the plasma glucose of individuals at risk. (Lemhadri et al., 2004) have shown that the aqueous extract of *O. vulgare*, commonly named "zaâtar" and growing wild in Tafilalet region of Morocco has an anti-hyperglycaemic activity in Streptozotocin-rats without affecting basal plasma insulin concentrations. Therefore, these studies provide a scientific basis to conduct clinical and randomized trials to assess the efficacy and the safety of these plants in humans. However, there was a report of the use of *Aristolochia longa* by one patient. *A. longa* is commonly used in traditional medicine (Bellakhdar et al, 1991). In 2001, Food and Drug Administration (FDA) published an alert about the safety of aristolochic acid, the active ingredient of *A. longa* (Food and Drug Administration (FDA), 2014). In 2002, the International Agency for Research on Cancer has classified products containing aristolochia species as a human carcinogen (IARC, 2002). Aristolochic acid is recognized to cause aristolochic acid nephropathy associated with a high long-term risk for renal failure and urothelial cancer (Al-Rowais, 2002; Zhou et al., 2010; Arlt VM et al., 2002) by DNA adduct formation (Allard et al., 2013).. From this scientific evidence-base, aristolochic acid-containing herbs should be banned in our country by health authorities as it is the case in many countries.

LIMITATIONS OF THE STUDY

The present study has several limitations. Firstly, the survey was carried out on patients attending the Department of Endocrinology and metabolism of a University Teaching hospital for treatment of diabetes and hence does not reflect the common practices in the general population. Secondly, we were unable to assess objectively and scientifically harmful or beneficial effects associated with HM use.

Conclusion

HM use among patients with diabetes mellitus in Oriental Morocco is very common. Menopausic and illiterate women with type 2 diabetes under both oral hypoglycaemic agents and insulin as a conventional treatment have a higher likelihood of HM use. Physicians should seek and discuss with their patients during diabetes education counseling the use of HM, their potential interactions and side-effects when used in conjunction with medicines.

ACKNOWLEDGMENTS

We would like to thank all survey respondents in this study and wish them a good control of their disease. Thank you to the members of the research group "Ethnopharmacologie au Service de la Phytothérapie" (Drs. Bahi Rachida, Imounachen Hassan, Imounachen Rachid, Karzazi Nissrine, Mahmoudi Omar, Nouar oussama) for their help in identifying some of the plants' use reported by our patients. We are also grateful to Prof. Intissar Haddiya for revising the English version of the manuscript.

REFERENCES

Alarcon-Aguilar FJ, Roman-Ramos R, Flores-Saenz JL, Aguirre-Garcia F (2002). Investigation on the hypoglycaemic effects of extracts of four Mexican medicial plants in normal and alloxan-diabeti mice. Phyto. Res. 16(4):383-386.

Ali-Shtayeh MS, Jamous RM, Jamous RM (2012). Complementary and alternative medicine use amongst Palestinian diabetic patients. Complement. Ther. Clin. Pract. 18(1):16-21.

Allard T, Wenner T, Greten HJ, Efferth T (2013). Mechanisms of herb-induced nephrotoxicity. Curr. Med. Chem. 20:2812-9.

Al-Rowais NA (2002). Herbal medicine in the treatment of diabetes mellitus. Saudi Med. J. 23:1327-31.

Arlt VM, Stiborova M, Schmeiser HH (2002). Aristolochic acid as a probable human cancer hazard in herbal remedies: a review. Mutagenesis 17:265-277.

Awad A, Al-Rabiy S, Abahussain E (2008). Self-medication practices among diabetic patients in Kuwait. Med. Princ. Pract. 17(4):315-20.

Baricevic D, Bartol T (2000). The biological/ pharmacological activity of the Salvia genus. In Sage-the Genus Salvia, [SE Kintzios, editor]. Amsterdam: Harwood Academic publishers. pp. 143-184.

Bellakhdar J, Claisse R, Fleurentin J, Younos C (1991). Repertory of standard herbal drugs in the Moroccan pharmacopoea. J. Ethnopharmacol. 35:123-143.

Ceylan S, Azal O, Taslipinar A, Türker T, Açikel CH, Gulec M (2009). Complementary and alternative medicine use among Turkish diabetes patients. Compl. Ther. Med. 17:78-83.

Chavez ML, Jordan MA, Chavez PI (2006). Evidence-based drug-herbal interactions. Life Sci. 78:2146-57.

Eddouks M, Maghrani M, Lemhadri A, Ouahidi ML, Jouad H (2002). Ethnopharmacological survey of medicinal plants used for the treatment of diabetes mellitus, hypertension and cardiac diseases in the south-east region of Morocco (Tafilalet). J. Ethnopharmacol. 82:97-103.

Eidi M, Eidi A, Zamanizadeh H (2005). Effect of Salvia officinalis L. leaves on serum glucose and insulin in healthy and streptozotocin-induced diabetic rats. J. Ethnopharmacol. 100:310-313.

Emslie M, Campbell M, Walker K (1996). Complementary therapies in a local healthcare setting Part 1. Is there real public demand? Complement Ther. Med. 4:39-42.

Food and Drug Administration. Dietary supplements: aristolochic acid. http://www.fda.gov/Food/RecallsOutbreaksEmergencies/SafetyAlerts Advisories/ucm096388.htm . Accessed on May 28th, 2014.

Hamza N, Berke B, Cheze C, Le Garrec R, Lassalle R, Agli AN, Robinson P, Gin H, Moore N (2011). Treatment of high fat diet induced type 2 diabetes in C57BL/6J mice by two medicinal plants used in traditional treatment of diabetes in the east of Algeria. J. Ethnopharmacol. 133:931-933.

Hamza N, Berke B, Cheze C, Agli AN, Robinson P, Gin H, Moore N (2010). Prevention of type 2 diabetes induced by high fat diet in the C57BL/6J mouse by two medicinal plants used in traditional treatment of diabetes in the east of Algeria. J. Ethnopharmacol. 128:513-518.

Hmamouchi M. Plantes médicinales et aromatiques du Maroc.2nd Edition, 2001.

IARC monographs on the evaluation of carcinogenic risk of chemicals to humans. Volume 82. Lyons, France: IARC Press, 2002.Some traditional herbal medicines, some mycotoxins, naphthalene and styrene. International Diabetes Federation, IDF, Diabetes Atlas. 6th Ed.: International Diabetes Federation; 2012.

Jouad H, Haloui M, Rhiouani H, El Hilaly J, Eddouks M (2001). Ethnobotanical survey of medicinal plants used for the treatment of diabetes, cardiac and renal diseases in the North centre region of Morocco (Fez–Boulemane). J. Ethnopharmacol. 77:175-182.

Kabbaj F, Meddah B, Cherrah Y, Faouzi A (2012). Ethnopharmacological profile of traditional plants used in Morocco by cancer patients as herbal therapeutics. Phytopharmacology. 2:243-256.

Kaeidi A, Esmaeili-Mahani S, Sheibani V Abbasnejad M, Rasoulian B, Hajializadeh Z, Afrazi S (2011). Olive (Olea europea L.) leaf extract attenuates early diabetic neuropathic patin through prevention of high glucose-induced apoptosis : in vitro and in vivo studies. J. Ethnopharmacol. 136:188-196.

Kumar D, Bajaj S, Mehrotra R (2006). Knowledge, attitude and practice of complementary and alternative medicines for diabetes. Public Health.120:705-711.

Lemhadri A, Zeqqwagh A, Maghrani M, Jouad H, Eddouks M (2004). Anti-hyperglycaemic activity of the aqueous extract of Origanum vulgare growing winld in Tafilalet region. J. Ethnopharmacol. 92:251-256.

Lew-Ting CY (2003). Who uses non-biomedical, complement and alternative health care? Sociodemographic undifferentiation and the effects of health needs. Taiwan J. Public Health. 22:155-66.

Lima CF, Azevedo MF, Araujo R, Fernandes-Ferreira M, Pereira-Wilson C (2006). Metformin-like effect of Salvia officinalis (common sage): is it useful in diabetes prevention? Br. J. Nutr. 96:326-33.

Lim MK, Sadarangani P, Chan HL, Heng JY (2005). Complementary and alternative medicine use in multiracial Singapore. Complementery Ther. Med. 13:16-24.

MacLennan AH, Wilson DH, Taylor AW (1996). Prevalence and cost of alternative medicine in Australia. Lancet 347:569-573.

McFarland B, Bigelow D, Zani B, Newsom J, Kaplan M (2002). Complementary and alternative medicine use in Canada and the United States. Am. J. Public Health. 92:1616-1618.

Moradabadi L, Montasser Kouhsari S, Fehresti Sani M (2013). Hypoglycemic Effects of Three Medicinal Plants in Experimental Diabetes: Inhibition of Rat Intestinal α-glucosidase and Enhanced Pancreatic Insulin and Cardiac Glut-4 mRNAs Expression. Iran J. Pharm. Res.12:387-397.

Otoom SA, Al-Safi SA, Kerem ZK, Alkofahi A (2006). The use of medicinal herbs by diabetic Jordanian patients. J. Herb Pharmacother. 6:31-41.

Tindle HA, Davis RB, Phillips RS, Eisenberg DM (2005). Trends in use of complementary and alternative medicine by US adults: 1997-2002. Altern Ther Health Med. 13:16-24.

Wazaify M, FU. Afifi, M El-Khateeb, Ajlouni K (2011). Complementary and alternative medicine use among Jordanian patients with diabetes. Complementary Ther. Clin. Pract. 17:71-75.

World Health Organization (WHO). http://www.who.int/topics/traditional_medicine/en/. Accessed on March 16, 2014.

Xue WL, Li XS, Zhang J, Lliu YH, Wang ZL, Rui-Juan Zhang RJ (2007). Effect of Trigonella foenum-graecum (Fenugreek) extract on blood glucose, blood lipid and hemorheological properties in streptozocin-induced diabetic rats. Asia Pac. J. Clin. Nutr. 16 (Suppl 1):422-426.

Evaluation of the anthelmintic activity of pumpkin seeds (*Cucurbita maxima*) in mice naturally infected with *Aspiculuris tetraptera*

Erol Ayaz[1*], Cengiz Gökbulut[2], Hamit Coşkun[3], Arzu Türker[4], Şeyda Özsoy[5] and Kübra Ceylan[5]

[1]Department of Medical Parasitology, Faculty of Medicine, Abant İzzet Baysal University Bolu, Turkey.
[2]Department of Medical Pharmacology, Balıkesir University Faculty of Medicine, Balıkesir, Turkey.
[3]Department of Psychology, Faculty of Art and Science, Abant İzzet Baysal University, Bolu, Turkey.
[4]Department of Biology, Faculty of Art and Science, Abant İzzet Baysal University Bolu, Turkey.
[5]Department of Medical Microbiology, Faculty of Medicine, Abant İzzet Baysal University Bolu, Turkey.

The aim of this study was to investigate the anthelmintic effect of pumpkin seeds (*Cucurbita maxima*) against *Aspiculuris tetraptera* in naturally infected mice. For this purpose, the natural infection was determined by the cellophane tape (on the anal region), and the centrifugal flotation methods of stool samples in approximately 150 male Swiss albino mice (27 to 35 g). The infected mice (29 animals) were divided into four groups. The animals in the first (G_1) and second groups (G_2) received water and ethanol extracts of pumpkin seeds orally at the dose suggested for human for 7 days, respectively. The mice in the positive control group (G_3) were treated with ivermectin intramuscularly at a dose of 0.2 mg/kg body weight. The mice in fourth groups (G_4) received the same amount of serum physiologic orally. The mice were housed in clean polypropylene cages and maintained under standard laboratory conditions at an ambient temperature of 20±2°C with 45% relative humidity and a 12 h light dark cycle. At the eighth day of the study, all animals were killed humanly following inhalation anaesthesia. After euthanasia, the number of parasites in the intestine was counted. Data obtained from the treatment groups were compared using one-way ANOVA. The percentage efficacy of the drugs was calculated. The results of the study showed that the efficacies for water (G_1) or ethanol (G_2) extracts of pumpkin seed and ivermectin were 81, 85 and 91% compared with the negative control, respectively. These results revealed that pumpkin seed has high anthelmintic activity against nematodes as well as its continued use in traditional medicine for the treatment of helminthiasis.

Key words: *Aspiculuris tetraptera*, mice, anthelmintic effect, efficacy, *Cucurbita maxima*.

INTRODUCTION

The traditional medicinal plant use in all cultures is well documented. Plants have been the main component of

*Corresponding author. E-mail: erolayaz@ibu.edu.tr.

traditional pharmacopoeias for generations, and continue to supply new remedies for the treatment of various maladies. According to the data of the World Health Organisation, 80% of people use these treatment methods in developing countries and 3.3 billion people benefit from medical plants as treatment. In recent years, their usage in developed countries has increased dramatically (Baytop et al., 1999; Saraçoğlu et al., 2005; Mindell, 2003; Saraç, 2006). The medicinal plants such as garlic, black cumin, stinger and pumpkin seeds have been used extensively in the treatments of various maladies as traditional medicine (Beech et al., 2011).

Squash is a member of Cucurbitaceae family that includes plants such as melon, watermelon, cucumber and gherkin. There are two kinds of squash as pumpkin and vegetable marrow. *Cucurbita maxima* (Lam.) (Vegetable marrow, Pumpkin), *Cucurbita moschata* (Lam.) Poiret (Winter squash) and *Cucurbita pepo* L. (Summer squash) are cultivated in Turkey and generally, *C.maxima* is used as an anthelmintic for medical purpose (Baytop, 1999; Saraçoğlu, 2005). Pumpkin seed is very rich in terms of amino acids that are building blocks of proteins, especially the essential amino acids such as phenylalanine, tryptophan and methionine which are not produced in the human body (Saraçoğlu, 2005).

It has a very rich composition of vitamin E, especially gamma tocopherol, unsaturated fatty acids which carry importance in terms of human health and phytosterol (Baytop, 1999; Saraçoğlu, 2005). It is known that not only the fruit but also the pumpkin seed has many benefits, so it has been used for a long time in traditional medicine in many countries as well as in Turkey. Pumpkin seed has been used in different parts of the world as traditional medicine for treatments of gastrointestinal parasites as anthelmintic, urinary dysfunctions, hyperplasia of prostate as a supporter, dysuria, cardiovascular disease, enuresis nocturna in children and lowering blood glucose (Saraçoğlu, 2005; Srivastava and Singh, 1967; Lans et al., 2007; Weiss, 1988; Dreikorn et al., 2002; Winkler et al., 2005). Moreover, it has been reported that compounds in pumpkin seed have an immune potential role (Winkler et al., 2005).

Despite the increase in scientific studies about pumpkin, there is a paucity of data available in the literature on its antiparasitic property. Especially the seeds of *C. maxima*, known as winter squash, are widely used to treatment of gastrointestinal parasites as an anthelmintic. It has been reported that a handful of pumpkin seed kernel was effective especially for the treatment of Taeniasis (Baytop, 1999; Cappelletti, 1985; Gonzales et al., 1974). It is known that the anthelmintic effect of pumpkin seed comes from cucurbitine, and is effective on turbellaria by paralyzing them (Asımgil, 2004; Baytop, 1999; Gonzales et al., 1974; Guarrera, 1999; Pieroni et al., 2005; Saraçoğlu, 2005). Díaz et al. (2004), reported that 1g meshed pumpkin seed displayed a high efficacy against turbellarias in dogs (Lans et al., 2007).

The purpose of this study was to evaluate the anthelmintic efficacy of pumpkin seeds (*Cucurbita maxima*) in mice naturally infected with *Aspiculuris tetraptera*. Hence, the results obtained from this trial could be extrapolated to human and other animal species.

MATERIALS AND METHODS

Experimental animals

One hundred and fifty (150) five-week-old male Swiss albino mice (27 to 35 g) were used in this study. They were housed in clean polypropylene cages and maintained under standard laboratory conditions at an ambient temperature of 20±2°C with 45% relative humidity and a 12 h light dark cycle. They were allowed free access to a standard pellet diet and water *ad libitum*. All animals were fed equally by 1/10 of their approximate body weights. Parasitological examinations of animals were made by centrifugal flotation techniques that were prepared by salt water and cellophane band method. The rats naturally infected by *A. tetraptera* were identified and used in the study. Before starting the study, the investigation was approved by the Experimental Animal Ethics Committee of the Abant İzzet Baysal University, Bolu, Turkey.

The mice (29 mice) naturally infected with *A. tetraptera* were divided into four groups (G_1, G_2, G_3 and G_4) according to the egg burden of the animals, and each group comprises 6 to 10 animals. The animals in G1 and G2 were given water and ethanol extracts of pumpkin seeds orally at a dose suggested for a human for 7 days. The animals in G_3 (positive control) were administered ivermectin intramuscularly at a dose of 0.2 mg/kg bodyweight. The rats in the control group (G_4) were given the same amount of water orally.

Preparation of pumpkin seed extract

The pumpkin seeds were bought from the local market in Bolu and taxonomically identified and authenticated by a taxonomist at the Department of Biology, Faculty of Art and Science, Abbant İzzet Baysal University, Bolu, Turkey. Approximately 200 g of pumpkin seed was milled fine and then water and ethanol extracts were prepared as follows.

Preparation of water extract

Pumpkin seed kernel (100 g) was milled and mixed with the addition of 300 ml distilled water at 40°C for 18 to 24 h. The obtained mixture was filtered and the liquid part (water) was evaporated by using a freeze dryer and pumpkin seed extract was obtained as pulverized.

Preparation of ethanol extract

Pumpkin seed kernel (100 g) was milled and extracted by adding 300 ml ethanol with a soxhlet extractor at 75°C for 24 h. At the end of this period, the mixture was filtered and the liquid part was evaporated by using a rotary evaporator. The remaining part of the pumpkin seed kernel extract was dissolved in 20 to 30 ml distilled water and the ethanol extraction of pumpkin seed was obtained as pulverized by evaporating the liquid part (water) by using freeze dryer. All the obtained extracts were dissolved by using sterile distilled water and the concentration to be given to rats, was prepared as 100 mg/ml. The water and ethanol extracts given orally were prepared every day for a week with a dose of 100 mg/kg by using an injector.

The treatment of rats with ivermectin in the positive control group

Ivermectin was administered to each rat in the positive control group at a dose of 0.2 mg/kg by diluting ethanol and distilled water. For this, 0.5 ml of mixture which was obtained by mixing 100 ml ethanol and 400 ml distilled water with 0.5 ml of ivermectin, was given to each rat by single i.m. injection.

Treatment

All the rats were examined parasitiologically by saturated saltwater floatation method. On the same day, the water and ethanol extracts of pumpkin seeds were given to rats every day for a week with a dose of 100 mg/kg. On the first day of the study, the rats infected with *A. tetraptera* in the positive control group was treated with a single dose of 0.2 mg/kg of ivermectin following i.m. injection.

Autopsy

The next day of starting and giving the last pumpkin seed, all the rats were killed by inhalation anaesthesia. The intestines of rats in all groups were opened and washed with a saline solution. The parasites were collected and identified under a stereomicroscope. The worm burden were compared between groups.

Statistical analysis

The results were evaluated statistically by using the statistical package for social sciences (SPSS) statistical programme. The significance of difference between groups was calculated statistically by using One-Way Analysis of Variance (ANOVA) and these differences were compared with Benferonni test. The percentage treatment efficacy (%) was calculated using the formula:

$$\text{Efficacy } (\%) = [(Cg - Tg) / Cg] \times 100$$

Where Cg is the geometric mean of parasites counted from the control group, Tg is the geometric mean of parasites counted from the treatment group.

RESULTS

Clinically no adverse reactions were observed in any of the rats treated with extracts given during the study. The number of parasites collected from the intestines of rats in control and the experiment groups, min-max values, geometrical means and percentages of efficacy were given in Table 1. The total parasite numbers in control, ivermectin and ethanol and water extract groups of pumpkin seed were 249, 29, 60 and 107 respectively. The geometric means of parasite numbers obtained in the negative control group were significantly higher than those obtained in the experimental groups. The efficacies for ivermectin (G_3), water (G_1) and ethanol (G_2) extracts were 91, 85 and 81% compared to the negative control group (G_4), respectively.

It was obtained that extra treatment had an important effect on the number of parasites, $F (3, 25) = 9.89$, $p = 0.0001$, $\eta^2 = 0.54$. This treatment or try had an effect on explaining 54% of the change (variance) in parasite numbers. According to Benferonni test which kept the type I error constant, when compared to control group (M= 10.70, S.D. = 4.15), the number of parasites statistically low between ivermectin (M= 6.33, S.D.=3.88), ethanol (M= 8.57, S.D. = 4.96) and water extract (M= 10.70, S.D. = 4.15) groups with these last groups being not significantly different from each other. As a result, when compared to control group, it was obtained that ivermectin with pumpkin seed water and ethanol extracts importantly decrease parasite numbers (Table 1).

DISCUSSION

Medicinal plants such as onion, thyme, sweet balm, black cumin and stinger have been used widely as a traditional treatment. Pumpkin seeds have been used for traditional treatment worldwide especially in the Far East. According to the data transferred from generation to generation and scientific researches, pumpkin seed has been used in traditional treatment for especially urinary diseases, diabetes, prostate and parasitic infections. It has been reported that in the last ten years, pumpkin seeds has been used for antitumor, antidiabetics, antihypertensive, antibacterial, anti-inflammatory, immunostimulant and analgesic purposes (Jafarian et al., 2012).

Díaz et al. (2004), reported that the minimal effective amount of the seeds from *C. maxima* was 23 g (approximately 73 pumpkin seeds) in rats. Moreover, they observed that the pumpkin seeds displayed proteolytic effect and destructions on tegument including base membrane and cause reduction in the number of eggs of reproduction of parasite rings. It was also obtained that pumpkin seeds caused erosive gastritis in rats at 9 g/kg pumpkin seed. In another study, (Díaz et al., 2004), 23 g pumpkin seed in 100 ml distilled water showed antihelmintic activity such as changes in the parasite movements and destruction in tegumentine and eggs in reproduction rings of parasites. In Italy, it was reported that an anthelmintic activity was observed against tenias in dogs when 1 g of meshed pumpkin seed was mixed and given with 250 ml distilled water (Lans et al., 2007). In the present study, it was found that the anthelmintic activities of water and ethanol extracts on *A. tetraptera* were considerably high (81 and 85%, respectively).

Moreover, Mahmoud et al. (2002) reported that pumpkin seed extract prepared with boiled water caused destruction on parasite eggs after administration orally to the puppies infected with *Heterophyes heterophyes* for two weeks (Mahmoud et al., 2002). Similarly, *C. maxima* was given to winged animals at 50, 100 and 200 mg/kg doses for 10 days for investigation of its anthelmintic activity, but no activity was observed (Lahon et al., 1978). They only reported that 2 ml ethanol extraction (300

Table 1. Control and experimental groups, the number of parasites collected from the intestines of rats, min-max values and influence the geometric mean of the percentages.

Groups	No	Number of parasite after the autopsy	Total	Min-max	Geo-mean±SD	% Efficacy
Control group (G_4) (n:6)	1	17	249	17-84	35.84±25.40	-
	2	26				
	3	34				
	4	84				
	5	60				
	6	28				
Ivermectin (G_3) group (n:6)	1	5	29	1-10	3.32±3.88	91
	2	1				
	3	3				
	4	10				
	5	9				
	6	1				
Ethanol extract (G_2) (n:7)	1	16	60	1-16	5.44±6.34	85
	2	1				
	3	14				
	4	9				
	5	1				
	6	5				
	7	14				
Water extract (G_1) (n:10)	1	1	107	1-27	6.78±9.27	81
	2	23				
	3	4				
	4	27				
	5	15				
	6	2				
	7	6				
	8	9				
	9	17				
	10	3				

mg/ml) causes an 8.69% reduction in *Raillietina cesticillus* in the animals. In this previous study, it was obtained that water and ethanol extractions of pumpkin seed is effective as 81 and 85% respectively against *A. tetrapteraya* in the intestines of rats. It was observed that its effect is more when ethanol extract is compared to water extract. These obtained results have a quality that supports the general usage of pumpkin seed in treatment of parasite infections.

It has been reported that the types of extraction play an important role at the level of antiparasitic activity. In a previous study, Amorim et al. (1991) investigated that the antimalarial effect of ethanol extracts of *C. maxima* seeds against *Plasmodium berghei* ans 50% reduction in the blood parasite amount was observed in the infected rats given the extracts at a dose of 250/500 mg/kg. Antigiardial effects of petroleum ether and methanol extract of *C. maxima* and *C. pepo* seeds at doses of 250, 500 and 1000 ppm were investigated by Elhadi et al. (2013). The extract dose of *C. maxima* obtained after petroleum ether extraction at 500 and 1000 ppm have 48 h, whereas 250 ppm concentration has 100% activity against giardia in 72 h. Moreover, *C. pepo* has 83.7% activity against giardia in 96 h at a concentration of 500 ppm. It was reported that *C. maxima* can be used as a good anti giardial agent. They thought the anti giardial effect of *C. maxima* depends on the existence of triterpens (Cucurbitacin E and Cucurbitacin L 2-0-β glucoseids). In addition, Marie-Magdeleine et al. (2009) studied three different extractions (water, methanol and dichloromethane) of *C. moschata in vitro* against *Haemoncus contortus*. They found that only water extract inhibited the larval developments of the parasite. It was reported that the pigs experimentally infected with *Oesophagostomum* sp. larvas were treated with pumpkin seeds following administration three times in a week at a dose of 5 g/kg and the results were compared with ivermectin treatment (Magi et al., 2005). The anthelmintic activity of pumpkin seeds (96.1%) was found similar to ivermectin treatment (97.5%).

With this study both in our country and in different parts of the world the anthelmintic effect of pumpkin seed (C. Maxima Lam) which is used in treatments of many parasitic diseases such as *Taenia saginata, Enterobius vermicularis ve Ascaris lumbricoides* was searched on *Enterobius vermicularis* and *A. tetraptera* in human as well as in natural infected rats.

Conclusion

The present study indicated that both water and ethanol extracts of pumpkin seeds were effective and displayed high anthelmintic efficacy (81 and 85%, respectively) against *A. tetraptera* in rats. Hence, the results obtained from this trial could be extrapolated to other animal species and human for the treatment of helminthiasis.

REFERENCES

Amorim CZ, Marques AD, Cordeiro RS (1991). Screening of the antimalarial activity of plants of the Cucurbitaceae family. Mem. Inst. Oswaldo Cruz 86(Suppl 2):177-180.

Asımgil A (2004). Şifalı Bitkiler. Timaş Yayınları, İstanbul. ISBN: 975-362-085-3.

Baytop T (1999). Türkiye'de Bitkiler ile Tedavi. İ. Ü. Yay. NO: 3255, İstanbul.

Beech RN, Skuce P, Bartley DJ, Martin RJ, Prichard RK, Gilleard JS (2011). Anthelmintic resistance: markers for resistance, or susceptibility? Parasitology 138(2):160-174.

Cappelletti EM (1985). Antifungal, parasiticide, insecticide, and anthelmintic herbal remedies in the traditional medicine of North-Eastern Italy. Curare 3:39-47.

Díaz OD, Lloja LL, Carbajal ZV (2004). Preclinical studies of cucurbita maxima (pumpkin seeds) a traditional intestinal antiparasitic in rural urban areas. Rev. Gastroenterol Peru 24(4):323-327.

Dreikorn K, Berges R, Pientka L, Jonas U (2002). Phytotherapy of benign prostatic hyperplasia. Current evidence-based evaluation. Article in German Urologe A. 41(5):447-451.

Elhadi IM, Koko WS, Dahab MM, El Imam YM, El Mageed MAEA (2013). Antigiardial Activity of some *Cucurbita* Species and Lagenaria Siceraria. J. For. Prod. Ind. 2(4):43-47.

Gonzales AE, Bravo OR, Garcia MH, Santos de la R and Tomas del ML (1974). Pharmacological (anthelmintic) study of Cucurbita maxima seeds and their active principle, cucurbitin. Ann. Real. Acad. Pharmaceut. 40:475-486.

Guarrera PM (1999). Traditional antihelmintic, antiparasitic and repellent uses of plants in Central Italy. J. Ethnopharmacol. 68(1-3):183-192.

Jafarian A, Zolfaghari B, Parnianifard M (2012). The effects of methanolic, chloroform, and ethylacetate extracts of the *Cucurbita pepo L.* on the delay type hypersensitivity and antibody production. Res. Pharm. Sci. 7(4):217-224.

Lahon LC, Khanikor HN, Ahmad N, Gogoi AR (1978). Preliminary and pharmacological and anticestodal screening of Curcurbita maxima. Indian J. Pharmacol. (4):315-317.

Lans C, Turner N, Khan T, Brauer G (2007). Ethnoveterinary medicines used to treat endoparasites and stomach problems in pigs and pets in British Columbia, Canada. Vet. Parasitol. 148(3-4):325-340.

Magi E, Talvik H, Jarvis T (2005). In vivo studies of the effect of medicinal herbs on the pig nodular worm (*Oesophagostomum* spp.). Helminthologia 42(2):67-69.

Mahmoud LH, Basiouny SO, Dawoud HA (2002). Treatment of experimental heterophyiasis with two plant extracts, areca nut and pumpkin seed. J. Egypt Soc. Parasitol. 32(2):501-506.

Marie-Magdeleine C, Hoste H, Mahieu M, Varo H, Archimede H (2009). In vitro effects of Cucurbita moschata seed extracts on Haemonchus contortus. Vet. Parasitol. 161(1-2):99-105.

Mindell E (2003). Mucize Bitkiler. Yeni ve Geleneksel Bitkisel İlaçların Bestseller Rehberi. Prestij yayınları, İstanbul. ISBN: 975-6435-05-4.

Pieroni A, Dibra B, Grishaj G, Grishaj I, Gjon Maçai S (2005). Traditional phytotherapy of the Albanians of Lepushe, Northern Albanian Alps. Fitoterapia 76(3-4):379-399.

Saraç EM (2006). Doğanın Şifalı Eli. Doğan Ofset Matbaacılık Aş.

Srivastava MC, Singh SW (1967). Anthelmintic activity of Cucurbita maxima (kaddu) seeds. Indian J. Med. Res. 55(6):629-632.

Weiss RF (1988). Herbal Medicine. Beaconsfield, England. Beaconsfield Publishers.

Winkler C, Wirleitner B, Schroecksnadel K, Schennach H and Fuchs D (2005). Extracts of Pumpkin (*Cucurbita pepo* L.) Seeds Suppress Stimulated Peripheral Blood Mononuclear Cells in vitro. Am. J. Immunol. 1:6-11.

Phytochemical analysis of *Urtica dioica* leaves by fourier-transform infrared spectroscopy and gas chromatography-mass spectrometry

Huda Jasim Al-Tameme, Mohammed Yahya Hadi and Imad Hadi Hameed*

Department of Biology, Babylon University, Hilla City, Iraq.

Phytochemicals are chemical compounds formed during the plants normal metabolic processes. These chemicals are often referred to as secondary metabolites. The objective of this research was to determine the chemical composition of leaves extract from methanol. The phytochemical compound screened by gas chromatography-mass spectrometry (GC-MS) method. Fifteen bioactive phytochemical compounds were identified in the methanolic extract of *Urtica dioica*. The identification of phytochemical compounds is based on the peak area, retention time molecular weight, molecular formula, mass spectrometry (MS) fragment-ions and pharmacological actions. GC-MS analysis of *U. dioica* revealed the existence of the Oxime- methoxy-phenyl, 2, 6,-Nonadienal, 3, 7-dimethyl, 1, 2, 3-Butanetriol, Silane, triethyl(2-phenylethoxy), Benzofuran, 2,3,-dihydro, 2,5,5,8a-Tetramethyl-1,2,3,5,6,7,8, 8a-octahydronaphthalen-1-ol, 2H-Indeno[1,2-b]furan-2-one, 3,3a, 4,5,6,7,8, 8b-octahydro-8,8-dimet, 1-Dodecanamine, N, N-dimethyl, 2(3H)-Naphthalenone, 4, 4a,5,6,7,8-hexahydro-1-methoxy, D-Fructose, diethyl mercaptal, pentaacetate, [1,1-Bicyclopropyl-2-octanoic acid 2hexyl-methyl ester, Estra-1,3,5(10)-trien-17B-ol, Cyclopropaneoctanoic acid, 2-[2-pentylcycloproyl)methyl]-methyl, 1-Hydroxy-2-(2,3,4,6-tetra-O-acetyl-beta-d-glucopyranosyl)-9H-xanthe and Ethyl iso- allochlate. The FTIR analysis of *U. dioica* leaves proved the presence of aromatic rings, alkenes, aliphatic fluoro, alcohols, ethers, carboxlic acids, esters, nitro compounds, hydrogen bonded alcohols and phenols. It contain chemical constitutions which may be useful for various herbal formulation as anti-inflammatory, analgesic, antipyretic, cardiac tonic and antiasthamatic.

Key words: GC-MS analysis, fourier-transform infrared, phytochemicals, *Urtica dioica*.

INTRODUCTION

Phytochemicals are defined as bioactive non-nutrient plant compounds in fruits, vegetables, grains, and other plant foods that have been linked to reducing the risk of major chronic diseases (Hai, 2004; Magee and Rowland, 2004; Altameme et al., 2015; Hameed et al., 2015a). General description of *Urtica dioica* erect perennial, 50 to 300 cm tall with 4-sided stems, armed with stinging hairs, opposite leaves, 7 to 15 cm long, the stalks from about 1/10 as long to nearly 1/2 as long as the blades, depending on variety. The stipules prominent, mostly 10

*Corresponding author. E-mail: imad_dna@yahoo.com.

to 15 mm long. Fruits are achenes, lens-shaped, flattened, about 1.5 mm long, enclosed by the 2 inner sepals. *U. dioica* has many hollow stinging hairs called trichomes on its leaves and stems, which act like hypodermic needles that inject histamine and other chemicals that produce the stinging sensation when contacted by humans and other animals (Kavalali, 2003; Petlevski et al., 2003; Gulcin, 2004).

The other compounds isolated are derivatives of the terpenoids previously isolated from the roots and flowers of *U. dioica* (Gozum et al., 2003; Luo, 2009), and they include stigmasterol derivative, sitosterol derivative and ethyl cholestanol (Belyakova et al., 2002; Benkeblia, 2004; Golalipour et al., 2009).

This study aims to analyze the chemical compounds of *U. dioica* leaves by fourier-transform infrared (FT-IR) spectroscopy and gas chromatography-mass spectrometry (GC-MS).

MATERIALS AND METHODS

Collection and preparation of plant material

The leaves were dried at room temperature for seven days and when properly dried then powdered using clean pestle and mortar, and the powdered plant was size reduced with a sieve (Hameed et al., 2015). The fine powder was then packed in airtight container to avoid the effect of humidity and then stored at room temperature (Hussein et al., 2015).

Preparation of sample

About 9 g of the plant sample powdered were soaked in 100 ml methanol individually. It was left for 72 h so that alkaloids, flavonoids and other constituents if present will get dissolved. The methanol extract was filtered using Whatman's No.1 filter paper and the residue was removed (Jasim et al., 2015).

Gas chromatography-mass spectrum analysis

The GC-MS analysis of the plant extract was made in a (Agilent 7890 A) instrument under computer control at 70 eV. About 1 μL of the methanol extract was injected into the GC-MS using a micro syringe and the scanning was done for 45 min. As the compounds were separated, they eluted from the column and entered a detector which was capable of creating an electronic signal whenever a compound was detected (Mohammed and Imad, 2013; Kareem et al., 2015; Imad et al., 2014). The greater the concentration in the sample, bigger was the signal obtained which was then processed by a computer. The time from when the injection was made (Initial time) to when elution occurred is referred to as the retention time (RT). While the instrument was run, the computer generated a graph from the signal called chromatogram. Each of the peaks in the chromatogram represented the signal created when a compound eluted from the gas chromatography column into the detector. The X-axis showed the RT and the Y-axis measured the intensity of the signal to quantify the component in the sample injected. As individual compounds eluted from the gas chromatographic column, they entered the electron ionization (mass spectroscopy) detector, where they were bombarded with a stream of electrons causing them to break apart into fragments. The fragments obtained were actually charged ions with a certain mass .The mass/charge (M/Z) ratio obtained was calibrated from the graph obtained, which was called the Mass spectrum graph which is the fingerprint of a molecule (Imad et al., 2014).

Before analyzing the extract using GC-MS, the temperature of the oven, the flow rate of the gas used and the electron gun were programmed initially. The temperature of the oven was maintained at 100°C. Helium gas was used as a carrier as well as an eluent. The flow rate of helium was set to 1 ml per min. The electron gun of mass detector liberated electrons having energy of about 70eV. The column employed here for the separation of components was Elite 1 (100% dimethyl poly siloxane) (Imad et al., 2014). The identity of the components in the extracts was assigned by the comparison of their retention indices and mass spectra fragmentation patterns with those stored on the computer library and also with published literatures.

RESULTS AND DISCUSSION

GC-MS analysis of compounds was carried out in methanolic leaves extract of *U. dioica*, as shown in Table 1. The GC-MS chromatogram of the 15 peaks of the compounds detected was shown in Figure 1. Chromatogram GC-MS analysis of the methanol extract of *U. dioica* showed the presence of fifteen major peaks and the components corresponding to the peaks were determined as follows. The first set up peak was determined to be Oxime- methoxy-phenyl (Figure 2). The second peak indicated to be 2, 6,-Nonadienal, 3, 7-dimethyl (Figure 3). The next peaks considered to be 1, 2, 3-Butanetriol, Silane, triethyl(2-phenylethoxy), Benzofuran, 2,3,-dihydro, 2,5,5,8a-Tetramethyl-1,2,3,5,6,7,8, 8a-octahydronaphthalen-1-ol, 2H-Indeno[1,2-b]furan-2-one, 3,3a, 4,5,6,7,8, 8b-octahydro-8,8-dimet, 1-Dodecanamine, N, N-dimethyl, 2(3H)-Naphthalenone, 4, 4a,5,6,7,8-hexahydro-1-methoxy, D-Fructose, diethyl mercaptal, pentaacetate, [1,1-Bicyclopropyl-2-octanoic acid 2hexyl-methyl ester, Estra-1,3,5(10)-trien-17B-ol, Cyclopropaneoctanoic acid, 2-[2-pentylcycloproyl)methyl]-methyl, 1-Hydroxy-2-(2,3,4,6-tetra-O-acetyl-beta-d-glucopyranosyl)-9H-xanthe and Ethyl iso- allochlate. (Figure 4-16).

The FTIR analysis of *U. dioica* leaves proved the presence of aromatic rings, alkenes, aliphatic fluoro, alcohols, ethers, carboxlic acids, esters, nitro compounds, hydrogen bonded alcohols and phenols which shows major peaks at 891.11, 958.69, 1010.70, 1091.71, 1242.16, 1319.31, 2686.84 and 3363.86 (Table 2; Figure 17). Polar extract of the *U. dioica* contains lignans +)-neoolivil, (-)-secoisolariciresinol, Dehydrodiconiferyl alcohol, isolariciresinol, pinoresinol, and 3,4divanillyltetrahydrofuran, and has antiinflammatory effects and stimulates the proliferation of human lymphocytes (Obertreis et al.,1996; Harput et al.,2005; Kanter et al., 2005; Hameed et al., 2015c). Traditionally, it has been used for uterine hemorrhage, cutaneous eruption, infantile and psychogenic eczema, epistaxis, and melena and specifically for nervous eczema (Bandow et al., 2003; Burt, 2004; Banso and

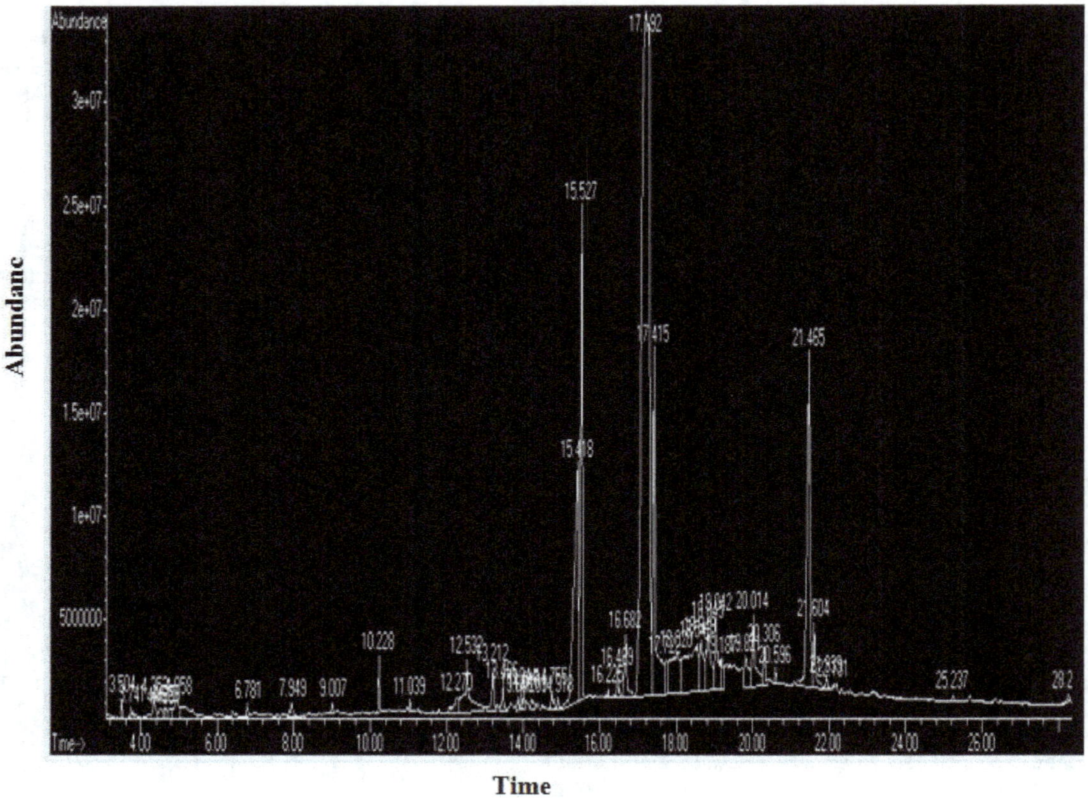

Figure 1. GC-MS chromatogram of methanolic leaves extract of *U. dioica* .

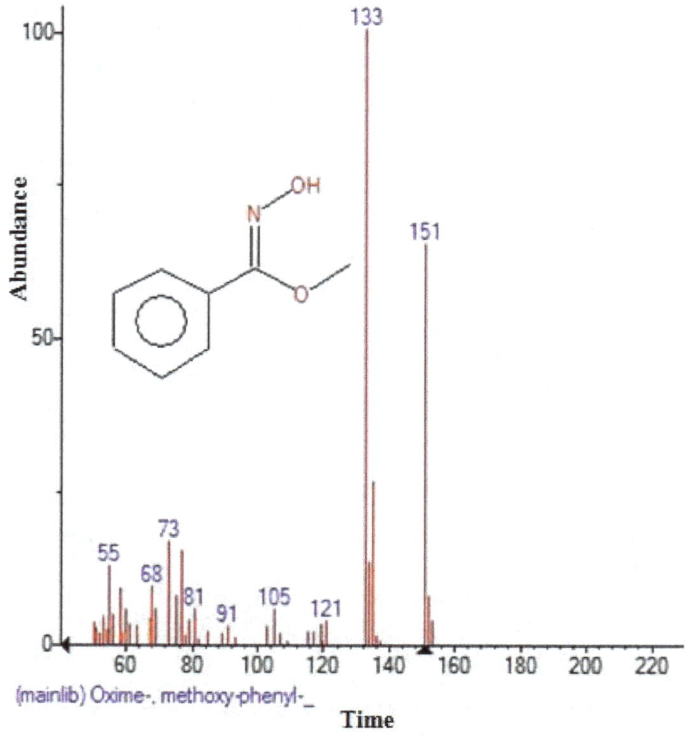

Figure 2. Mass spectrum of Oxime- methoxy-phenyl with retention time (RT) = 3.504.

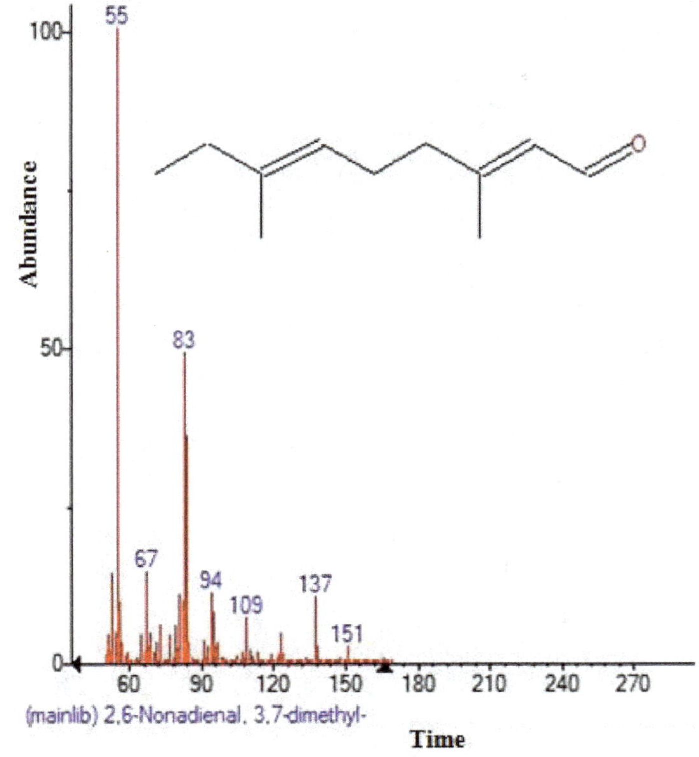

Figure 3. Mass spectrum of 2,6,-Nonadienal,3,7-dimethyl with retention time (RT)= 3.739.

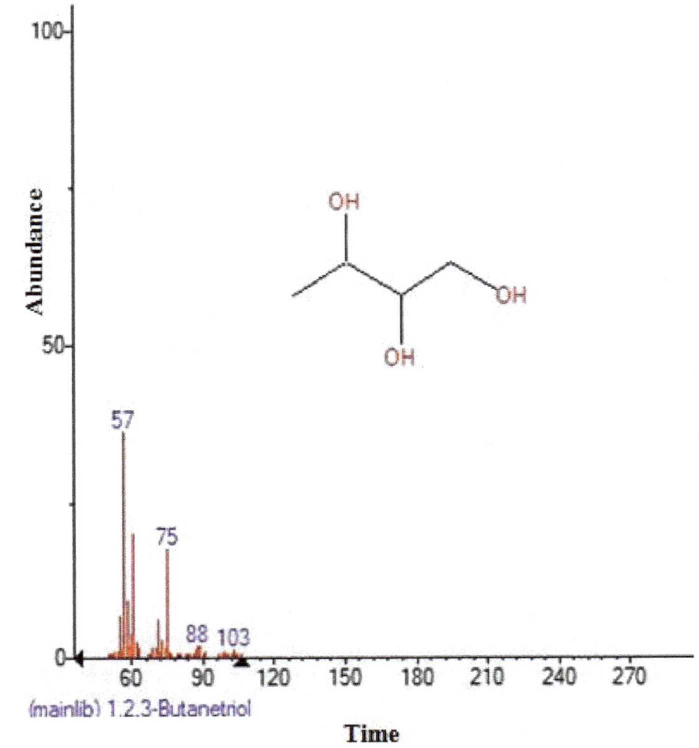

Figure 4. Mass spectrum of 1, 2, 3-Butanetriol with retention time (RT)= 4.380.

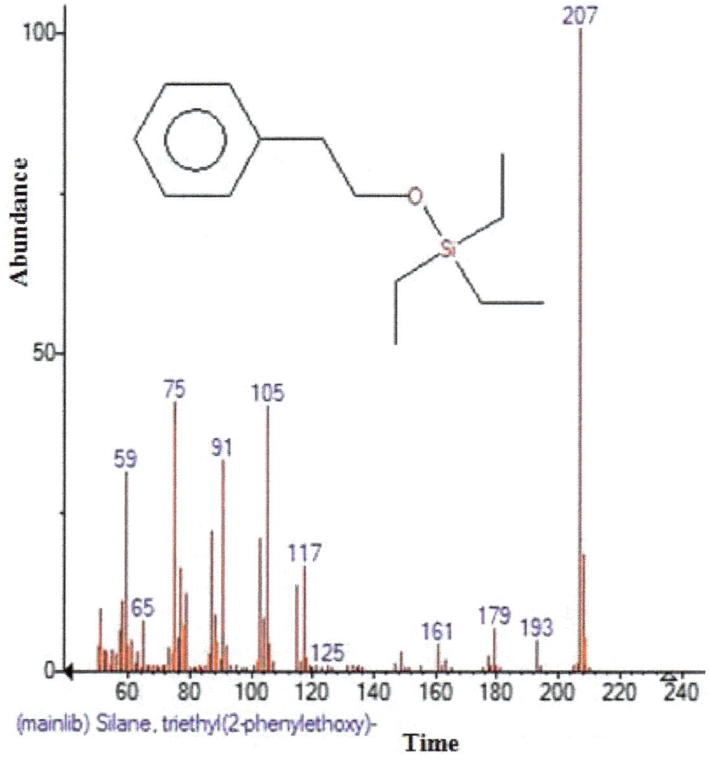

Figure 5. Mass spectrum of Silane, triethyl(2-phenylethoxy) with retention time (RT)= 4.975.

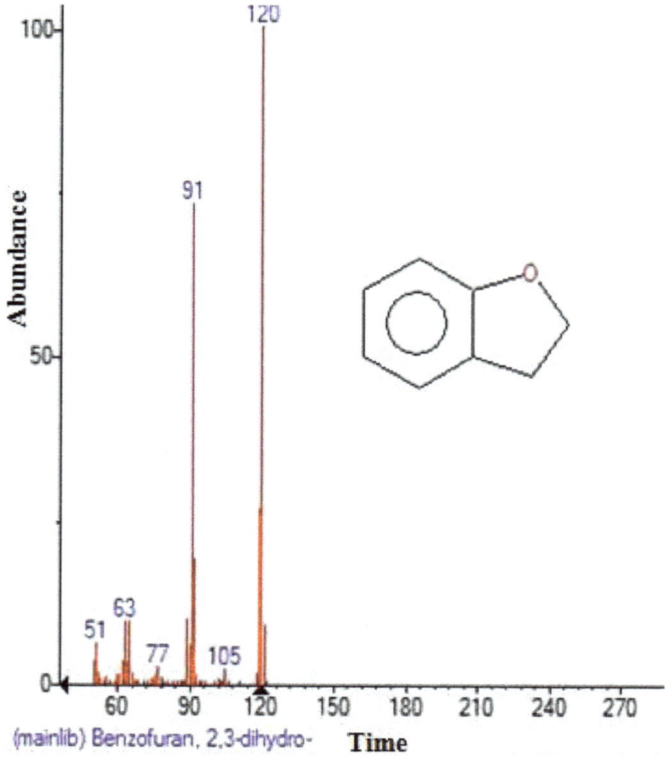

Figure 6. Mass spectrum of Benzofuran, 2,3,-dihydro with retention time (RT)= 6.777.

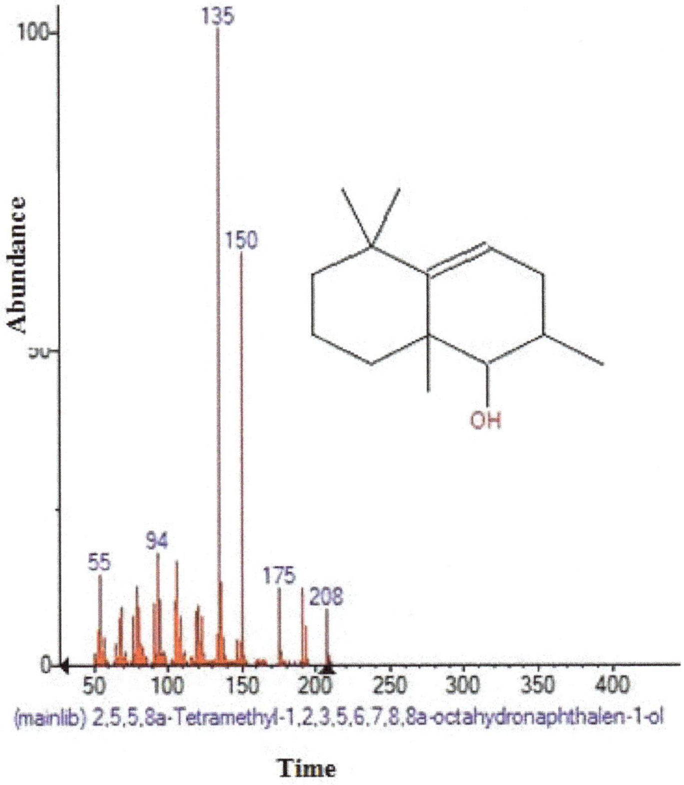

Figure 7. Mass spectrum of 2,5,5,8a-Tetramethyl-1,2,3,5,6,7,8, 8a-octahydronaphthalen-1-ol with retention time (RT)= 7.939.

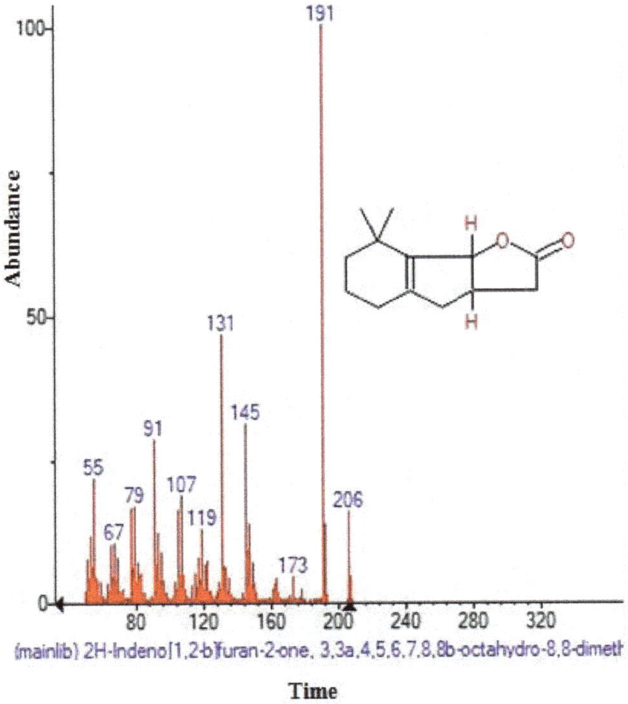

Figure 8. Mass spectrum of 2H-Indeno[1,2-b]furan-2-one, 3,3a, 4,5,6,7,8, 8b-octahydro-8,8-dimet with retention time (RT)= 8.992.

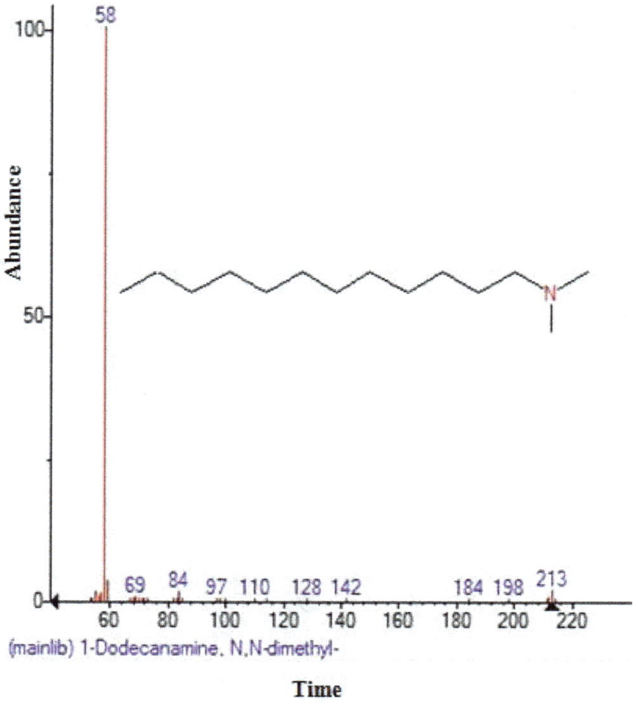

Figure 9. Mass spectrum of 1-Dodecanamine, N, N-dimethyl with retention time (RT)= 10.228.

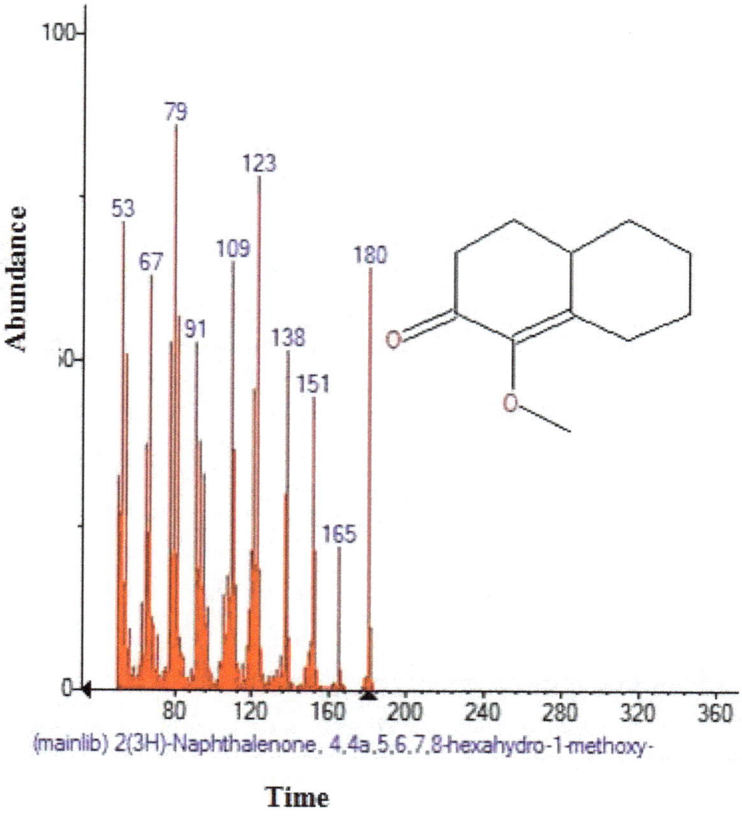

Figure 10. Mass spectrum of 2(3H)-Naphthalenone, 4, 4a,5,6,7,8-hexahydro-1-methoxy with retention time (RT)= 11.029.

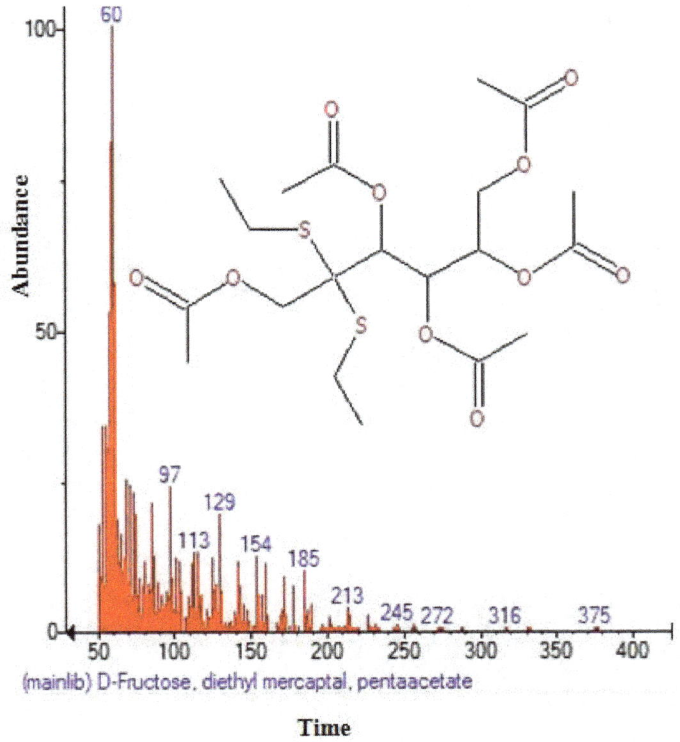

Figure 11. Mass spectrum of D-Fructose, diethyl mercaptal, pentaacetate with retention time (RT)= 13.243.

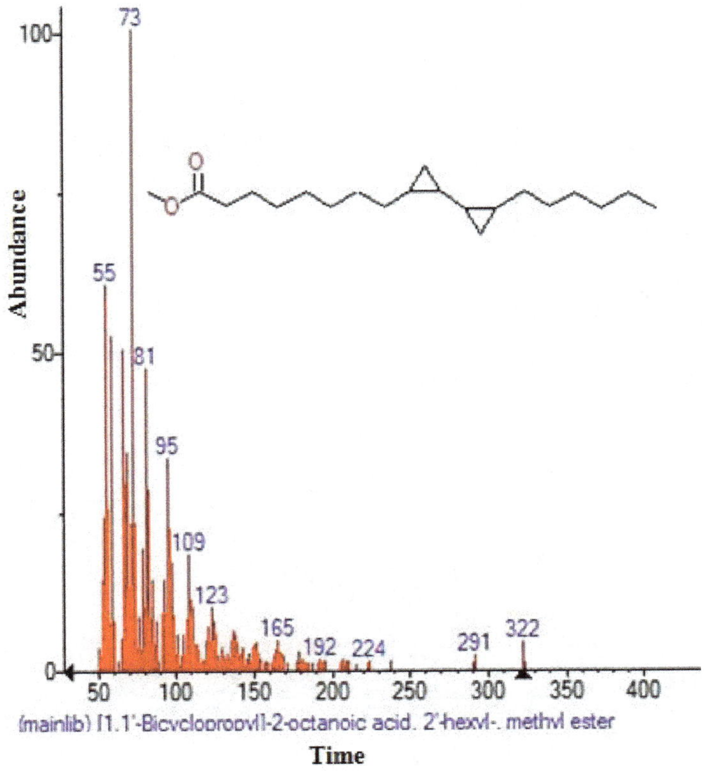

Figure 12. Mass spectrum of [1,1-Bicyclopropyl-2-octanoic acid 2hexyl-methyl ester with retention time (RT)= 13.501.

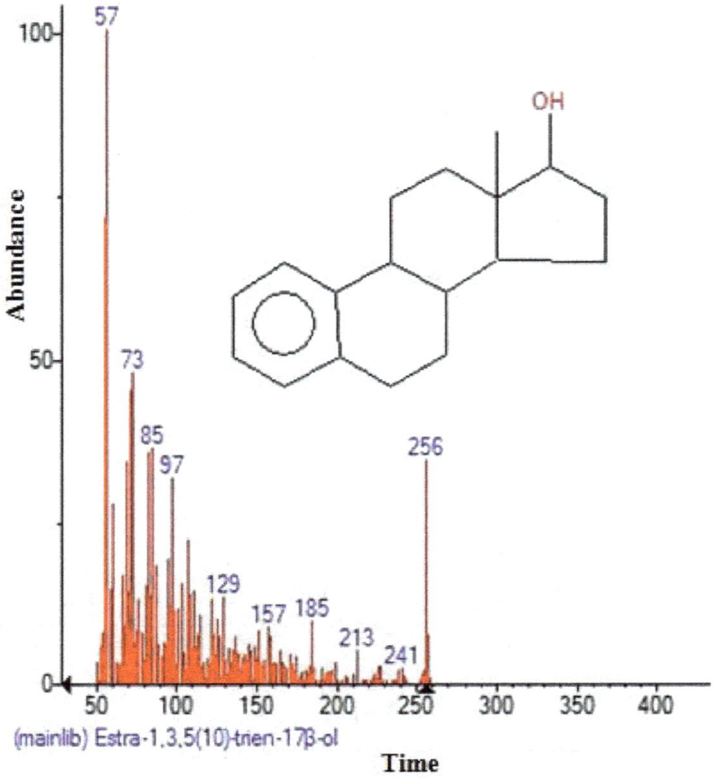

Figure 13. Mass spectrum of Estra-1,3,5(10)-trien-17B-ol with retention time (RT)= 15.561.

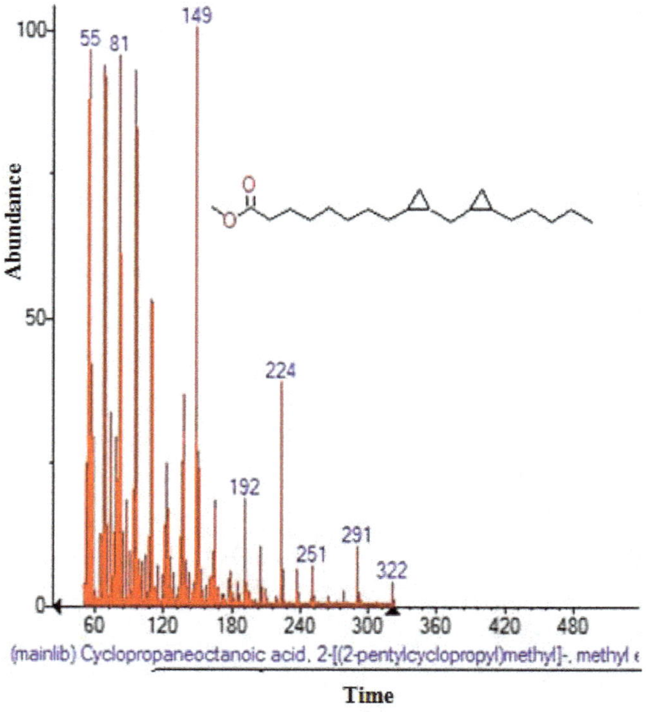

Figure 14. Mass spectrum of cyclopropaneoctanoic acid, 2-[2-pentylcycloproyl)methyl]-methyl with retention time (RT)= 20.327.

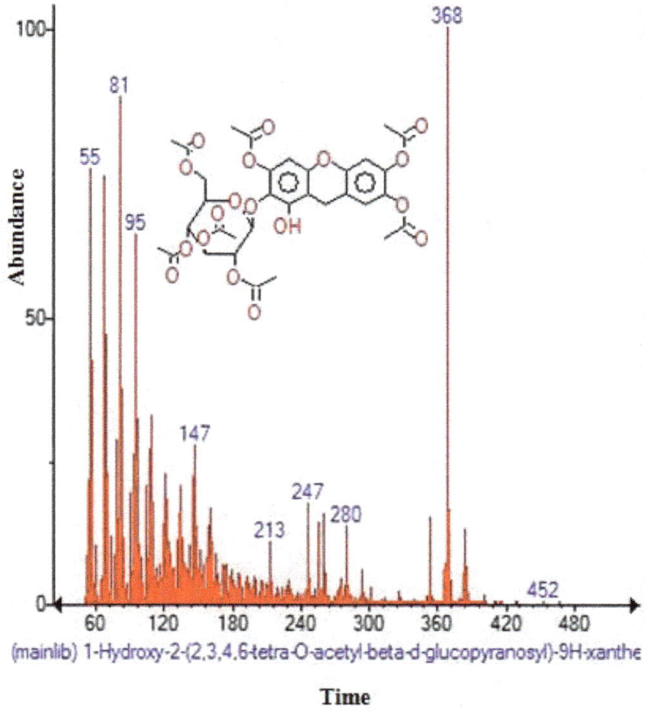

Figure 15. Mass spectrum of 1-Hydroxy-2-(2,3,4,6-tetra-O-acetyl-beta-d-glucopyranosyl)-9H-xanthe with retention time (RT)= 20.585.

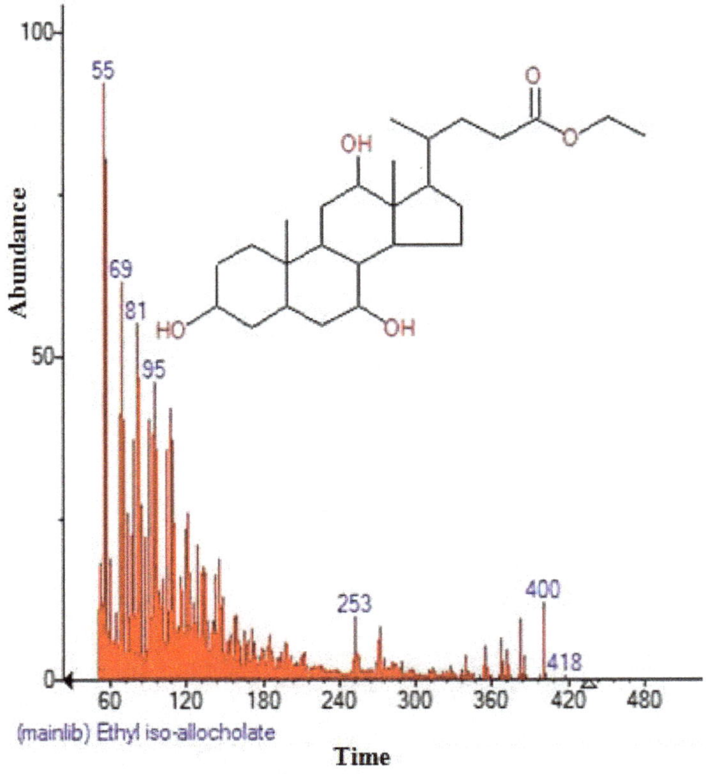

Figure 16. Mass spectrum of Ethyl iso- allochlate with retention time (RT)= 25.277.

Table 1. Major phytochemical compounds identified in methanolic leaves extract of *Urtica dioica*.

S/N	Phytochemical compound	RT(min)	Formula	Molecular weight	Exact mass	Chemical structure	MS Fragment- ions	Pharmacological actions
1.	Oxime- methoxy-phenyl	3.504	$C_8H_9NO_2$	151	151.063329	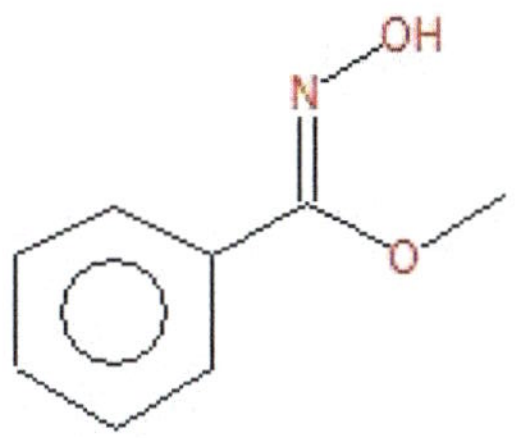	55,68,73,81,91,105,121,133,151	Antioxidant and antimicrobial activity
2.	2, 6,-Nonadienal, 3, 7-dimethyl	3.739	$C_{11}H_{18}O$	166	166.13576	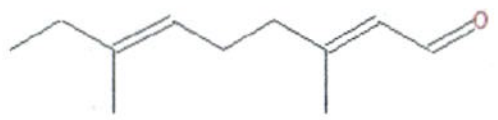	55,67,83,94,109,137,151	Anti-inflammatory and antioxidant activity
3.	1, 2, 3-Butanetriol	4.380	$C_4H_{10}O_3$	106	106.062994	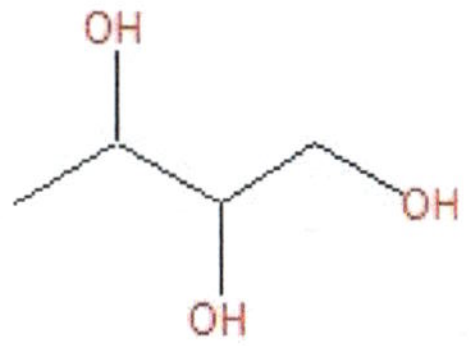	57,75,88,103	Wide range of biological properties including antitumor activity
4.	Silane, triethyl(2-phenylethoxy)	4.975	$C_{14}H_{24}OSi$	236	236.159642	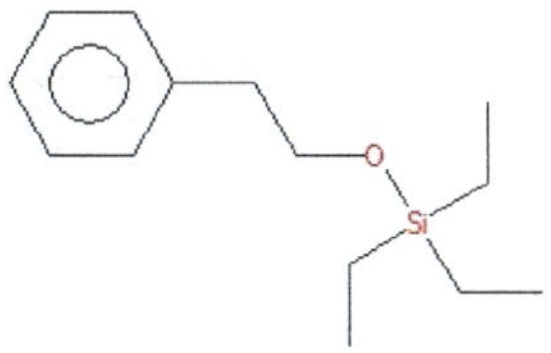	59,65,75,91,105,117,125,161,179,193	Biocontrol
5.	Benzofuran, 2,3,-dihydro	6.777	C_8H_8O	120	120.057514	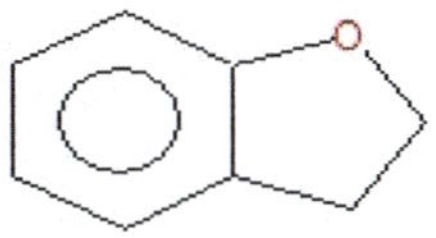	51,63,77,91,105,120	Antiarrhytmic, spasmolitic, antiviral

Table 1. Condt.

6.	2,5,5,8a-Tetramethyl-1,2,3,5,6,7,8, 8a-octahydronaphthalen-1-ol	7.939	$C_{14}H_{44}O$	208	208.182715	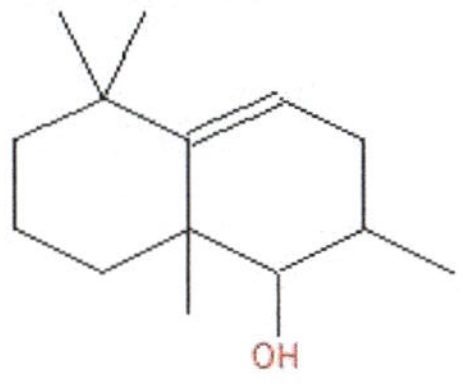	55,94,135,150,175,208	Pharmacological action of this product is unknown
7.	2H-Indeno[1,2-b]furan-2-one, 3,3a, 4,5,6,7,8, 8b-octahydro-8,8-dimet	8.992	$C_{13}H_{18}O_2$	206	206.13068	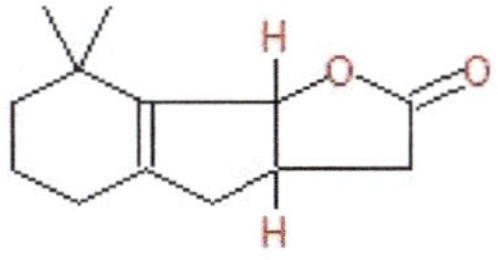	55,67,79,91,107,119,131,145,17 3,191,106	New chemical compound
8.	1-Dodecanamine, N, N-dimethyl	10.228	$C_{14}H_{31}N$	213	213.24565	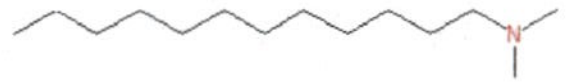	58,69,84,97,110,128,142,184,19 8,213	Anti-Staphylococcal Activity
9.	2(3H)-Naphthalenone, 4, 4a,5,6,7,8-hexahydro-1-methoxy	11.029	$C_{11}H_{16}O_2$	180	180.115029	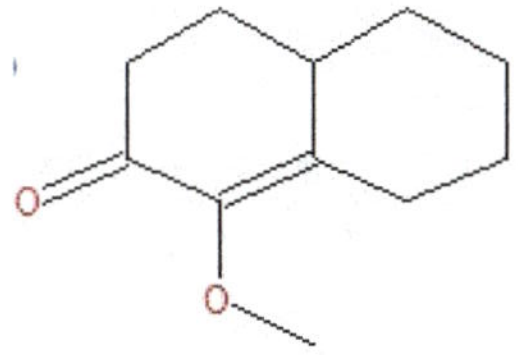	53,67,79,91,109,123,138,151,16 5,180	Pharmacological action of this product is unknown
10.	D-Fructose, diethyl mercaptal, pentaacetate	13.243	$_{20}H_{32}O_{10}S_2$	496	496.14369	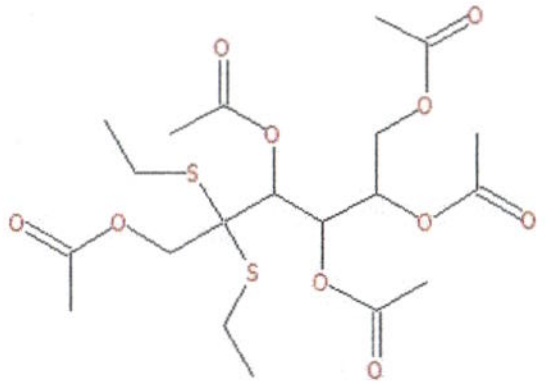	60,97,113,129,154,185,213,245, 272,316,375	Antitumor and antibacterial activity
11.	[1,1-Bicyclopropyl-2-octanoic acid 2hexyl-methyl ester	13.501	$C_{21}H_{38}O_2$	322	322.28718	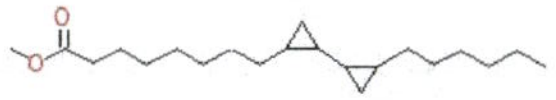	55,73,81,95,109,123,165,192,22 4,291,322	Anti-diabetic and anti-inflammatory and anti-inflammatory,

Table 1. Condt.

12.	Estra-1,3,5(10)-trien-17B-ol	15.561	$C_{18}H_{24}O$	256	256.18271	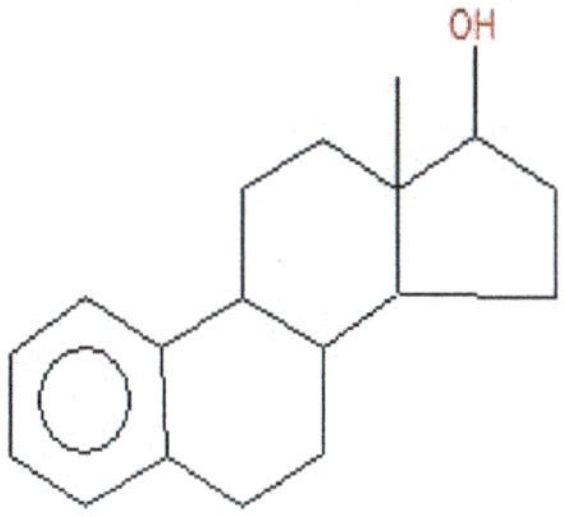	57,73,85,97,129,157,185,213,24 1,256	anti-proliferative effect
13.	Cyclopropaneoctanoic acid, 2-[2-pentylcycloproyl)methyl]-methyl	20.327	$C_{18}H_{20}O_3$	322	322.28718	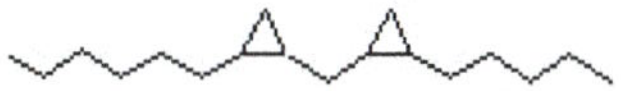	55,81,149,192,224,251,291,322	New chemical compound
14.	1-Hydroxy-2-(2,3,4,6-tetra-O-acetyl-beta-d-glucopyranosyl)-9H-xanthe	20.585	$C_{33}H_{34}O_{18}$	718	718.174515	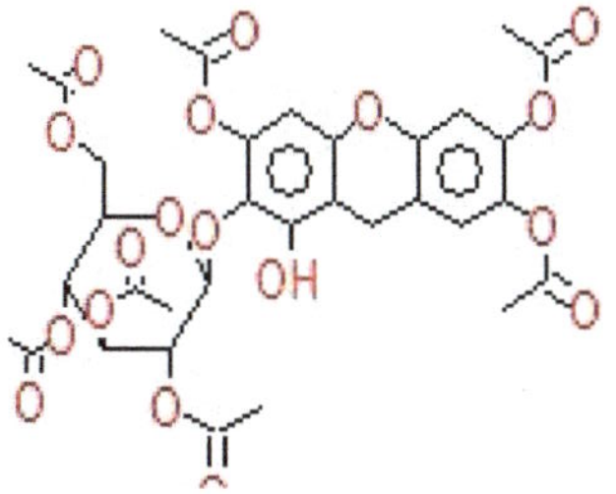	55,81,95,147,213,247,280,368,4 52	New chemical compound
15.	Ethyl iso- allochlate	25.277	$C_{26}H_{44}O_5$	436	436.31887	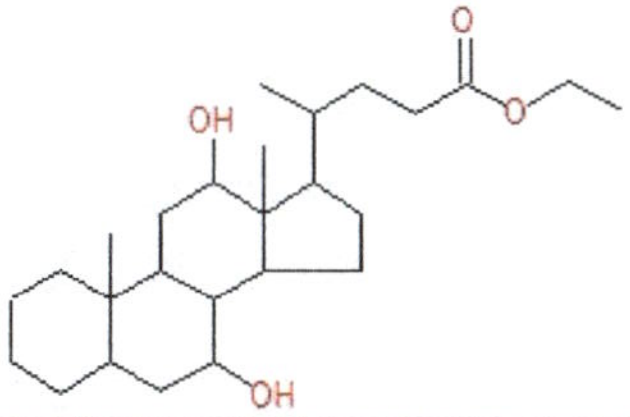	55,69,81,95,253,400	Antimicrobial. Antioxidant. Anti-inflammatory

Adeyemo, 2006). Among those identified, phytocompounds have the property of antioxidant and antimicrobial activities (Silva et al., 2004; Sein et al., 2008). Plant based antimicrobials have enormous therapeutic potential as they can serve the purpose with lesser side effects. Continued

Table 2. FT-IR peak values of *Urtica dioica* methanol leaf extract.

S/N	Peak (Wave number cm-¹)	Intensity	Bond	Functional group assignment	Group frequency
1.	891.11	74.304	C-H	Aromatic rings	690-900
2.	958.69	68.024	C-H	Alkenes	675-995
3.	1010.70	56.914	C-F stretch	Aliphatic fluoro compounds	1000-10150
4.	1091.71	61.891	C-F stretch	Aliphatic fluoro compounds	1000-10150
5.	1242.16	76.996	C-O	Alcohols, Ethers, Carboxlic acids, Esters	1050-1300
6.	1319.31	73.166	NO2	Nitro Compounds	1300-1370
7.	1338.60	71.524	NO2	Nitro Compounds	1300-1370
8.	1361.74	71.150	NO2	Nitro Compounds	1300-1370
9.	1373.32	70.723	C-H	Alkenes	1340-1470
10.	1539.20	73.241	NO2	Nitro Compounds	1500-1570
11.	1595.13	71.600	C-C	Aromatic rings	1500-1600
12.	2306.86	90.993	-	Unknown	-
13.	2686.84	89.928	O-H	Hydrogen bonded Carboxylic acids	2500-2700
14.	2752.42	89.287	-	Unknown	-
15.	2848.86	82.640	-	Unknown	-
16.	2918.30	79.097	C-H	Alkanes	2850-2970
17.	3064.89	84.666	H-O	H-bonded H-X group	2500-3500
18.	3182.55	81.242	H-O	H-bonded H-X group	2500-3500
19.	3246.20	80.081	O-H	Hydrogen bonded Alcohols, Phenols	3200-3600
20.	3273.20	79.592	O-H	Hydrogen bonded Alcohols, Phenols	3200-3600
21.	3363.86	80.541	O-H	Hydrogen bonded Alcohols, Phenols	3200-3600

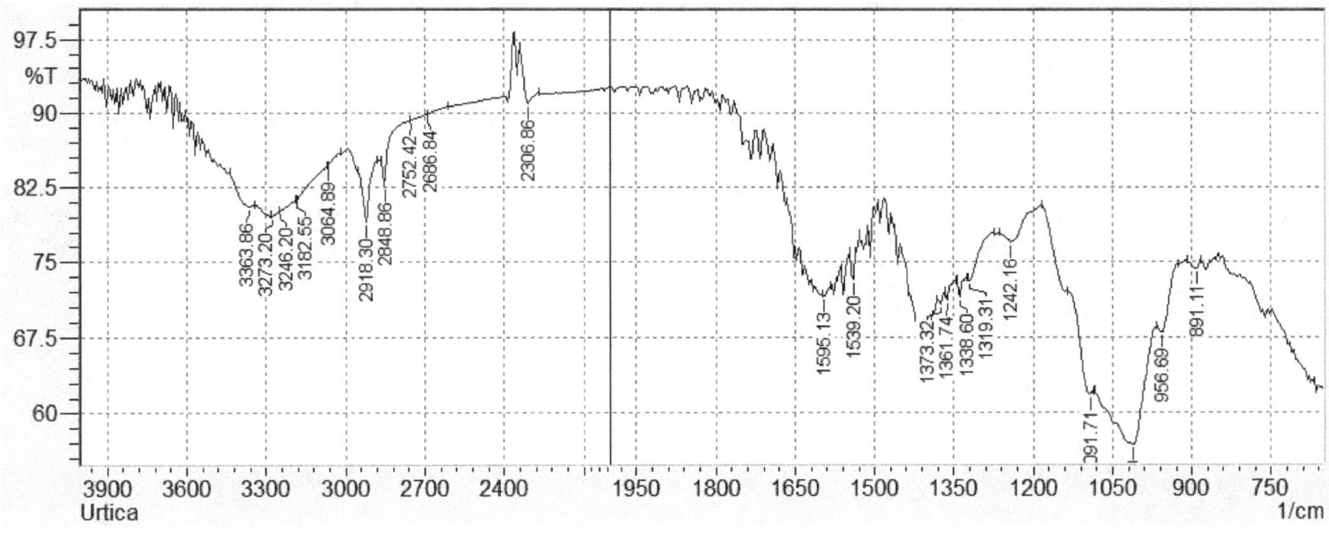

Figure 17. Fourier-transform infrared profile of leaves extract of *Urtica dioica*.

further exploration of plant derived antimicrobials is needed today.

Conclusion

U. dioica is native plant of Iraq. It contains chemical constitutions which may be useful for various herbal formulation as anti-inflammatory, analgesic, antipyretic, cardiac tonic and antiasthamatic properties.

ACKNOWLGEMENT

The authors wish to express their deepest gratitude to Prof. Dr. Adul-Kareem for his valuable contributions and support throughout this study. They would also like to express their gratitude to Dr. Ali for his valuable suggestions and comments.

REFERENCES

Altameme HJ, Hameed IH, Kareem MA (2015). Analysis of alkaloid phytochemical compounds in the ethanolic extract of *Datura stramonium* and evaluation of antimicrobial activity. Afr. J. Biotechnol.14(19):1668-1674.

Bandow JE, Brotz H, Leichert L (2003). Proteomic approach to understanding antibiotic action. Antimicrob. Agents Chemother. 47:948-955.

Banso A, Adeyemo S (2006). Phytochemical screening and antimicrobial assessment of Abutilon mauritianum, Bacopamonnifera and Daturastr-amonium. Biochemistry 18(1):39-44.

Belyakova VA, Vainshtein KV, Markova Y, Demchenko T, Chibilyaev TH (2002). Extraction of nettle leaves using synthetic esters of fatty acids. Pharm. Chem. J. 39(11):598-602.

Benkeblia N (2004). Antimicrobial activity of essential oil extracts of various onions (*Allium cepa*) and garlic (*Allium sativum*). Lebensm-Wiss u-Technol. 37:263-268.

Burt S (2004). Essentials oils: their antibacterial properties and potential applications in food: a review. Int. J. Food Microbiol. 94:254-259.

Golalipour MJ, Ghafari S, Farsi MM (2009). Effect of *Urtica dioica* extract on quantitative morphometric alterations of liver paranchymal cells in STZ diabetic rats. Int. J. Morphol. 27(4):1339-1344.

Gozum S, Tezel A, Koc M (2003). Complementary alternative treatments used by patients with cancer in eastern Turkey. Cancer Nurs. 26:230–236

Gulcin I (2004). Antioxidant, antimicrobial, antiulcer and analgesic activities of nettle (*Urtica dioica* L.). J. Ethnopharmacol. 90:205-215.

Hai LR (2004). Potential Synergy of Phytochemicals in Cancer Prevention: Mechanism of Action. J. Nutr. 134:3479-3485.

Hameed IH, Hussein HJ, Kareem MA, Hamad NS (2015a). Identification of five newly described bioactive chemical compounds in methanolic extract of *Mentha viridis* by using gas chromatography-mass spectrometry (GC-MS). J. Pharmacogn. Phytother. 7(7):107-125.

Hameed IH, Ibraheam IA, Kadhim HJ (2015b). Gas chromatography mass spectrum and fourier-transform infrared spectroscopy analysis of methanolic extract of *Rosmarinus oficinalis* leaves. J. Pharmacogn. Phytother. 7 (6):90-106.

Hameed IH, Jasim H, Kareem MA, Hussein AO (2015c). Alkaloid constitution of Nerium oleander using gas chromatography-mass spectroscopy (GC-MS). J. Med. Plants Res. 9(9):326-334.

Harput S, Saracoglu I, Ogihara Y (2005). Stimulation of Lymphocyte Proliferation and Inhibition of Nitric Oxide Production by Aqueous *Urtica dioica* Extract U. Phytother. Res.19:346–348.

Hussein AO, Hameed IH, Jasim H, Kareem MA (2015). Determination of alkaloid compounds of *Ricinus communis* by using gas chromatography-mass spectroscopy (GC-MS). J. Med. Plants Res 9(10):349-359.

Imad H, Mohammed A, Aamera J (2014a). Genetic variation and DNA markers in forensic analysis. Afr. J. Biotechnol. 13(31):3122-3136.

Imad H, Mohammed A, Cheah Y, Aamera J (2014b) Genetic variation of twenty autosomal STR loci and evaluate the importance of these loci for forensic genetic purposes. Afr. J. Biotechnol. 13:1-9.

Imad H, Muhanned A, Aamera J, Cheah Y (2014c). Analysis of eleven Y-chromosomal STR markers in middle and south of Iraq. Afr. J. Biotechnol. 13(38):3860-3871.

Jasim H, Hussein AO, Hameed IH, Kareem MA (2015). Characterization of alkaloid constitution and evaluation of antimicrobial activity of *Solanum nigrum* using gas chromatography mass spectrometry (GC-MS). J. Pharmacogn. Phytother. 7(4):56-72.

Kanter M, Coskun O, Budancamanak M (2005). Hepatoprotective effects of Nigella sativa L. and *Urtica dioica* L. on lipid peroxidation, antioxidant enzyme systems and liver enzymes in carbon tetrachloride-treated rats. World J. Gastroenterol. 42:6684–6688.

Kareem MA, Hussein AO, Hameed IH (2015). Y-chromosome short tandem repeat, typing technology, locus information and allele frequency in different population: A review. Afr. J. Biotechnol. 14(27):2175-2178.

Kavalali G (2003). Hypoglycemic activity of *Urtica pilulifera* in streptozotocin-diabetic rats. J. Ethnopharmacol. 84(2-3):241-5.

Luo JR (2009). Paleophytochemical components from Miocene-Fossil wood of *Pinus griffithii*. J. Chin. Chem. Soc. 56(3):600-605.

Magee PJ, Rowland IR (2004). Phyto-oestrogens, their mechanism of action: current evidence for a role in breast and prostate cancer. Brit. J. Nutr. 91:513-531.

Mohammed A, Imad H (2013). Autosomal STR: From locus information to next generation sequencing technology. Res. J. Biotechnol. 8(10):92-105.

Obertreis B, Ruttkowski T, Teucher T, Behnke B (1996). Ex-vivo in-vitro inhibition of lipopolysaccharide stimulated tumor necrosis factor-alpha and interleukin-1 beta secretion in human whole blood by extractum *Urticae dioicae* foliorum. Arzneimittelforschung 46(9):936.

Petlevski R, Hadzija M, Slijepcević M, Juretić D, Petrik J (2003). Glutathione S-transferases and malondialdehyde in the liver of NOD mice on short-term treatment with plant mixture extract. Phytother. Res. 17(4):311-4.

Sein TT, Spurio R, Cecchini C, Cresci A (2008). Screening for microbial strains degrading glass fiber acrylic composite filters. Int. Biodeterior. Biodegrad. 63:901–905.

Silva BM, Andrade PB, Valentão P, Ferreres F, Seabra RM, Ferreira MA (2004). Quince (*Cydonia oblonga* Miller) fruit (pulp, peel, and seed) and jam: antioxidant activity. J. Agric. Food Chem. 52:4405–4712.

Phytochemical studies and thin layer chromatography of leaves and flower extracts of *Senna siamea lam* for possible biomedical applications

Ismail Adamu Hassan[1], Idris Abdullahi Nasiru[2]*, Amina Muhammed Malut[1], Ibrahim Abdulkadir S.[1] and Audu Sani Ali[1]

[1]Faculty of Pharmacy, University of Maiduguri, PMB 1069, Maiduguri, Nigeria.
[2]Department of Medical Microbiology, University of Abuja Teaching Hospital, PMB 228 Gwagwalada, Abuja Nigeria.

***Senna siamea* is a medium-size, evergreen plant which has been utilized as a source of food, medicine and other agricultural purposes in different communities. However, there is dearth of information in regard to its possible biomedicinal uses, especially in Nigeria. Thus the preliminary phytochemical analysis and thin layer chromatography (TLC) separation was done using methanol, n-hexane and ethyl acetate (1:3:1) as solvent system while iodine vapour as spotting agent. The phytochemical screening of methanol extracts of leaves revealed the presence of cardiac glycoside, flavonoid, saponin, alkaloid and tannins while chloroform extracts of leaves revealed saponin only. Ethyl acetate and petroleum ether extracts revealed absence of all these phytochemicals. The chloroform, ethyl acetate and petroleum ether extracts of flower revealed absence of saponin, flavonoids, tannins and alkaloids but with traces of saponin and anthraquinones. TLC separation showed nine (9) spots each of chloroform and ethyl acetates, six (6) spots of methanol, three (3) spots of petroleum ether from leaves extracts. While, three (3) spots each of ethyl acetate and methanol, six (6) spots of chloroform were identified for flower extracts. No water spot separated from both leaves and flower extracts. From our findings, it can be concluded that *S. siamea lam* contains some significant phytochemicals that can exhibit desired therapeutic activities such as hypoglycemia, anti-arrthymia and antimicrobial. However, there is the need to conduct further pharmaceutical analyses on test extracts in order to establish these biomedical applications.**

Key words: *Senna siemea,* thin layer chromatography, antimicrobial, phytochemical.

INTRODUCTION

Plants have been found to be the source of energy for the animal kingdom. In addition, plant can synthesize a large variety of chemical substances that are of physiological significance (Kretovich, 2005). The active phytochemical principles produced by plants include, alkaloids, phenolic, anthraquinones, flavonoids, phenols, saponins, steroid, tannins, terpenes etc (Namukobea et al., 2011).

Medicinal plants are those that contains one or more of its phytochemicals that can be used for the synthesis of useful therapeutic agents (Sofowora, 2000). The wide

*Corresponding author. E-mail: eedris888@yahoo.com.

range of medicinal plant parts like flowers, leaves, barks, stems, fruits, roots extracts are used as powerful raw drug possessing a variety of pharmacological activities (Momin et al., 2012). In the last two centuries, there have been serious investigations into the chemical and biological activities of plants and these have yielded compounds for the development of synthetic organic chemistry and the emergence of medicinal chemistry as a route for the discovery of more effective therapeutic agents (Roja and Rao, 2000).

Senna siamea is native to Southeast Asia from India, Sri Lanka, and Thailand to Indonesia, Burma, and Malaysia and forms part of the warm and wet tropical forests. The species has been introduced in Africa and America. *S. siamea* is effective in managing constipation association with a number of causes including surgery, childbirth and the use of narcotic pain relievers (Hill, 1992). It is used locally as antimalarial drugs especially when decocted (the leaves and bark) (Lose et al., 2000). In traditional medicine, the fruit is used to charm away intestinal worms and to prevent convulsion in children. The young fruits and leaves are also eaten as vegetables in Thailand. The flowers and young fruits are used as curries (Kiepe, 2001) and as an antimalarial (Otimenyin et al., 2010). The stem bark extract was reported to have analgesic and anti-inflammatory effects (Ntandu et al., 2010). Isolated compounds, emodu and lupeol from the ethyl acetate fraction of the stem bark of *S. siamea* were reported to be the active principles responsible for the antiplasmodial property with IC_{50} values of 5 µg/ml, respectively (Ajaiyeoba et al., 2008). Sub-chronic studies of the aqueous stem bark extract of the plant in rats did not show significant toxic effect after seven weeks of administration (Mohammed et al., 2012)

This study was designed to determine the phytochemical compositions as well as to perform thin layer chromatography separation of the leaves and flowers extracts of *S. siamea* in order to create awareness of its possible medicinal and nutritional values.

MATERIALS AND METHODS

These include the test plant (the fresh leaf and flower of *S. siamea*), beaker, conical flask, measuring cylinder (large and small), glass funnel, glass stirrer, cotton wool, spatula, bunsen burner, top mettler weighing balance, test tubes, stainless steel tray, thermostat water bath, oven, syringe and needle, aluminum foil paper, hand gloves, mortar and pestle, analytical weighing balance, test-tube holder, refrigerator, meter rule, sieves (No. 5), bottles, UV fluorescence analysis cabinet tripod stand, wire gauze, capillary tubes, retort stand, thin layer chromatography (TLC) paper, TLC tank, test tube rack, tiles and filter paper.

Reagent used

Dragendoff's reagent, methanol, chloroform, 1% aqueous hydrochloric acid, Mayer's reagent, sodium chloride solution, glacial acetic acid, concentrated sulphuric acid, 10% Ferric chloride solution, Molisch's reagent, Fehling's solution A and B, lead sub-acetate solution, 10% sodium hydroxide, 10% ferric chloride in 95% alcohol, Barfoed's reagent, 3,5 dinitro benzoic acid I, iodine solution, dilute hydrochloric acid, Wagner's reagent, concentrated hydrochloric acid, 3.2% ferric chloride in glacial acetic acid, 10% lead acetate, 10% tannic acid, 1% w/v picric acid, 5% sodium hydroxide, bromine water, potassium iodide solution, 3% hydrogen peroxide, 1 M sodium hydroxide , acetic anhydride.

Sterilization

All work surfaces were comprehensively disinfected with cotton wool soaked in antiseptic fluid to minimize contamination during work process.

Dry heat sterilization

An hot air oven was used to sterilize the conical flasks, forceps, office punch, wire loop and filter paper discs (wrapped in foil paper) and beaker at 160°C for 45 min.

Moist heat sterilization

All materials used in the course of this research project that are not sensitive to moist heat sterilization were adequately sterilized using autoclave and detergents. Materials such as glass wares, beakers and conical flasks etc. were properly washed with detergent and water so as to remove dirt and contaminants and were allowed to dry prior to usage. These materials were then sterilized in a portable laboratory autoclave at 121°C for 15 min.

Collection, authentication and processing of plant materials

The fresh leaves and flowers of *S. siamea* were collected from the botanical garden of University of Maiduguri. Plant materials were identified and authenticated by a taxonomist, Professor S. S. Sanusi of the Department of Biological Sciences, University of Maiduguri, Nigeria in respect with the description in published literatures (Dalziel, 1958; Keay et al., 1989). The plant materials were dried under shade at our Pharmaceutical Chemistry Laboratory for about four weeks and then made into powdered form, using mortar and pestle and then sieved.

Extraction

The method of extraction in this experiment was by maceration. The general process on a small scale, consist of placing the powdered plant material (250 g) of leave was soaked in 500 ml methanol while that of flower was soaked with different solvents that is water, petroleum ether, methanol, chloroform and ethyl acetate (in order of decreasing polarity) in 1 L capacity conical flasks stopper and kept for 48 h with intermittent shaking. The cold extracts thus obtained were filtered with Whatman No. 1 filter paper into different conical flask and allowed to dry at room temperature under normal atmospheric pressure. 50 g of the powdered leaves were soaked in 100 ml distilled water and the extract was obtained using the aforementioned method.

Phytochemical analysis

Phytochemical analysis for the qualitative detection of alkaloids, anthraquinone, carbohydrates, flavonoids, tannins and saponins

Table 1. Leaves extraction results.

Parameter	Methanol	Chloroform	Ethyl acetate
Volume of solvent used (ml)	500	500	500
Weight of dried powdered (g)	200	200	200
Weight of solvent extract (g)	53.5	4.3	5
Extractive value (%)	26.8	2.15	2

Table 2. Leaves methanol extract partitioned

Parameter	Methanol/Water	Chloroform	Ethyl acetate	Petroleum ether
Volume of solvent used for partitioning (ml)	150	150	150	150
Weight of partitioned solvent extract (g)	47.6	18.8	9.9	20.8

was carried out on the extracts as described by Trease and Evans (2010), Sofowora (1993) and Harbone (1973).

Thin layer chromatography (TLC)

Commercially available standard TLC plate was used with standard particle size range to improve reproducibility. The absorbent silica gel coated on an aluminum foil of 22 cm length, 11.5 cm breadth and 0.3 cm thick plate for leaves while 22 cm length, 11.9 cm breadth and 0.3 cm thick plate for flower. Small spot of the solution containing the sample was applied on the plate 1.5 cm from the bottom marked by a line ruled using a pin. For a multiple spotted plate, the spots are applied 1 cm apart to avoid cross contamination and interference as they move up the plate.

Spotting and development

The sample spotted on the plate was allowed to dry before the plate was placed into the chromatographic tank which was covered immediately after which its atmosphere is completely saturated with solvent (mobile phase). The reaction was then monitored as the solvent moved up the plate (elutes the sample) using mobile phase solvent ratio 1:3:1 of methanol, n-hexane and ethyl acetate, respectively. When the solvent reaches the top of the plate, it is removed, marked and dried.

Visualization

Following separation of the solvent, the plate was removed and dried; the spots detected using various techniques and reagents. This includes visualization in daylight; viewing under UV at 254 and 366 nm i.e. short and long wavelengths and spraying with spotting reagent, using iodine vapor tank.

Findings

The phytochemical screening of methanol extracts of leaves revealed the presence of cardiac glycoside, flavonoid, saponin, alkaloid and tannins while chloroform extracts of leaves revealed saponin only. Ethyl acetate and petroleum ether extracts revealed absence of all these phytochemicals. The chloroform, ethyl acetate and petroleum ether extracts of flower revealed absence of saponin, flavonoids, tannins and alkaloids but with traces of saponin. Anthraquinones glycosides was absent in all the extracts.

Extraction process for leaves and flowers

This is seen in Tables 1 and 2.

Extractive value = weight of plant (part) extract/weight of dry powdered sample × 100

Volume of methanol used = 1 L.
Weight of dried powdered = 300 g.
Weight of methanol extract = 101 g.
Extractive value = 101/300 × 100 = 33.7%

Phytochemical screening results

This is seen in Tables 3 to 9.

Thin layer chromatography (TLC)

Extracts of leaves and flowers were individually applied on the origin, they dissolved and moved with the solvent, each extract separated into bio constituents and moved to different locations. After all the spots became clear. UV fluorescence lamp at 254 nm was used to visualize and identify all the various spots. However, at 366 nm and daylight, spots were not clearly visualized. On exposure to iodine vapour, spots of various extracts became darker. TLC separation showed nine (9) spots each of chloroform and ethyl acetates, six (6) spots of methanol, three (3) spots of petroleum ether from leaves extracts. While, three (3) spots each of ethyl acetate and methanol, six (6) spots of chloroform were identified for flower extracts. No water spot separated from both leaves and flower extracts.

Summary of TLC results

Leaves TLC

Length of the plate = 22 cm.
Breath of the plate =11.5 cm.
Thickness of the plate = 0.1 cm.

Table 3. Test for carbohydrate.

Tests	Extracts	Solvents used				
		Water	Methanol	Chloroform	Ethyl acetate	Petroleum ether
Molisches test (for carbohydrate)	leaves	++	++	-	++	+
	flowers	++	++	+	+	
Iodine test (for starch)	leaves	-	+	++	+	-
	flowers	-	+	++	+	
Fehling's test (for reducing sugar)	leaves	-	++	+	+	+
	flower	-	++	-	++	
Combined reducing sugar test	leaves	-	+	++	++	+
	flowers	+	++	-	+	
Barfoed test (for monosaccharides)	leaves	-	-	-	-	-
	flowers	-	-	-	-	-

++ More abundance, + Abundance, - Absence

Table 4. Tests for tannins (hydrolysable and condensed).

Tests	Extracts	Solvents used				
		Water	Methanol	Chloroform	Ethyl acetate	Petroleum ether
Lead sub- acetate test	Leaves	+	++	-	++	-
	Flowers	+	++	-	-	-
Ferric chloride test	Leaves	++	+	-	+	-
	Flowers	++	+	-	+	-
Bromine water test	Leaves	-	-	-	-	-
	Flower	-	-	-	-	-

++ More abundance, + Abundance, - Absence

Solvent front of the plate = 18.3 cm.
R_f value = distance move by the solute ÷ distance move by the solvent.

Tables 10 to 13 shows the TLC results of leaves.

Flowers TLC

Length of the plate = 22 cm.
Breath of the plate = 11.9 cm.
Thickness of the plate = 0.1 cm.
Solvent front of the plate = 17.9 cm.
R_f value = distance move by the solute ÷ distance move by the solvent.

Tables 14 to 16 shows TLC results of flowers.

DISCUSSION

S. siamea plants grow virtually everywhere in Nigeria and Maiduguri in particular. The plant has been used in this region for the treatment of typhoid fever and fever related conditions. Traditionally, it has also been used for treatment of jaundice, abdominal pain, menstrual pain, and hypoglycemic agent among diabetics. Ethno medicinally, *S. siamea* is used as laxative, blood cleaning agent, cure for digestive system and genitourinary

Table 5. Tests for anthraquinones glycosides.

Tests	Extracts	Solvents used				
		Water	Methanol	Chloroform	Ethyl acetate	Petroleum ether
Borntrager's Test	Leaves	-	-	-	-	-
	Flowers	-	-	-	-	-

++ More abundance, + Abundance, - Absence

Table 6. Tests for cardiac glycosides.

Tests	Extracts	Solvents used				
		Water	Methanol	Chloroform	Ethyl acetate	Petroleum ether
Burchard test (for glycosides steroids)	Leaves	-	-	-	+	++
	Flowers	-	-	-	+	-
Salkwoskii test (for steroidal nucleus)	Leaves	-	++	-	+	+
	Flowers	-	+	-	+	-
Keller killiani's test	leaves	++	+	-	-	++
	flower	++	-	+	+	-
Kedde test	leaves	-	-	-	-	-
	flowers	-	-	-	-	-

++ More abundance, + Abundance, - Absence

Table 7. Tests for Saponin.

Tests	Extracts	Solvents used				
		Water	Methanol	Chloroform	Ethyl acetate	Petroleum ether
Frothing test	Leaves	++	+	++	-	-
	Flowers	+	-	-	-	-
Haemolysis test	Leaves	+	+	+	-	-
	Flowers	+	+	-	-	-

++ More abundance, + Abundance, - Absence

disorders, herpes and rhinitis (Aliyu, 2006). When decocted, *S. siamea* leaves are locally used as anti-malaria drug (Lose et al., 2000). Previous studies on *S. siamea* extracts have confirmed some of the traditional uses: antiplasmodial activity (Gbeassor et al., 1990; Nsonde-Ntandou et al., 2005; Mbatchi et al., 2006). Antibacterial activities of the extract were tested against thirteen pathogenic bacteria and were compared with the standard antibiotic, kanamycin by measuring the zone of inhibition diameter and expressed in millimeter (mm) (Hailu et al., 2005; Dahiru et al., 2013).

Phytochemical screening reveals that methanolic extract contains carbohydrate, cardiac glycosides, saponins, flavonoids, tannins and alkaloids. The extracting solvent used are decreasing order of polarity in which each of them extract a number of solvent to their own polarity depending on the active metabolites the plant contained. Based on this experiment the alkaloid, tannins and saponins content of this can be responsible for its antibacterial activity (Dahiru et al., 2013)

Preliminary phytochemical analysis showed that leaf extracts of *S. siamae* possesses alkaloids, saponins, tannins and glycosides which is in support with studies done by Momin et al. (2012), Edeoga et al. (2005) and Bukar et al. (2009). Phytoconstituents such as saponins, phenolic compounds and glycosides when present in *S.*

Table 8. Tests for Flavonoids.

Tests	Extracts	Solvents used				
		Water	Methanol	Chloroform	Ethyl acetate	Petroleum ether
Shinoda's test	Leaves	-	+	-	-	-
	Flowers	-	+	-	-	
Ferric chloride test	Leaves	++	+	+	+	-
	Flowers	+	-	-	-	-
Lead acetate test	Leaves	+	++	-	-	-
	Flower	+	++	-	-	-
Sodium hydroxide test	Leaves	+	-	-	-	-
	Flowers	+	-	-	-	-

++ More abundance, + Abundance, - Absence

Table 9. Tests for alkaloids.

Tests	Extracts	Solvents used				
		Water	Methanol	Chloroform	Ethyl acetate	Petroleum ether
Mayers reagent	Leaves	-	-	-	-	-
	Flowers	-	-	-	-	-
Dragendorff A × B	Leaves	-	-	-	-	-
	Flowers	-	-	-	-	
Wagners reagent	Leaves	+	+	-	-	-
	Flower	+	+	-	-	-
10% w/v tannic acid	Leaves	-	+	-	-	-
	Flowers	-	-	-	-	-
1% w/v picric acid	Leaves	-	+	+	-	+
	Flowers	-	+	-	-	-

++ More abundance, + Abundance, - Absence

Table 10. Leaves methanol extract TLC results.

Spots positions (cm)	R_f values (cm)	Day light	UV-254 nm	UV-366 nm	Iodine vapour
16.3	0.89	Green	Green	Blue black	Light Green
15.2	0.83	Green	Green	Blue black	Light Green
14.1	0.77	Light green	Light green	Blue black	Yellow
11.5	0.62	Light yellow	Light yellow	-	Yellow
10.8	0.59	Yellow	Light brown	-	White
9.3	0.50	White	White	-	Brown

- No colour

siamea have been reported to inhibit bacterial growth and to be protective to plants against bacterial and fungal infections (Gonzalel and Mather, 1982; Okwute, 1992). Cardiac glycosides have also been found useful in

Table 11. Leaves Chloroform extract TLC results.

Spots positions (cm)	R_f values (cm)	Day light	UV-254 nm	UV-366 nm	Iodine vapour
16.8	0.91	White	White	White	Yellow
16.1	0.87	Green	Violet	Blur black	Green
14.6	0.79	Green	Green	Blue black	Green
14.4	0.78	Light green	Green	-	Yellow
13.7	0.74	Light green	Light green	-	Yellow
13.5	0.73	Light brown	White	-	Yellow
11.9	0.65	White	Violet	-	Brown
10.8	0.59	Light brown	Light brown	-	Brown
9.8	0.53	Light yellow	Violet	-	Brown

- No colour

Table 12. Leaves ethyl acetate extract TLC results.

Spots positions (cm)	R_f values (cm)	Day light	UV-254 nm	UV-366 nm	Iodine vapour
15.9	0.86	Green	Light green	Blue black	Yellow
14.8	0.80	Green	Green	Blur black	Green
13.9	0.75	Light green	Green	Blue black	Green
13.1	0.71	Light green	Light brown	-	Yellow
11.3	0.61	Light green	Light brown	-	Yellow
10.5	0.57	Yellow	Light brown	-	Yellow
9.4	0.51	Brown	Brown	-	Yellow
8.7	0.47	Green	Brown	-	Brown
7.6	0.41	Light green	Violet	-	Brown

- No colour

Table 13. Leaves petroleum ether extract TLC results.

Spots positions (cm)	R_f values (cm)	Day light	UV-254 nm	UV-366 nm	Iodine vapour
16.3	0.89	Green	Green	Blue black	Green
15.0	0.81	Green	Green	-	Light green
14.6	0.79	Yellow	Violet	-	Yellow

- No colour

Table 14. Flowers methanol extract TLC results.

Spots positions (cm)	R_f values (cm)	Day light	UV-254 nm	UV-366 nm	Iodine vapour
11.9	0.66	Yellow	Violet	Blue black	Brown
10.8	0.60	Light brown	Brown	-	Brown
9.7	0.54	Yellow	Violet	-	brown

- No colour

treatment of heart failure and supraventricular arrhythmias (Zamotaev et al., 2005). The traditional uses indicate that both the leaves and flowers have been used together for therapeutic purposes. From this study, findings showed that the leaves have more phyto-chemicals than the flowers and since all active metabolites in the flowers are also present in the leaves, using leaves alone might suffice for treatments.

Presence of alkaloids, tannins, saponins, glycosides, steroids, phenolic compounds and flavonoids in all the

Table 15. Flowers chloroform extract TLC results.

Spots positions (cm)	R_f values (cm)	Day light	UV-254 nm	UV-366 nm	Iodine vapour
15.9	0.88	Green	Light green	White	Brown
15.5	0.86	Light green	Yellow	White	Brown
14.5	0.81	White	White	White	Brown
12.9	0.72	Yellow	Violet	White	Brown
11.9	0.66	Yellow	Violet	White	Brown
8.9	0.49	Light brown	Brown	White	brown

- No colour

Table 16. Flowers ethyl acetate extract TLC results.

Spots positions (cm)	R_f values (cm)	Day light	UV-254 nm	UV-366 nm	Iodine vapour
15.9	0.88	Light green	Green	-	Brown
15.5	0.86	Yellow	Yellow	-	Brown
14.6	0.81	Light yellow	Violet	-	brown

- No colour, Solvent system- methanol: n-hexane: ethyl acetate (20: 60: 20), Running time- 53 min, Adsorbent used- silica aluminum sheet, Locating reagent- Day light, UV 254 nm, UV 366 nm and iodine vapour

extracts confirmed the presence of rich bioactive principles in the leaf. Tannins, steroids and glycosides had been reported in ethanol extract of the leaf of *S. siamea* (Bukar et al., 2009; Muhammad et al., 2012) while alkaloids, saponins, phenolics and flavonoids by Momin et al. (2012). Secondary metabolites are mostly produced by plant during adverse condition for protection against herbivores (Chitra et al., 1999). Alkaloids, flavonoids, tannins and saponins were known to show medicinal activity as well as exhibiting physiological activity (Edeoga et al., 2005). The presence of phenolic group in plants is to protect them from microbial, insect and herbivores damage (Conco, 2000). Many of these active compounds also possess other functional attributes like anti-inflammatory, antimutagenic, hypocholestemic and antiplatelet aggregation properties (Praveena et al., 2012). These phytochemical compounds carry out their activity by combining with protein, lipids or other components of the bacterial cell membrane that are relevant to one or more vital physiological roles thereby disrupting the integrity and functional behaviour of the membrane (de Kruijff et al., 2000).

Conclusion

From our findings, it can be concluded that *S. siamea lam* contains some significant phytochemicals that can exhibit desired therapeutic activities such as hypoglycemia, anti-arrthymia and antimicrobial. However there is the need to conduct further pharmaceutical analyses on test extracts in order to establish these biomedical applications.

REFERENCES

Ajaiyeoba EO, JS Ashidi, Okpako LC, PJ Houghton, CW Wright (2008). Antiplasmodial compounds from Cassia siamea stem bark extract. Cassia siamea L. (Fabaceae). Phytother. Res. 22(2):254-255.

Aliyu BS (2006). West African Ethnomedicinal Plants. Triumph Publishing Company, Kano, Nigeria.

Bukar A, Mukhtarand MD, Hassan AS (2009). Phytochemical screening and antibacterial activity of leaf extracts of *Senna siamea* (lam) on *Pseudomonas aeruginos*". Bayero J. Pure Appl. Sci. 2(1):139-142.

Chitra S, Patil MB, Rav K (2009). Wound healing activity of Hyptissuaveolens (L) Poit (Laminiaceae). Int. J. Pharm. Tech. Res. 1: 737-744.

Conco WZ (1999). Zulu Traditional Medicine, its role in modern society. Comm. Health 5: 8-13.

Dahiru D, Malgwi AR, Sambo HS (2013). Growth Inhibitory Effect of Senna siamea Leaf Extracts on Selected Microorganisms. Am. J. Med. Med. Sci. 3(5):103-107.

Dalziel JM (1958). Flora of West Tropical Africa. Vol. I Part II, R. W. J. Keay (Ed.). Crown Agents, London pp. 485-503.

de Kruijff B, Cullis RP,Verkelij JA, Hope JM,Van Echteld AJC, Taraschi FT (2000). Lipid polymorphism and membrane function. Enzym of Biol Membranes. (Martonosi, A. N.,Ed.), 2nd ed. Plenum Press, New York pp. 131-204.

Edeoga HO, Okwu DE, Mbaebie BO (2005). Phytochemical consttituent of some Niger ian Medicinal plants. Afr. J. Biotechnol. 4(7):685-688.

Gbeassor M, Kedjagni AY, Koumaglo K, de Souza C, Agbo K, Aklikokou K, Amegbo KA (1990). *In vitro* Antimalarial Activity of Six Medicinal Plants. Phytother. Res. 4(3):115-117.

Gonzalel L, Mather S (1982). Identification of terpenoids from leaves of

Piptocarphaperitora and their biological activities. J. Nat. Prod. 45:495-496
Hailu T, Endris M, Kaleab A, Tsige G (2005). Antimicrobial activities of some selected traditional Ethiopian medicinal plants used in the treatment of skin disorder. J. Ethnopharmacol. 100:168-175.
Harbone JB (1973). Phytochemical methods. London, Chapman and Hall Ltd. pp 49-188
Hill AR (1992). Medicinal plants and tradition medicine in Africa. J. Int. Med. 39:42-45.
Keay RWJ (1989). Trees of Nigeria. Clarendon Press, Oxford. Medicine in Africa 2nd edition Spectrum Books Ltd, Sunshine House, Ibadan Nigeria pp. 81-93, 134-156.
Kiepe P (1995). Effects of Cassia siamea hedgerow barriers on soil physical properties. Geoderma 66:113-120.
Kretovich UL (2005). Principles of plant biochemistry permagon. Oxford Press. J. Food Sci. 54:254-260.
Lose GA, Bernard SJ, Leihner DE. (2000). Studies on agro forestry hedgerow system with Senna siamea rooting patterns and competition effects. J. Ethnopharmacol. 38, 57-60.
Mbatchi SF, Mbatchi B, Banzouzi JT, Bansimba T, Nsonde-Ntandou GF, Ouamba JM, Berry A, Benoit-Vica LF (2006). *In vitro* antiplasmodial activity of 18 plants used in Congo Br-azzaville traditional medicine. J. Ethnopharmacol. 104:168-174.
Mohammed A, Mada SB, Yakasai HM. (2012). Subchronic study of aqueous stem bark extract of Senna siamea in rats". Asian J. Biol. Sci. 5(6):314-321
Momin MAM, Bellah SF, Afrose A, Urmi KF, Rana MS (2012). Phytochemical Screening and Cytotoxicity Potential of Ethanolic Extracts of Senna siamea Leaves". J. Pharm. Sci. Res. 4(8):1817-1879.
Namukobea J, Kaseneneb JM, Kiremere BT In. Amukama M, Kamatenesi-Mugisha S, Krief V, Dumontet DJ, Kabasa JD (2011). Traditional plants used for medicinal purpose by local communities around northern sector of KiboleNational park, Uganda. J. Ethnopharmacol. 136:236-255.
Nsonde-Ntandou GF, Ndounga M, Ouamba JM, Gbeassor M, Etou-Ossibi A, Ntoumi F, Abena AA (2005). Ethnobotanical survey, chemical screening and effective treatment of certain plants used in traditional medicine to treat malaria in Brazzaville. Phytotherapia 1: 13-18.
Nsonde Ntandou GF, Banzouzi JT, Mbatchi B, Elion-Itou RD, Etou-Ossibi AW, Ramos S, Benoit-Vical F, Abena AA, Ouamba JM (2010). Analgesic andanti-inflammatory effects of Cassia siamea Lam. stem bark extract. J. Ethnopharmacol. 127:108-111.
Okwute SK (1992). Plant derived pesticidal and antimicrobial agents for use in Agriculture. A review of phytochemical and biological studies on some Nigerian plants. J. Agric. Sci. Technol. 2(1):62-70.
Otimenyin SO, Kolawole JA, Nwosu M (2010). Pharmacological basis for the use of the root of Senna siamea in traditional medicine. Int. J. Pharm. Biosci. 1:1-9.
Praveena B, Pradeep SN (2012). Antioxidant and Antibacterial Activities in the Leaf Extracts of Indian Borage (Plectranthusamboinicus). Food Nutr. Sci. 3:146-152.
Roja G, Rao PS (2000). Anticancer compound from tissue cultures of medicinal plant. J. Herbs Spices Med. Plants 7:71-102.
Sofowora A (1993). Medicinal plants and Traditional Medicines in Africa. Spectrum Books Ltd, Ibadan, Nigeria p 289
Sofowora A (2000). Phytochemical screening of Nigerian medicinal plants. J. Integr. Med. 41:234-246.
Trease GE, Evans MC (2008). A textbook of Pharmacognosy. BuillerTindall and Causel London 13th Edition 1978, pp 176-180.
Zamotaev IUN, Kremnev IUA, Podshibiakin SE (2005). Cardiac glycosides in complex treatment of patients with heart failure and supraventricular arrhythmias. Klin. Med. (83)7:59-63.

12

Design and optimisation of novel Huperzine A analogues capable of modulating the acetylcholinesterase receptor for the management of Alzheimer's disease

Sara Bonavia* and Claire Shoemake

Department of Pharmacy, University of Malta, Msida MSD 2080, Malta.

This is a *de novo* drug design study that aimed to create novel structures based on the alkaloid Huperzine A, capable of inhibiting the acetylcholinesterase (AChE) enzyme ligand binding pocket (AChE_LBP) for the management of Alzheimer's disease. The X-ray crystallographic model of the Torpedo Californica AChE complexed to Huperzine A was identified from the Protein Data Bank (PDB ID 1VOT). Molecular visualisation and modelling was carried out using SYBYL® 1.2, *in silico* predicted ligand binding affinity (LBA) was quantified using XSCORE_V1.3 and *de novo* drug design was carried out using LIGBUILDER®V1.2. Two seed structures were constructed in SYBYL® 1.2 according to a methodology that took into account the relationship between molecular structure and biological activity as described in the literature. Based on SAR data derived from Huperzine A, the points considered to be critical for binding were retained in each seed and planted into the AChE_LBP with growth being allowed according to defined parameters of LIGBUILDER®V1.2. The implication of this study consequently is that novel structures compliant to Lipinski's Rule of 5 may be promoted to second level drug design which could lead to identification of novel AChE inhibitors with better potency and a low side effect profile.

Key words: *de novo* drug design, Huperzine A, acetylcholinesterase, Alzheimer's disease, Lipinski's Rule of 5.

INTRODUCTION

Alzheimer's disease is the most common cause of dementia (Akhondzadeh and Abbasi, 2006) characterised by the build-up in the brain of protein rich plaques and leading to decreased cerebral nerve cell connectivity culminating in the death of nerve cells and loss of brain tissue (Wang et al., 2006a). It is also

*Corresponding author. E-mail: sbon121@gmail.com.

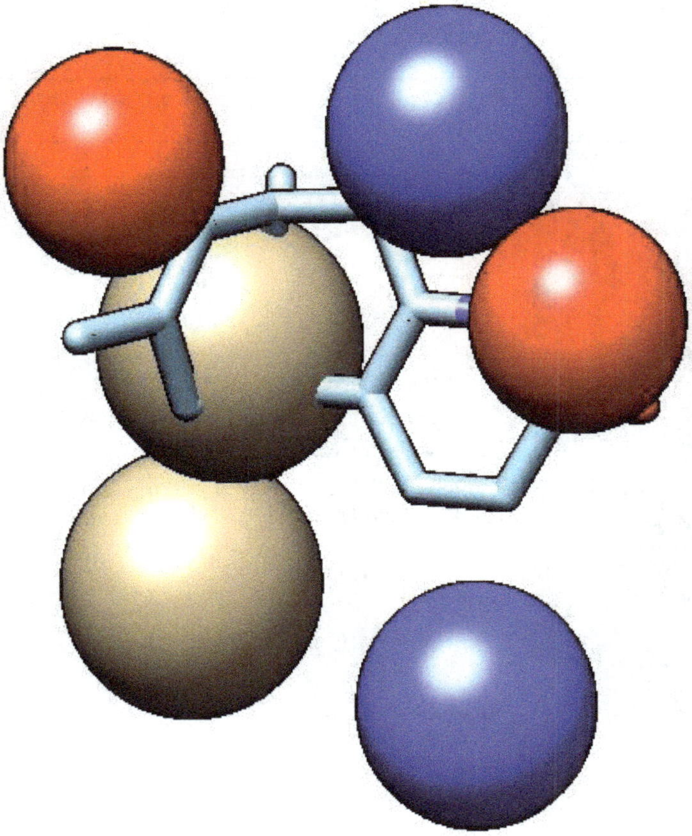

Figure 1. Huperzine A onto its pharmacophore shown in beads rendered in Chimera®v.1.7.

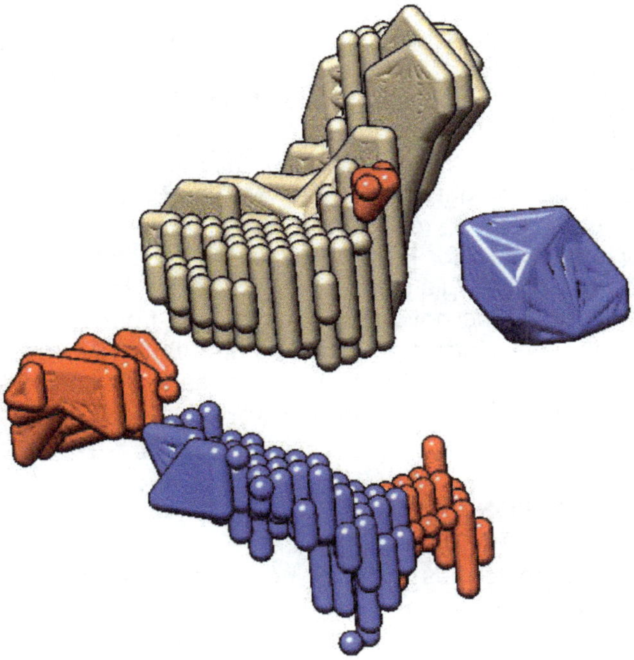

Figure 2. Huperzine A key interaction sites rendered in Chimera® v.1.7 based on the coordinates of PDB ID 1VOT (Raves et al., 1997).

associated with decreased acetylcholine (Ach) levels, due to the fact that this is broken down at a higher than average rate by the acetylcholinesterase (AChE).
This also contributes to incomplete transmission of nerve impulses (Picoulin, 2002).

The naturally occurring alkaloid Huperzine A has been shown to be a potent inhibitor of the transport of choline through cholinesterase inhibition consequently resulting in an increase in ACh. AChE inhibition also results in a slower rate of breakdown of acetylcholine and in nerve impulses of strength and duration consequently enhancing cerebral performance (Zangara, 2003).

In this study, an analysis of the binding modality of Huperzine A within the AChE Ligand Binding Pocket and the use of the Huperzine A scaffold to generate analog series of lead molecules for further optimisation using a static algorithm were reported.

METHODOLOGY

Molecular modelling

X-ray crystallographic deposition 1VOT describing the bound co-ordinates of the Torpedo Californica AChE bound to the nootropic alkaloid Huperzine A was identified from the Protein Data Bank and used as a template for this study (Raves et al., 1997).

Molecular modelling was carried out in Sybyl®-X, Ligand Binding Affinity (LBA) was quantified in X-Scorev1.2, and *de novo* ligand generation was carried out using LigBuilderv2.0. VMD® v.1.9 (Humphrey et al., 1996) and Chimera® v.1.7 were used for image generation.

Protein Data Bank crystallographic deposition 1VOT was then read into Sybyl®-X and all water molecules at a distance ≥5Å from the Ligand Binding Pocket were removed. The bound ligand, Huperzine A was extracted from the AChE Ligand Binding Pocket. The now *apo*-AChE and the extracted ligand were saved in PDB and *mol2* format, respectively.

Quantifying the binding affinity (p*K*d) of huperzine A for the AChE

The apo-AChE (saved in pdb format) and the extracted ligand (saved in mol2 format) were used as input files for X-Score®v1.2, which quantified, based on atomic interactions, the affinity(p*K*d) of the bioactive conformer of Huperzine A for its co-crystallised Ligand Binding Pocket (Wang et al., 1998). This procedure was considered as vital in the establishment of a baseline affinity against which that of the *de novo* generated Huperzine A analogs could be compared.

AChE ligand binding pocket mapping

The POCKET module of LIGBUILDER® v2.0 (Wang et al., 2000) was used to generate a pharmacophore and a 3-Dimensional map of the AChE Ligand Binding Pocket as circumscribed around the bioactive conformation of Huperzine A. Both the general pharmacophoric structure and the 3-Dimensional map of the AChE Ligand Binding Pocket were colour coded by atom type, with hydrogen bond donors and acceptors being coloured blue and red, respectively and with hydrophobic sites being coloured cyan. These are described in Figures 1 and 2, respectively.

The output file in each case was in pdb format and could be

Table 1. The 2-dimensional and 3-dimensional structure of Huperzine A as rendered in Symyx® Draw 4.0 and VMD®[1] v1.9, along with its predicted *in silico* ligand binding affinity to its cognate receptor 1VOT, as calculated in X-Score® v1.3.

2-Dimensional Structure	3-Dimensional Structure	Predicted *in silico* LBA within cognate receptor
	Huperzine A within 1VOT	
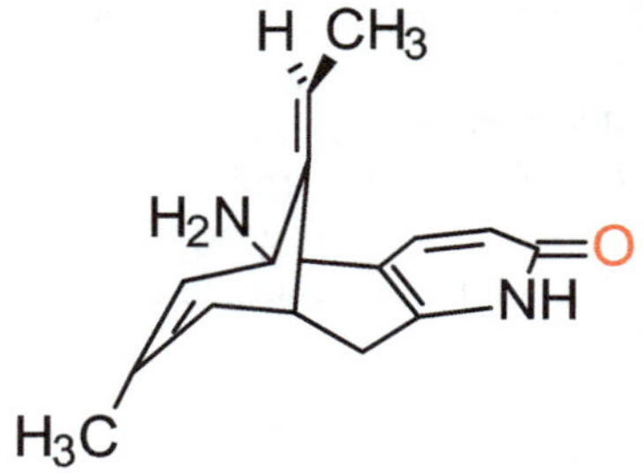 	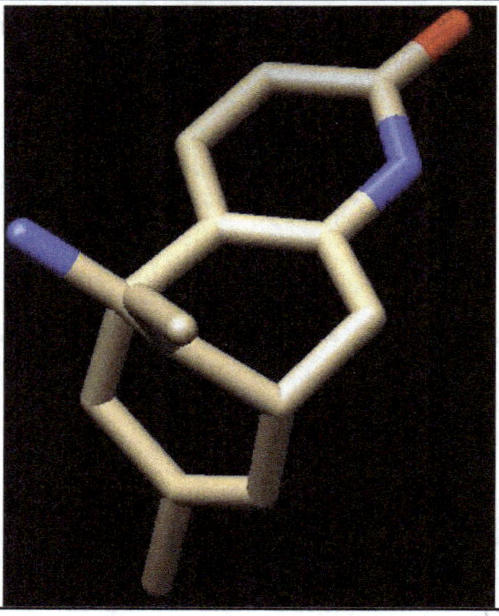	HPScore –log(Kd) = 6.41 HMScore –log(Kd) = 6.41 HSScore –log(Kd) = 6.54 Predicted average –log(Kd) = 6.45 Predicted binding energy = -8.80 kcal/mol

visualised in VMD® v.1.9 (Humphrey et al., 1996) and Chimera® v.1.7. This process was important because it established the pharmacophoric space available for de novo ligand construction, as well as the general pharmacophoric structure to which all the de novo generated ligands must necessarily comply for efficient binding.

Seed structure construction

A seed structure is essentially a molecular scaffold that is capable of sustaining molecular growth at user directed pre-designated growing sites. For this study, two seed structures were constructed in Sybyl®-X according to a methodology that took into account the relationship between molecular structure and biological activity as described in the literature. Seed A was created by removing the methyl group at the 15-position and the carbon group at the 14-position thereby opening the last ring of Huperzine A.

Seed B was created by removing the fused cyclic rings and retaining solely the aromatic ring bearing the carbonyl group and two methyl groups at the 6 and 12 positions. The carbonyl group was retained in both seeds because the pyridone oxygen forms a strong hydrogen bond with a protein residue of the ligand binding pocket. In Seed A, atoms 8 and 13 were designated as growing sites (*H.spc*) whereas in Seed B, atoms 6 and 12 were designated as growing sites (*H.spc*).

de Novo ligand design

The modelled seed structures were successively docked into the AChE Ligand Binding Pocket 3-Dimensional map, with which molecular growth was sustained according to the generic algorithm embedded in the GROW module of LigBuilder®V2.0.

The PROCESS module of LigBuilder®V2.0 was used to organise the de novo generated structured into families based on pharmacophoric similarity, and ranked in order of Ligand Binding Affinity (p*K*d).

RESULTS

The *in silico* LBA (p*K*d) of Huperzine A to its cognate receptor was predicted to be 6.45 as shown in Table 1. The algorithm embedded in the PROCESS module of LIGBUILDER®V2.0. This process resulted in 200 and 600 molecules to be generated from Seeds A and B, respectively. These *de novo* structures were divided into a number of families whose *in silico* affinity (p*K*d), molecular weight (Daltons/Da) and logP are displayed in Figures 3 to 8, respectively. Each molecular structure was assessed for Lipinski rule of 5 (predictors of *in vivo* bioavailability) rule compliance (Lipinski et al., 1997). The p*K*d for the *de novo* molecules ranged from 6.30 to 10, while molecular weight ranged from 300 to 526 and the LogP ranged from 3 to 5.99. A summary of all the values in each seed may be seen in Table 2.

DISCUSSION

All 15 molecules chosen from Seed A and all 45 molecules chosen from Seed B were Lipinski rule compliant. In an ideal scenario, the molecules with the highest LBA (p*K*d) would also have the lowest LBE (kcal mol^{-1}). The best molecule from the top 15 molecules chosen from Seed A is molecule number 6 having a p*K*d of 8.82 and a LBE of 126.999 kcal mol^{-1}. Moreover, the

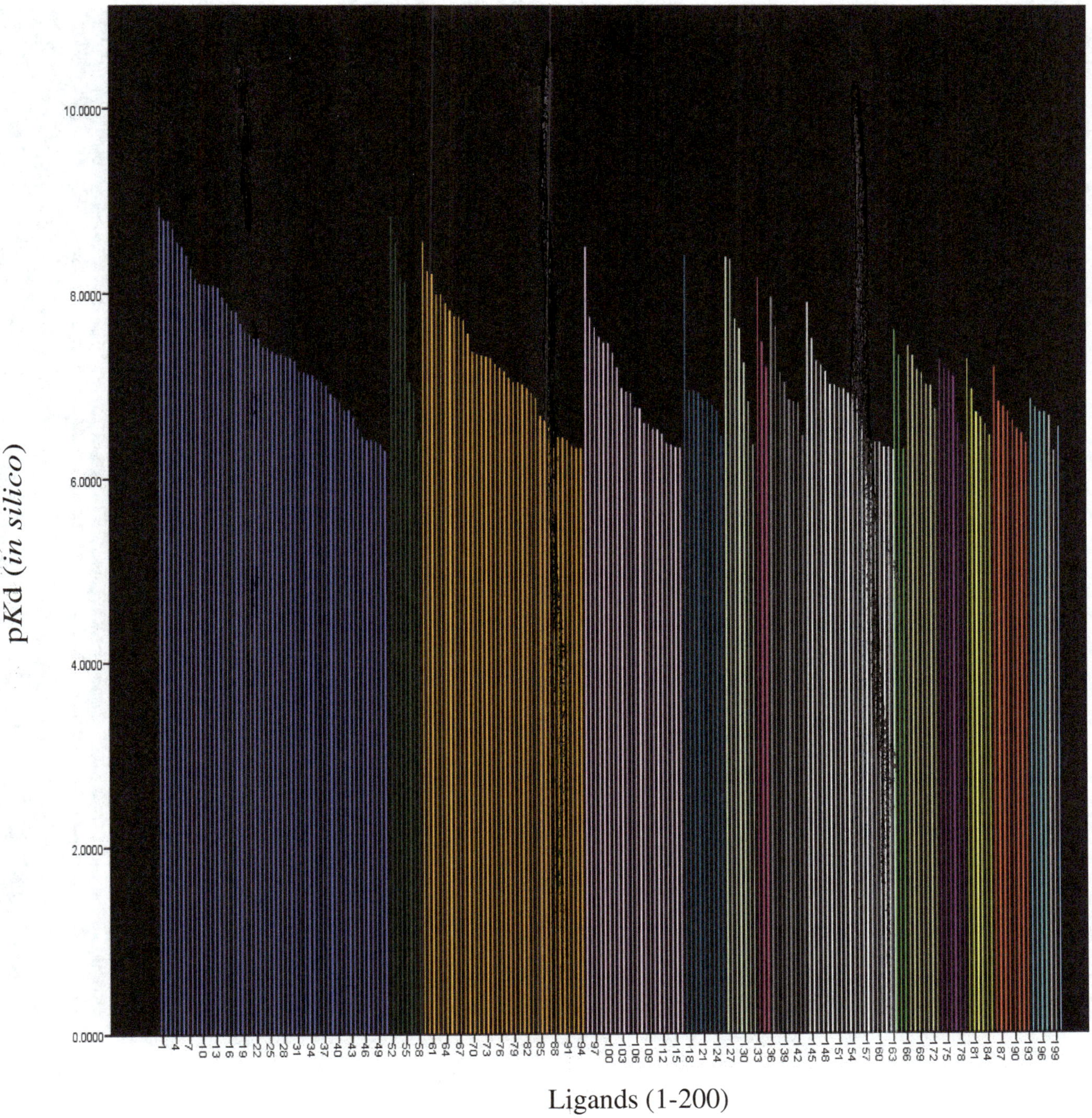

Figure 3. A graph showing the p*K*d (*in silico*) for the 200 *de novo* designed ligands from Seed A; the 17 different colours imply the 17 family series.

best molecule from the top 45 molecules chosen from Seed B is molecule number 3 having a p*K*d of 9.37 and a LBE of 45.796 kcal mol^{-1}. The binding poses of molecules 6 and 4 are superimposed onto the bound co-ordinates of Huperzine A as shown in Figures 9 and 10.

From this *de novo* study, the following relationships between structure and activity have been identified:

1) Ligands having two aromatic rings connected by an aliphatic chain have a high LBA (p*K*d) and a low LBE (kcal mol^{-1}). This was evident from molecules generated from Seed B.

2) Molecules with an aromatic ring directly attached to a pyridine ring bearing a negatively charged oxygen atom have been observed to have a lower LBA (p*K*d) and a higher LBE (kcal mol^{-1}). This was apparent from ligands generated from Seed A.

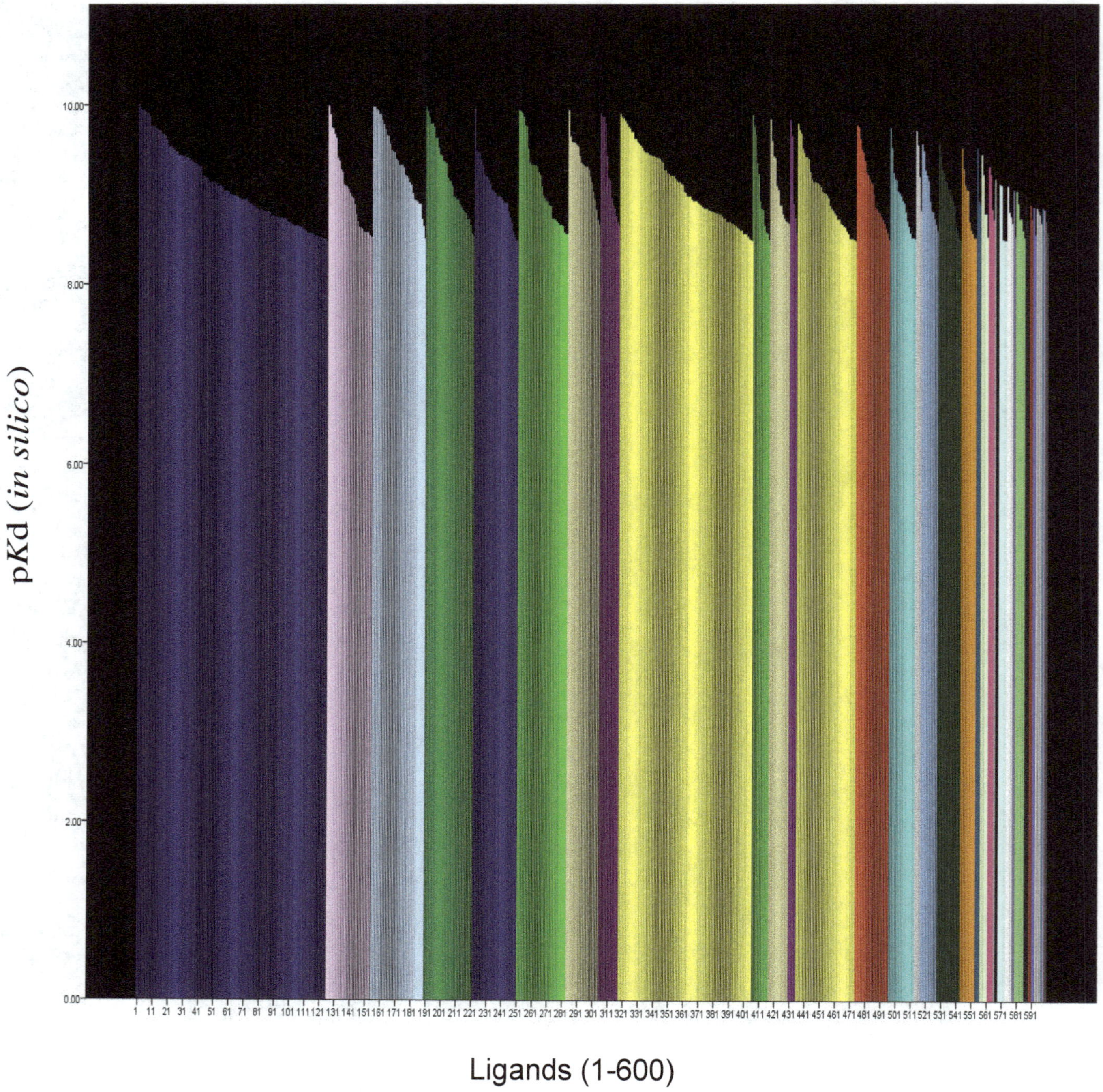

Figure 4. A graph showing the p*K*d (*in silico*) for the 600 *de novo* designed ligands from Seed B; the 35 different colours imply the 35 family series.

(3) Ligands with lateral branching ending in an acidic group (specifically the carboxyl group) from the pyridine bearing the carbonyl group have a higher LBA (p*K*d) than those which did not have an acidic group.
(4) Molecules having an aromatic ring linked to a pyridine bearing a negatively charged oxygen group exhibited a lower LBA (p*K*d) than molecules not having a negatively charged oxygen group connected to the pyridine ring.
(5) Ligands having an aromatic ring bearing a carboxylate anion had a higher LBA (p*K*d) than those without the carboxylate anion.

The implication of this study is that all the novel molecules sampled from both seeds which are also compliant to Lipinski's Rule of 5, are candidates for subsequent iterative rounds of rational drug design and *in vitro* validation.

The best two ligands identified from this study may be considered as viable leads for further optimisation studies. Comparative molecular dynamics studies could shed further light on the way that these ligands interact

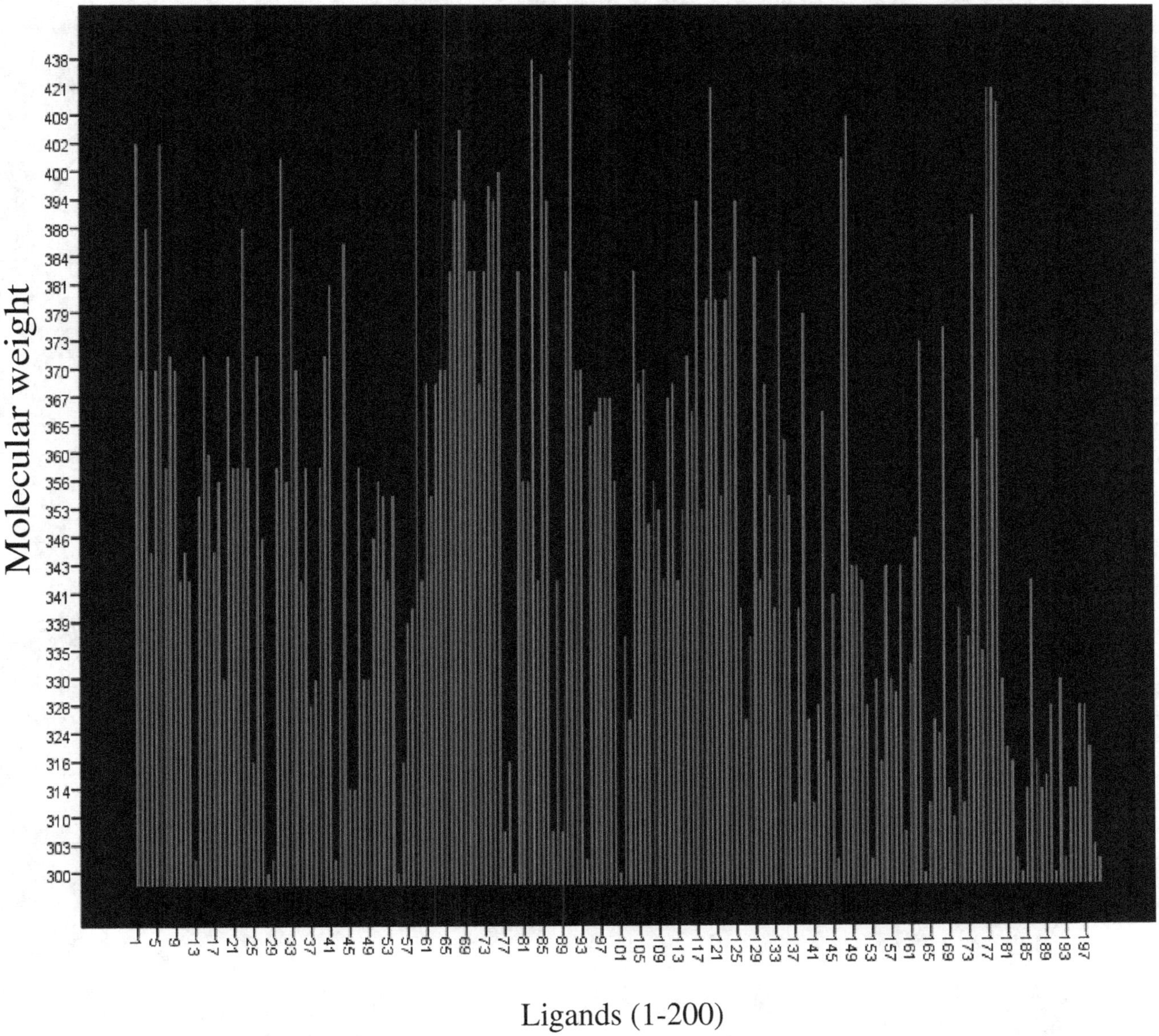

Figure 5. A graph showing the molecular weight for the 200 *de novo* designed ligands from Seed A. All ligands have a molecular weight of less than 500 and therefore are Lipinski rule of 5 compliant with respect to molecular weight only.

Table 2. Summary of important parameters of all the *de novo* molecules generated within LigBuilder® v2.0.

AChE_LBP	Seed A	Seed B
Total number of molecules	200	600
No. of families	17	35
Maximum number of molecules per family	51	125
Minimum number of molecules per family	1	1
Maximum p*K*d	8.92	10
Minimum p*K*d	6.30	8.47
Maximum molecular weight	438	526
Minimum molecular weight	300	326
Maximum LogP	5.43	5.99
Minimum LogP	3	3.01

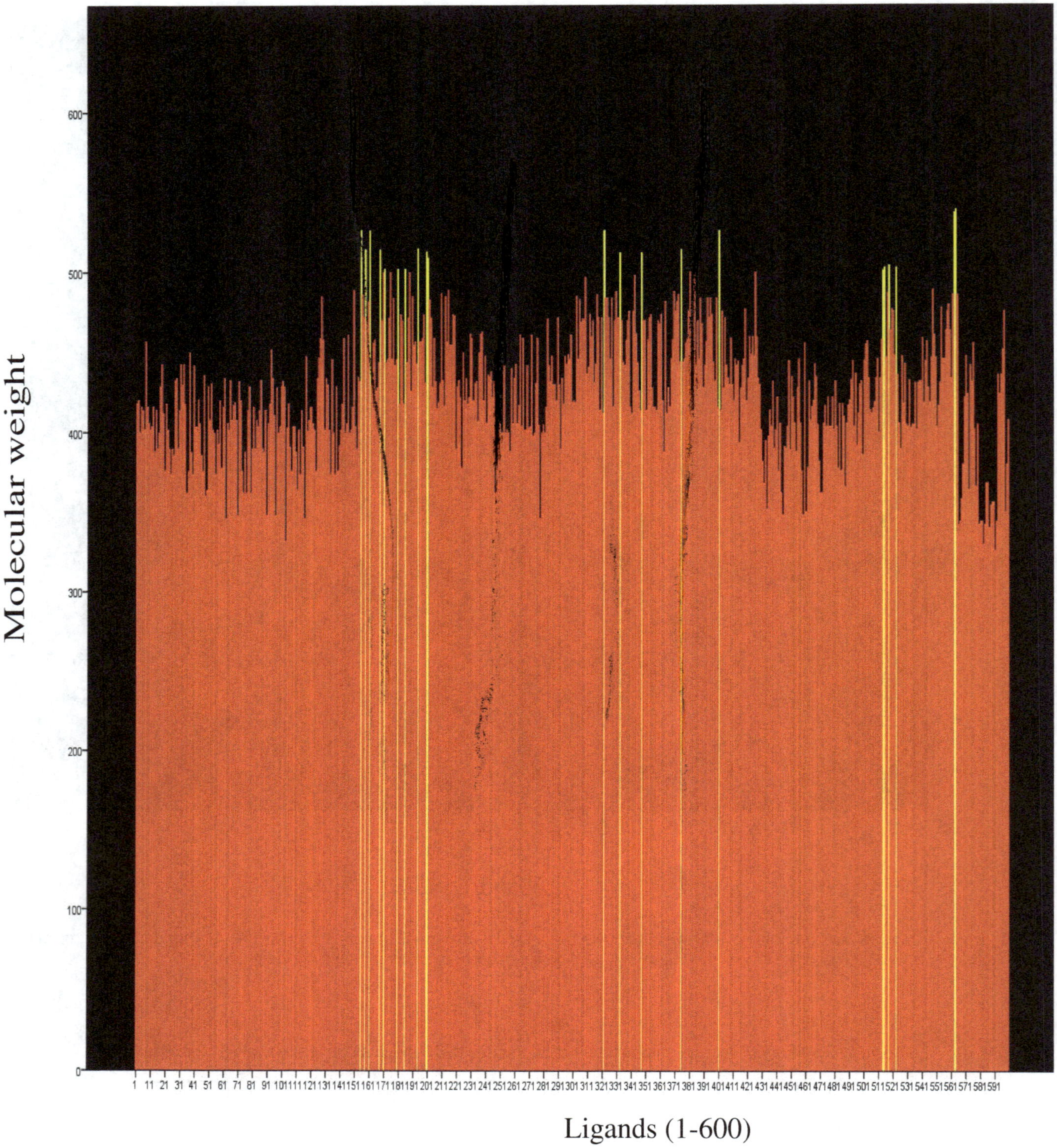

Figure 6. A graph showing the molecular weight for the 600 *de novo* designed ligands from Seed B. The red colour indicates a molecular weight of less than 500 and therefore these ligands are Lipinski rule of 5 compliant with respect to molecular weight only. The yellow colour indicates a molecular weight exceeding 500 and thus such ligands are not Lipinski rule of 5 compliant with respect to molecular weight only.

with the AChE Ligand Binding Pocket relative to Huperzine A, with Principal Component Analysis indicating the most significant ligand driven conformational changes which could be exploited in *in silico* attempts to identify novel entities with higher LBAs(pKd) and lower LBEs (kcal mol^{-1}). This could lead

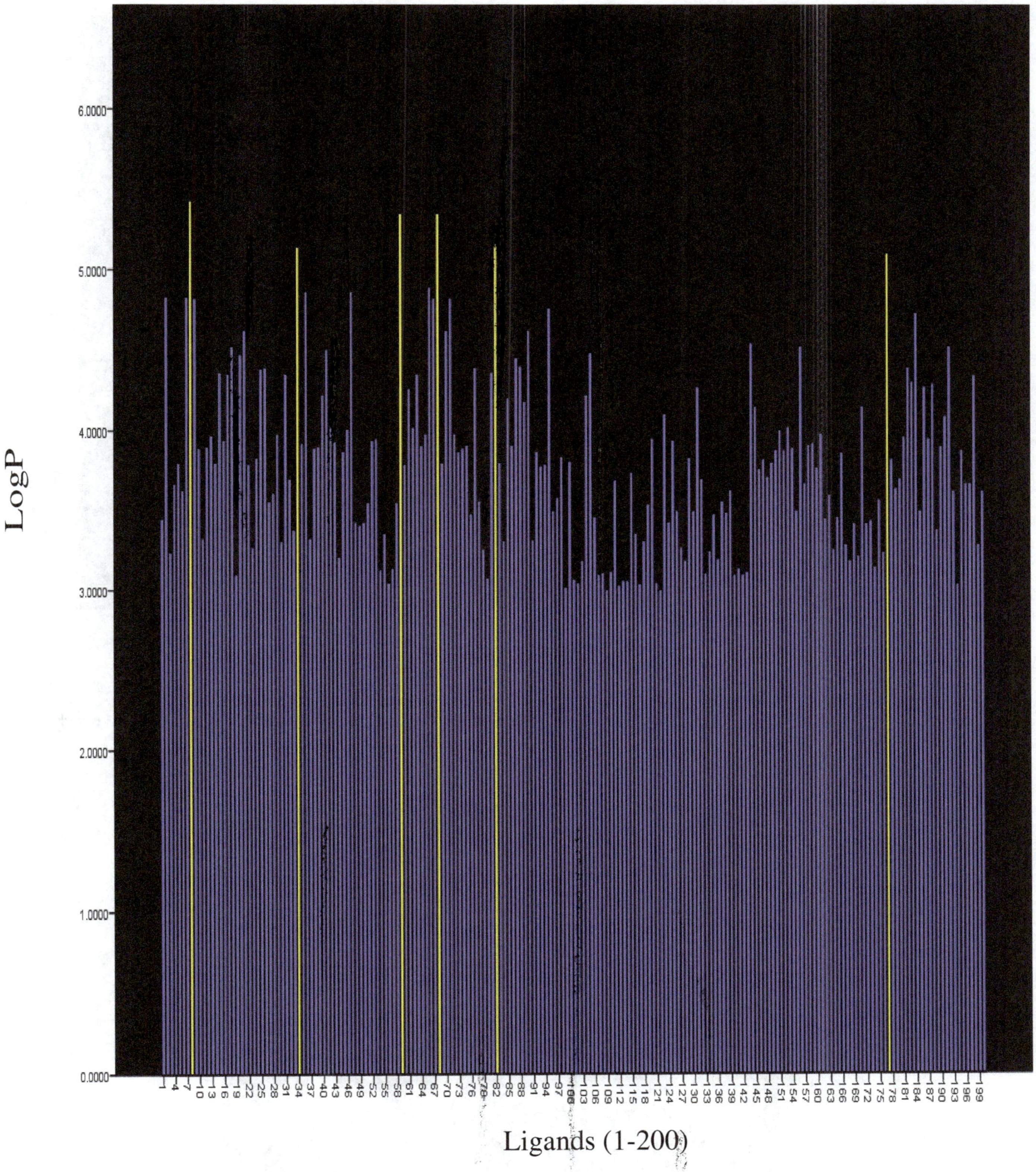

Figure 7. A graph showing the value of LogP for the 200 *de novo* ligands generated from Seed A. The yellow colour indicates a value of more than 5 and therefore such molecules are non-compliant with the Lipinski Rule of 5 with respect to LogP only.

to the identification of innovative AChE inhibitors with better potency and a low side effect profile. AChE inhibitors will continue to be developed, because this class of drugs has shown promise in symptomatic

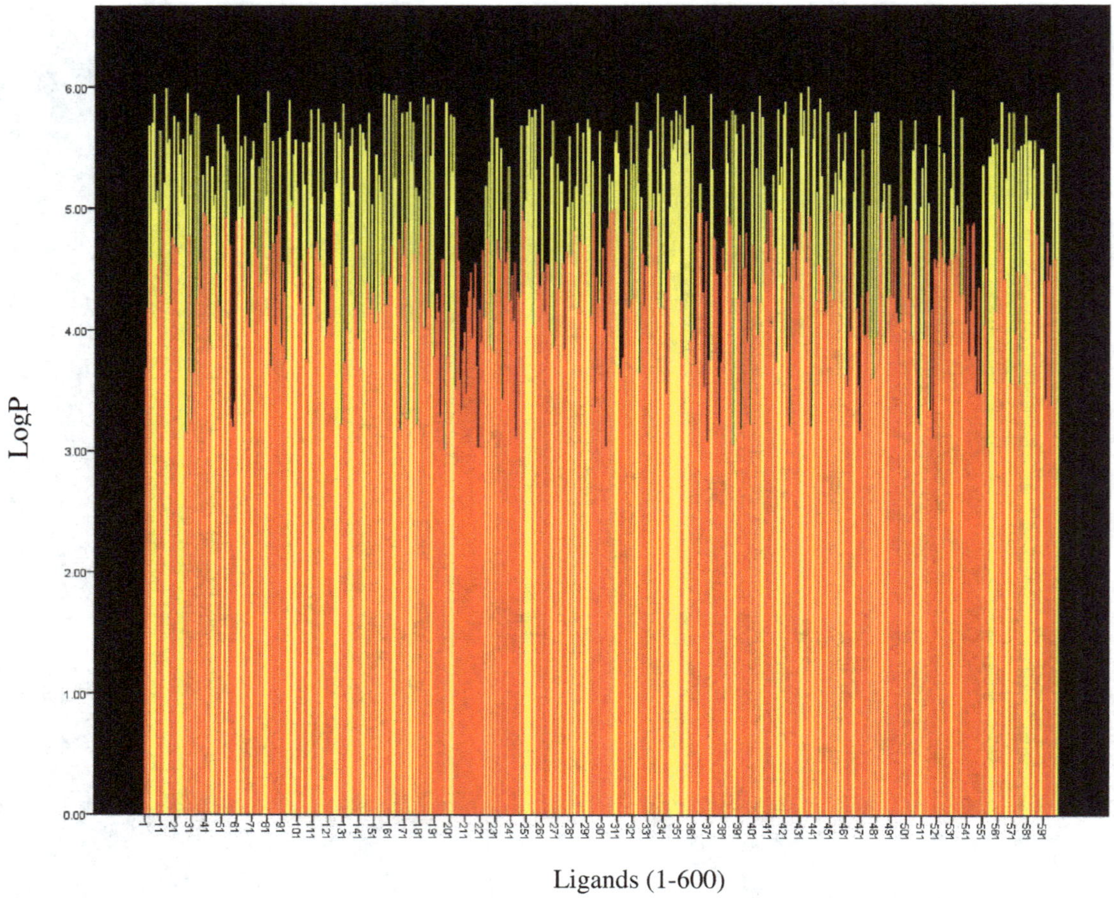

Figure 8. A graph showing the value of LogP for the 600 *de novo* ligands generated from Seed B. The yellow colour indicates a value of more than 5 and therefore such molecules are non-compliant with the Lipinski Rule of 5 with respect to LogP only.

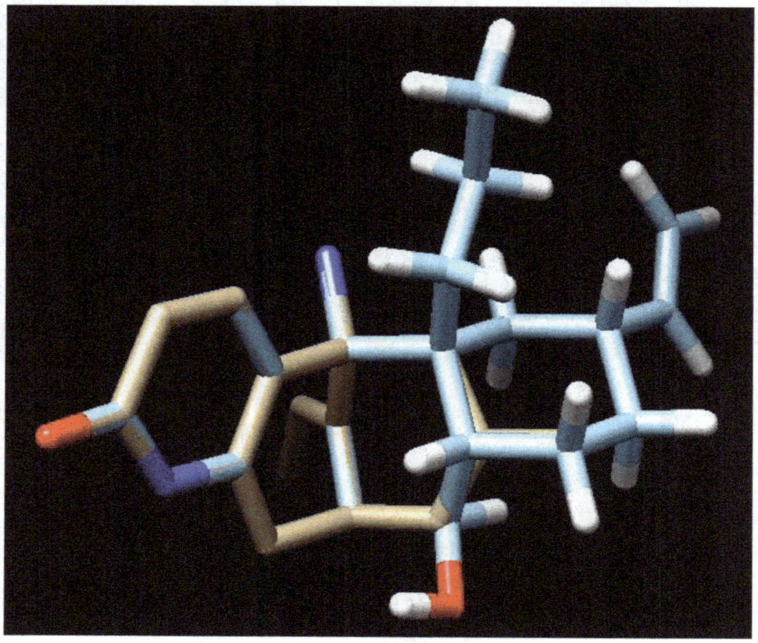

Figure 9. Superimposition of Molecule 6 (shown in light blue and white) onto Huperzine A (shown according to molecular type).

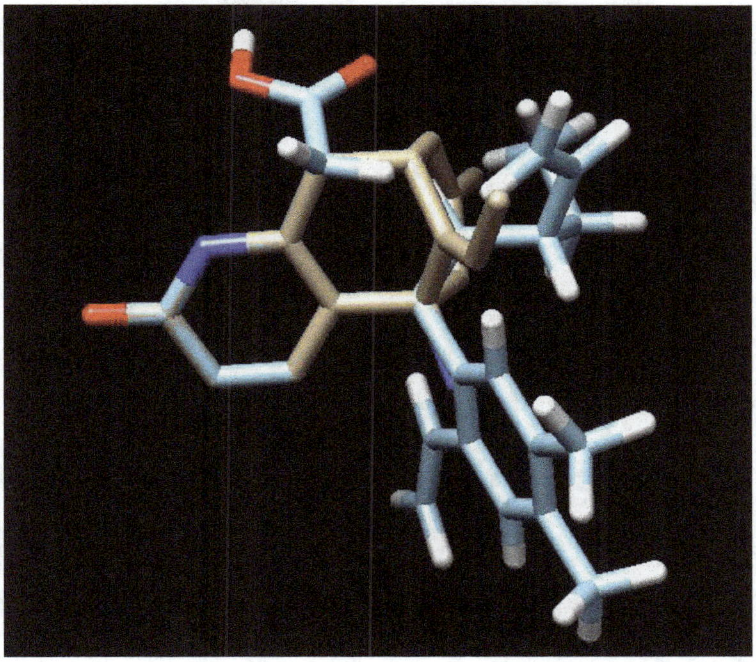

Figure 10. Superimposition of Molecule 4 (shown in light blue and white) onto Huperzine A (shown according to molecular type).

therapy (Mehta et al., 2011).

ACKNOWLEDGEMENT

"This submission is sponsored by APL Swift Services (Malta) Limited, a subsidiary of Aurobindo Pharma Limited."

REFERENCES

Akhondzadeh S, Abbasi SH (2006). Herbal medicine in the treatment of Alzheimer's Disease and Other Dementias. Am. J. Alzheimers Dis. Other Demen. 21:113-118.

Humphrey WF, Dalke A, Schulten K (1996). VMD - Visual Molecular Dynamics. J. Mol. Graphics 14:33-38.

Lipinski CA, Lombardo F, Dominy BW, Feeney PJ (1997). Experimental and computational approaches to estimate solubility and permeability in drug discovery and development settings. Adv. Drug Delivery Rev. 23(1-3):3-25.

Mehta M, Adem A, Sabbagh M (2011). New Acetylcholinesterase Inhibitors for Alzheimer's Disease. Int. J. Alzheimers Dis. 728983.

Picoulin K (2002). Reversing Alzheimer's Naturally. Canada: Auburn Hill Publishing Co.

Raves ML, Harel M, Pang YP, Silman I, Kozikowski AP, Sussman JL (1997). Structure of acetylcholinesterase complexed with the nootropic alkaloid, (-)-huperzine A. Nat. Struct. Biol. 4:57-63.

Wang R, Gao Y, Lai L (2000). LigBuilder: A multi-purpose program for structure-based drug design. J. Mol. Model. 6(7-8):498-516.

Wang R, Liu L, Lai L, Tang Y (1998). Score: A New Emperical Method for Estimating the Binding Affinity of a Protein-Ligand Complex. J. Mol. Model 4:379-394.

Wang R, Yan H, Tang XC (2006a). Progress in studies of Huperinze A, a natural cholinesterase inhibitor form Chinese herbal medicine. Acta Pharmacologica Sinica 27:1-26

Zangara A (2003). The psychopharmacology of huperzine A: an alkaloid with cognitive enhancing and neuroprotective properties of interest in the treatment of Alzheimer's disease. Pharmacol. Biochem. Behav. 75(3):675-86.

Antiprotozoal and cytotoxic activities, and the acute toxicity of extracts from of *Brucea sumatrana* Roxb. (Simaroubaceae) leaves collected in Mai-Ndombe, Democratic Republic of Congo

Cimanga R. Kanyanga[1,3]*, Tshodi M. Ehata[1], Nsaka S. Lumpu[1], Kikweta C. Munduku[1], Mbenza A. Phuati[1], Kambu O. Kabangu[1], Cos, P.[2], Maes, L.[2], Apers, S.[3], Vlietinck, A. J. and Pieters, L.[3]

[1]Faculty of Pharmaceutical Sciences, University of Kinshasa, P.O. Box 212, Kinshasa XI, Democratic Republic of Congo.
[2]Faculty of Pharmaceutical Sciences, Biomedical and Veterinary Sciences, Laboratory of Microbiology, Parasitology and Hygiene, University of Antwerp, Universisteitsplein 1, B-2610 Antwerp, Belgium.
[3]Department of Pharmaceutical Sciences, Laboratory of Natural Products and Food-Research and Analysis (NatuRa), University of Antwerp, Universiteitsplein 1, B-2610, Antwerp, Belgium.

Results from the *in vitro* evaluation of the antiprotozoal activity of the aqueous extract, the 80% methanol extract and its fractions from the leaves of *Brucea sumatrana* against *Trypanosoma brucei brucei*, *Trypanosoma cruzi*, *Lesihmania infantum*, the multidrug-resistant K1 and chloroquine-sensitive NF54 strains of *Plasmodium falciparum* indicated that all samples from the leaves extract presented interesting antiprotozoal activity at different extents. The 80% methanol extract, its chloroform acid, petroleum ether and 80% methanol soluble fractions and the aqueous extract exhibited strong activity against *Trypanosoma b. brucei*, *T. cruzi*, *L. infantum* and the multidrug-resistant K1 strain of *P. falciparum* with IC_{50} values from < 0.25 to 4.35 µg/ml as well as against chloroquine-sensitive NF54 strain of *P. falciparum* with IC_{50} values ranging from < 0.02 to 2.0.4 µg/ml. Most samples were cytotoxic against MRC-5 cell lines (0.2 < cytotoxic concentration 50 (CC_{50}) < 24.5 µg/ml) and showed good selective effect against all tested parasites. In acute toxicity, the aqueous extract was found to be non-toxic and its LD_{50} was estimated to be greater than 5 g/kg. In addition, it did not significantly modify the concentration levels of some evaluated biochemical and hematological parameters in rats. These results constitute a scientific validation supporting and justifying the traditional use of the leaves of *B. sumatrana* for the treatment of malaria, sleeping sickness and at some extent Chaga disease.

Key words: *Brucea sumatrana*, Simaroubaceae, leaves, extracts, antiprotozoal activity, cytotoxic activity, acute toxicity.

INTRODUCTION

Brucea sumatrana Roxb. (synonyms: *Brucea amarissima* Desv. ex Gomes, *Brucea javanica* (L.) Merr., Gonusamarissimus Lour or Loussaamarissma O. Ktze) (Simaroubaceae) is a medicinal plant mainly growing in some Asian countries, such as Cambodia, China, Indonesia and Thailand. It is also found in Panama

(South America). In these countries, the fruit of this medicinal plant is used for the treatment of various ailments such as cancer, malaria and amoebic dysentery (O'Neill et al., 1987; Wright et al., 1988).

Different biological activities of extracts and quassinoids isolated the Asian *B. javanica* fruits including anti-plasmodial (O'Neill et al., 1985, 1987; Pavanand et al., 1986), antileukemic (Lee et al., 1979), antiamoebic (Wright et al., 1988), antiprotozoal (Wright et al., 1993; Bawm et al., 2008), antinematodal (Alen et al., 2000), antidiarrhoeal, (Sawangjaroen and Sawangjaroen, 2005), antibabesial (Subeki et al., 2007) activities were previously reported. This plant species is also found in some African countries and its seeds, leaves and stem bark are used for treatment of various ailments among them protozoal diseases such as malaria, amoebic dysentery and sleeping sickness (Biruniya, 1993; Ngoma and Bikengeli, 1993; Neuwinger, 2000).

In Democratic Republic of Congo (DR Congo), to treat malaria, 4 or 5 seeds are chewed 2 to 3 times per day for the treatment of malaria crisis, while an aqueous decoction of leaves or stem bark is drunk three times/day until the disappearance of fever (Biruniya, 1993). During our ethnopharmacological and ethnobotanical studies conducted in Mai-Ndombe, Bas-Congo province of Democratic republic of Congo (RD Congo) near traditional healers about their knowledge to treat parasitic diseases, the leaves of *B. sumatrana* were frequently cited as starting plant materials used to prepare traditional remedies to treat malaria, amoebiasis and sleeping sickness or human african Trypanosomiasis (HAT) (Musuyu Muganza et al., 2006).

On the basis of the aforementioned ethnopharmacological information and the lack of an investigation conducted in this field, it was decided to evaluate *in vitro* the antiprotozoal activity of aqueous extract, 80% methanol extract and its fractions from leaves of *B. sumatrana* against *T. brucei brucei*, *T. cruzi*, *L. infantum*, the multi-resistant K1 and chloroquine-sensitive NF54 strains of *P. falciparum*. The potential cytotoxic effects against MRC-5 cell line (human lung fibroblasts) of all samples as well as the acute toxicity of the aqueous extract which is the used traditional preparation were also assessed.

MATERIALS AND METHODS

Reagents

Methanol from Fischer Scientific (UK) was of high performance liquid chromatography (HPLC) grade. Chloroform and petroleum ether of HPLC grade were obtained from Across Organics (USA). Distilled water was used for the preparation of an aqueous decoction.

Plants

Leaves of *B. Sumatrana* Roxb. (Simaroubaceae) were collected in the district Mai-Ndombe's province Bandundu in DR Congo in December, 2009. The plant was identified by Mr. Bavukinina of the Institut de Recherches en Sciences de la Santé (I.R.S.S.) of Kinshasa, DR Congo. A voucher specimen (B 20122009BSL) was deposited in the herbarium of this institute. Leaves were dried at room temperature and reduced to powder.

Preparation of crude extracts, fractions and subfractions

A 150 g of dried powdered leaves of *B. sumatrana* were submitted to a Soxhlet extraction with 80% methanol (500 ml) for 2 h. The extractive solvent was evaporated *in vacuum* yielding corresponding dried 80% methanol extract denoted as ME-1 (12.53 g). 5 g of this dried 80% methanol extract were dissolved in 100 ml distilled water and fractionated according to the Mitscher's procedure (Figure 1) (Mitscher et al., 1978). The obtained fractions and sub-fractions were treated as described, yielding the corresponding dried extracts denoted as ME-1.1 to ME-1.6. On the other hand, 20 g of the powdered plant material were mixed with 150 ml distilled water and boiled at 100°C for 15 min. After cooling and filtration, the filtrate was treated as described, yielding the dried aqueous extract denoted as AE-1 (5.89 g). The total alkaloids extract (ME-2, 3.06 g) of plant part was obtained using the acid/base procedure described in the literature (Harborne, 1998).

Phytochemical screening

This study was performed by thin layer chromatography (TLC) on precoated silica gel plates F_{254} (thickness later 0.25, mm, Merck, Germany) using different reagents and mobile phases described in the literature to identify major chemical groups such as alkaloids, anthraquinones, coumarins, flavonoids, terpenes and steroids. Hydrochloride acid 0.2 N (aqueous solution of the sample anthocyanins. Froth test and Stiasny's reagent were used to detect saponins and tannins, respectively (Harborne, 1998).

Evaluation of biological activities

The antiprotozoal activity of all the samples obtained from the leaves of *B. sumatrana* was tested *in vitro* against *T. b. brucei*, *T. cruzi* and *L. infantum* from the laboratory of Microbiology, Parasitology and Hygiene of Prof. L. Maes,

*Corresponding author. E-mail: kanyanga.cimanga@ua.ac.be, rkcimanga@gmail.com.

University of Antwerp, Belgium according to the respective procedures previously described by Kuypers et al. (2006) and Tshodi et al. (2012). The antiplasmodial activity against chloroquine and pyrimethamine-resistant K1 strain of *P. falciparum* obtained from the same laboratory, and chloroquine-sensitive NF54 from Tropical Medicine Institute of Antwerp, Belgium, was evaluated according to the lactate deshydrogenase procedure previously described by Makler et al. (1993) with some modifications (Kuypers et al., 2006). The cytotoxic effect against MRC-5 cell lines (human lung fibroblasts) was assessed using the MTT assay previously described by Kuypers et al. (2006). The selective index (SI) as a ratio cytotoxic concentration 50/inhibitory concentration 50 (CC_{50}/IC_{50}) was calculated for each sample to appreciate its effect against the tested parasites and MRC-5 cell lines. SI < 1 indicated a selective effect against the cell line while SI > 1 indicated a selective action against the tested parasite (Camacho et al., 2003; Tshodi et al., 2012). For the purpose of this *in vitro* antiprotozoal screening study, the following criteria were adopted: $IC_{50} \leq 5$ µg/ml: strong activity; $5 < IC_{50} \leq 10$ µg/ml: good activity; $10 < IC_{50} \leq 20$ µg/ml: moderate activity; $20 < IC_{50} \leq 40$ µg/ml: weak activity; $IC_{50} > 40$ µg/ml: inactive.

Acute toxicity

In the present study, only the acute toxicity of the aqueous extract was investigated in Wistar rats according to the procedure described by the Organization for Economic Co–operation and Development (OECD) guideline for testing chemicals, TG420 (OECD, 2001). Briefly, groups I (2 rats) orally received 5 ml distilled water and constituted the negative control groups. After, fifteen Wistar rats of either sex, (body weight: 130 to 150 g, aged 8 to 10 weeks) were divided in three groups of 5 rats each noted as groups II, III and IV which orally received a single oral dose of 500, 1000 and 5000 mg/kg body weight (bw), respectively. The animals were observed for toxic symptoms continuously for the first 4 h dosing and were daily weighted. Finally, all animals were then maintained in daily observation and the number of toxic effects and survivor were recorded for 14 days and further 28 days.

Biochemical and hematological parameters analysis

Blood from rats having received 5 g/kg of the aqueous extract (AE-1) was collected from tail vein on Day 28 for analysis. For biochemical parameters, blood was centrifuged at 4000 g for 5 min to obtain plasma, which was stored at –20°C. Glucose, creatinin, aspartate aminotransferase (ASAT), alanine aminotransferase (ALAT), serum glutamo pyruvate transferase (SGPT), serum glutamo oxalate transferase (SGOT), uric acid, total cholesterol, triglycerides, high-density lipoproteins (HDL), low-density lipoproteins (LDL), total and direct bilirubin were quantified using Architect (Abottâ) automation with Boehringen Ingelheim biochemical kits. Total proteins were estimated using Biuret's method. Hematological parameters analysis was carried out using an automatic hematological analyzer (Coulter STK, Beckam) with appropriated kits. The differential leucocyte count was performed with an optical microscopy after staining and, in each case, 100 cells were counted.

RESULTS AND DISCUSSION

Antiprotozoal and cytotoxic effects

Table 1 represents the antiprotozoal activity and the cytotoxicity of samples from the leaves of *B. sumatrana*. All samples were tested *in vitro* against *T. b. brucei*, *T. cruzi*, *L. infantum*, chloroquine and pyrimethamine-resistant K1 while Table 2 represents the activity of the samples against chloroquine-sensitive NF54 strains of *P. falciparum*. The cytotoxic effects of all samples against MRC-5 cell lines (human lung fibroblasts) (Table 1) and the acute toxicity only of the aqueous extract as the used traditional preparation were also evaluated.

The obtained results indicated that all samples exhibited the evaluated biological activities at different extents. The 80% methanol extract (ME-1) exhibited good activity against *T. cruzi* (6.15 µg/ml) and weak activity against *L. infantum* (24 µg/ml), while it showed strong activity against *T. b. brucei* and the multidrug-resistant K1 strain of *P. falciparum* with IC_{50} values of 4.35 and < 0.25 µg/ml, respectively (Table 1). Interestingly, its chloroform soluble fraction (ME-1.1) rich in waxes, steroids and terpenes and its petroleum ether soluble subfraction (ME-1.2) rich in waxes and lipids had the same antiprotozoal spectra of activity and presented strong activity against all selected protozoa with IC_{50} values ranging from < 0.25 to 1.70 µg/ml (Table 1). The 80% methanol soluble subfraction (ME-1.3) rich in steroids and terpenes exhibited strong activity against *T. b. brucei* and *T. cruzi* with IC_{50} value < 0.25 µg/ml for both parasites, weak activity against chloroquine and pyrimethamine-resistant K1 strain of *P. falciparum,* and was inactive against *L. infantum* (Table1).

The aqueous acid soluble fraction (ME-1.4), its chloroform base soluble subfraction (ME-1.5) rich in alkaloids and aqueous alkaline soluble subfraction (ME-1.6) rich in phenolic compounds had also the same antiprotozoal spectra of activity. All samples displayed good activity

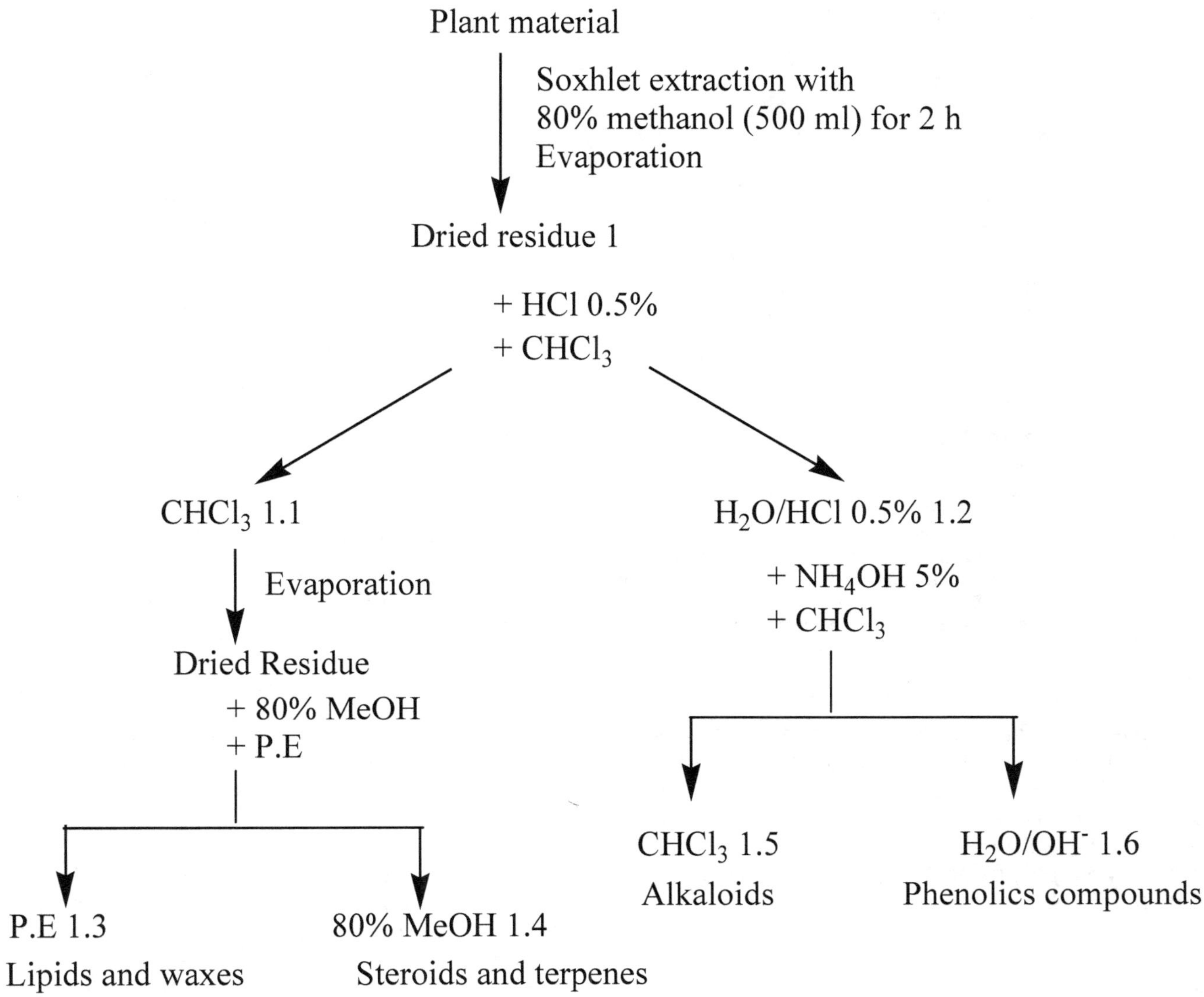

Figure 1. Fractionation of the 80% methanol extract.
Source: Mitcher et al. (1978).

against *T. b. brucei* and the multidrug-resistant K1 strain of *P. falciparum*, weak activity against *T. cruzi* and were inactive against *L. infantum* (Table 1). The aqueous extract (AE-1) which is the used traditional remedy exhibited strong activity against *T. b. brucei*, *T.cruzi* and the multidrug-resistant K1 strain of *P. falciparum* with IC_{50} values ranging from < 0.25 to 0.70 µg/ml (Table 1) and good activity against *L. infantum* (IC_{50} = 5.06 µg/ml). The total alkaloids extract (ME-2) showed good, moderate and weak activity against *T. b. brucei*, *T. cruzi*and *L.* infantum, respectively (Table 1). In addition, it however exhibited strong activity against the multidrug-resistant k1 strain of *P. falciparum* with IC_{50} value of 1.80 µg/ml.

All samples from *B. sumatrana* leaves exhibited strong activity against chloroquine-sensitive NF54 strain of *P. falciparum* with IC_{50} values from < 0.02 to 2.04 µg/ml. The most active samples were ME-1, ME-1.1, ME-1.4, ME-1.5, ME-2 and AE-1 inhibiting its growth with IC_{50} value < 0.25 µg/ml. In addition, ME-1.3 and ME-1.4 also showed strong activity against this *P. falciparum* strain with IC_{50} values of 1.04 and 1.55 µg/ml, respectively. In general, all samples showed strong antiplasmodial activity against this strain of *P. falciparum* (IC_{50} < 5 µg/ml) (Table 2).

With regards to the activity showed by the reference products, it is important to point out that ME-1.1, ME-1.2 and ME-1.5 exhibited higher activity (0.25 ≤ IC_{50} < 0.70 µg/ml) than benznidazol against *T. cruzi* (IC_{50} = 2.65 µg/ml) whereas the antiplasmodial activity of ME-1, ME-1.1, ME-1.1 and AE-.1 (IC_{50} < 0.25 µg/ml) against the multidrug-resistant K1 strain of *P. falciparum* was

Table 1. Antiprotozoal and cytotoxic activities of samples from *Brucea sumatrana* leaves.

Code sample	MRC-5	*T. b. brucei*	*T. cruzi*	*L. infantum*	*P. falc.* K1
ME-1	2.34	4.35	6.15	24.00	< 0.25
ME-1.1	< 0.25	< 0.25	< 0.25	0.32	< 0.25
ME-1.4	< 0.25	< 0.25	0.31	1.70	< 0.25
ME-1.3	> 64	< 0.25	< 0.25	> 64	35.33
ME-1.4	34.24	12.35	27.57	> 64	10.00
ME-1.5	10.32	8.11	21.22	> 64	7.05
ME-1.6	24.05	10.04	25.06	> 64	8.15
ME-2	7.00	8.30	12.70	24.00	1.80
AE-1	0.46	0.57	0.70	5.06	< 0.25
Tamoxifen	10.5				
Metarsoprol		0.02			
Benznidazol			2.65		
Multeforine				3.56	
Chloroquine	> 64				0.18

ME-1 : 80% methanol extract, ME-1.1 : chloroform acid soluble fraction, ME-1.2 : petroleum ether soluble subfraction, ME-1.3 : methanol 80% soluble subfraction, ME-1.4 : aqueous acid soluble fraction, ME-1.5 : chloroform base soluble subfraction, ME-1.6 : aqueous alkaline soluble subfraction, ME-2 : totum alkaloids extract,AE-1 : aqueous (decoction) extract, *T.b. brucei: Trypanosome bruceibruce, T. cruzi: Trypanosome cruzi, I. infantum: leishmania infantum, P. falc. K1: Plasmodium falciparum K1.*

comparable to that of chloroquine used as an antimalarial reference product (IC_{50} = 0.18 µg/ml). In addition, samples ME-1, ME-1.1, ME-1.2 and AE-1 were the most cytotoxic samples and were 4.49, < 42, < 42 and 23 times more cytotoxic, respectively (CC_{50} = 2.34, < 0.25, < 0.25 and 0.46 µg/ml, respectively) than tamoxifen (CC_{50} = 10.5 µg/ml) (Table 1).

Cytotoxic effects of samples of *B. sumatrana* leaves against MRC-5 cell line

In the cytotoxic studies, it was observed that except ME-1.3 and ME-1.4 samples devoid of cytotoxic effect against MRC-5 cell line (CC_{50} > 64 and 34.24 µg/ml, respectively) since their CC_{50} were greater than 32 µg/ml, the remaining samples were cytotoxic against this cell line with CC_{50} values ranging from < 0.25 to 24.05 µg/ml, since they were lower than 32 µg/ml (Kuypers et al., 2006). By assessing their respective selectivity index (SI), it was observed that the activities of ME-1, ME-1.1, ME-1.2, MS-2 and AE-1 against *T. b. brucei*, *T. cruzi* and *L. infantum* were correlated to their cytotoxic effect against MRC-5 cell line, since their SI were lower than 1 (Camacho et al., 2003; Tshodi et al., 2012). They however presented good selective action against the multidrug-resistant K1 strain of *P. falciparum,* since their respective SI were greater than 1 (Camacho et al., 2003; Tshodi et al., 2012) (Table 3). ME-1.3 had the highest selectivity index against *T. b. brucei* and *T. cruzi* since its SI value was > 256. Its selective action against *L. infantum* and the strain K1 of *P. falciparum* was also appreciable (Table 3).

Against chloroquine-sensitive NF54 of *P. falciparum*, most samples showed good selective action. The best selective action was observed with ME-1.4 (SI = 1721), followed by ME-1.5 (SI = 516), ME-2 (SI = 350) and ME-1 (SI ≥ 117). The inhibitory effect of ME-1.2 on the growth of this parasite was correlated to its cytotoxic effect since it SI was lower than 1 (SI < 0.24) (Table 2) (Camacho et al., 2003; Tshodi et al., 2012).

Effects of the aqueous extract of *B. sumatrana* leaves on the concentration levels of haematological parameters

The hematological parameter profile is presented in Table 4. The reported results indicated that the oral administration of the aqueous extract of *B. sumatrana* leaves (AE-1) at the oral dose of 5 g/kg bw in acute toxicity, did not affect concentration levels of evaluated hematological parameters and no significant difference between the treated animals compared to untreated was deduced ($p > 0.005$). They remained all in normal limits and presented no sign of a particular pathologic state.

Table 2. Antiplasmodial activity of samples from *B. sumatrana* leaves against chloroquine-sensitive NF54 strain of *P. falciparum.*

Code sample	MRC-5	*P. falciparum. NF54*	*Selectivity index*
ME-1	2.34	< 0.02	> 117
ME-1.1	< 0.25	< 0.02	< 12.5
ME-1.4	< 0.25	1.04	< 0.24
ME-1.3	> 64	1.55	> 41.29
ME-1.4	34.24	< 0.02	> 1712
ME-1.5	10.32	< 0.02	> 516
ME-1.6	24.05	2.04	11.79
ME-2	7.00	< 0.02	> 350
AE-1	0.46	< 0.02	> 23
Chloroquine	> 64	0.15	> 426.67

ME-1 : 80% methanolextract, ME-1.1 : chloroform acid soluble fraction, ME-1.2 : petroleum ether soluble subfraction, ME-1.3 : methanol 80% soluble subfraction, ME-1.4 : aqueous acid soluble fraction, ME-1.5 : chloroform base soluble subfraction, ME-1.6 : aqueous alkaline soluble subfraction, ME-2 : totumalkaloidsextract,AE-1 : aqueous (decoction) extract, *T.b. brucei: Trypanosome bruceibruce, T. cruzi: Trypanosome cruzi, I. infantum: leishmania infantum, P. falc. K1: Plasmodium falciparum K1.*

Table 3. Selectivity index (SI= CC_{50}/IC_{50}) of samples from*Brucea sumatrana* leaves.

Code sample	MRC-5/*T.b.brucei*	MRC-5/*T. cruzi*	MRC-5/*L. infantum*	MRC-5/*P. falc.*K1
ME-1	0.53	0.38	0.10	> 9.36
ME-1.1	< 1	<1	< 0.80	< 1
ME-1.2	< 1	< 080	> 0.14	< 1
ME-1.3	> 256	> 256	ND	> 1.81
ME-1.4	2.77	1.24	ND	4.86
ME-1.5	1.27	0.48	ND	1.46
ME-1.6	2.40	0.96	ND	2.95
ME-2	0.84	0.55	0.29	3.89
AE-1	0.80	0.66	0.09	< 1.84
Chloroquine	> 64	-	-	> 355.55

ME-1 : 80% methanol extract, ME-1.1 : chloroform acid soluble fraction, ME-1.2 : petroleum ether soluble subfraction, ME-1.3 : methanol 80% soluble subfraction, ME-1.4 : aqueous acid soluble fraction, ME-1.5 : chloroform base soluble subfraction, ME-1.6 : aqueous alkaline soluble subfraction, ME-2 : totumalkaloidsextract,AE-1 : aqueous (decoction) extract, *T.b. brucei: Trypanosome bruceibruce, T. cruzi: Trypanosome cruzi, L. infantum: Leishmania infantum, P. falc. K1: Plasmodium falciparum K1.* ND: not determined because the tested sample was inactive.

Effects the aqueous extract of *B. sumatrana* leaves on the concentration levels of evaluated biochemical parameters

Table 5 shows the effects of the oral administration of the aqueous extract (decoction, AE-1) of *B. sumatrana* leaves on the concentration levels of some biochemical parameters of Wistar rats. The obtained results indicated that the oral administration of the extract at the highest oral dose of 5 g/kg bw in acute toxicity test produced significant decrease of the concentration level of glucose in treated groups compared to untreated groups ($p < 0.05$). This decrease may be due to the hypoglycaemic and antidiabetic properties of the extract as also previously reported for other plant extracts (Okoli et al., 2010; Luka et al., 2012).

Alanine amino transferase (ALAT) also called alanine transaminase (ALT) and aspartate transaminase (AST) also known as aspartate amino transferase (ASAT/AspAT/AAT) are two liver enzymes associated in the hepatocellular damages and thus considered as indicators of liver damages. ALAT is only specific for liver functions and ASAT is mostly found in the myocardium, skeletal muscle, kidneys and brain (Wasan et al., 2001; Crook et al., 2006). Although a slight decrease was observed, the results reported here indicated that

Table 4. Effects the aqueous extract of *B. sumatrana* leaves (AE-1) at oral dose of 5 g/kgbw on the concentration levels of haematological parameters.

Parameter	Negative control	*B. sumatrana*: 5g/kgbw	*Reference values*
RBC (×10^6 µME-1)	8.1 ± 0.8	8.4 ± 1.2	7.6-10.29
Hemoglobin (g/dl)	14.2 ± 0.2	16.4 ± 1.2	15-18.2
Hematocrit (%)	43.2 ± 0.1	47.2 ± 2.0	40.7-50
Platelets (×10^3 µME-1)	1421.0 ± 0.2	1404.2 ± 0.2	995-1713
WBC (x10^3 µME-1)	13.3 ± 0.3	16.0 ± 0.5	6.6-20.5
Neutrophils (%)	18.8 ± 0.7	23.2 ± 1.2	3-24.7
Basophils (%)	0.0	0.0	0.0
Eosinophils (%)	1.5 ± 0.1	1.5 ± 0.4	0-2
Lympocytes (%)	89.2 ± 1.1	88.3 ± 0.1	58.8-94
Monocytes (%)	3.4 ± 1.1	3.6 ± 1.2	0-4
Segmented leucocytes (%)	15.1 ± 0.6	19.3 ± 2.1	-

RBC; red blood cells, WBC : white blood cells

Table 5. Effects the aqueous extract of *B. sumatrana* leaves (AE-1) at oral dose of 5 g/kgbw on the concentration levels of biochemical parameters.

Parameters	Negative control	*B. sumatrana*: 5 g/kg bw
Glucose (mg/dl)	245.5 ± 0.4	206.3 ± 1.4
Creatinin (mg/dl)	0.90 ± 0.05	0.87 ± 0.02
AST (UI/L)	180.6 ± 0.3	178.2 ± 0.5
ALT (UI/L)	52.2 ± 2.2	53.5 ± 1.2
Totalcholesterol (mg/dl)	54.2 ± 1.1	53.3 ± 2.2
Triglycerides (mg/dl)	47.7 ± 1.8	46.3 ± 3.5
Total bilurbin (mg/dl)	0.6 ± 0.1	0.6 ± 0.1
Direct bilurbin (mg/dl)	0.2 ± 0.0	0.2 ± 0.0
Total proteins (g/dl)	8.0 ± 0.3	8.4 ± 1.1
Albumin (g/dl)	3.6 ± 0.5	3.5 ± 0.6
ALP (IU/L)	148.4 ± 1.6	146.3 ± 2.4
HDL (mg/dl)	65.3 ± 1.3	65.6 ± 1.3
LDL (mg/dl)	39.5 ± 2.1	38.5 ± 0.4
Uric acid (mg/dl)	1.8 ± 0.1	2.2 ± 0.5
SGOT (UI/L)	128.3 ± 1.6	126.4 ± 0.2
SGPT (UI/L)	32.7 ± 2.3	33.3 ± 1.2
Urea (mmol/L)	6.1 ± 0.8	6.6 ± 1.6

AST: aspartate transferase, ALT : alanine transferase, ALP : alkalinephospahte, HDL : hight-densitylipoproteins, LDL : low-densitylipoproteins, SGOT : serumglutamoxatetransferase, SGPT : serum glutamate transferase

concentration levels of these both enzymes in treated animals did not show a significant difference compared to the negative control ($p > 0.05$). This finding showed that the aqueous leaf extract at this tested oral dose may not cause liver, heart or kidney damages as also previously reported by Pieme et al. (2006) and Lima et al. (2009). Moreover, the hepatic function of these animals can be considered to be maintained (Arüjo et al., 2005). In addition, the concentration levels of creatinin and SGPT which did not show significant difference in treated rat groups compared to untreated rat groups ($p > 0.05$) well support this observation.

The slight decrease of the concentration levels of cholesterol and triglycerides in treated rat groups was not significant ($p > 0.05$) (Table 5). This effect may be due to the hypolipidimic property of the aqueous leaves extract and to the increased secretion of thyroid hormones T3 and T4 (Arüjo et al., 2005). A slight decrease in concentrations of high density lipoprotein (HDL) and low density lipoprotein (LDL) in treated animals was also observed, but, it did not show significant difference compared to the control groups ($p > 0.05$). It can be considered as a consequence of the decrease of total cholesterol. These results suggest that the extract has some beneficial effects by reducing some risk factors related to cardiovascular diseases (Ameyaw and Owusu-Ansah, 1998).

Albumin is a protein with high concentration in plasma. Since it is produced in the liver, its decrease in serum may arise from liver and kidney diseases (Lima et al., 2009). Fortunately, a slight decrease of the concentration level of albumin was observed, but did not show significant difference compared to untreated groups ($p > 0.05$). In addition, although a slight decrease for the concentration levels of the total and direct bilirubin was observed, there was no significant difference of this biochemical parameter in treated animals compared to control groups ($p > 0.05$). The level of total proteins slightly increased ($p < 0.05$), suggesting an external supply. A slight increase of the concentration level of SGOT and SGPT in treated animals was observed. Nevertheless, it did not show significant difference compared to the control groups ($p > 0.05$) indicating that the heart and liver were not affected. No significant difference in the concentration level of ALP in treated rat groups compared to untreated groups was recorded although a slight decrease or increase in treated groups according to the case was observed ($p > 005$) (Table 5). As the presence of infiltrative diseases of the liver and all bones diseases is associated with osteoplastic activity, it is likely seen that the oral dose used in this study for the aqueous extract of *B. sumatrana* leaves did not abnormally interfere with the calcification or metabolic activities involving the liver. The intrahepatic and extrahepatic bile functions did not know an obstruction (Vasudevan and Sreekumari, 2005). This finding is in good agreement with results reported concerning the effect of other plant extracts on ALP concentration level in animals (Pieme et al., 2006; Eden and Usoh, 2009).

As urea production in mammals occurs specially in liver, its concentration level could also be used as an indicator of hepatic function. In our study, the urea concentration level significantly increased in treated groups compared to untreated groups ($p < 0.02$), but this observation was not found as a sign of insufficiency renal because its concentration level remained within the normal limits (2.5 to 7.5 mmol/L). Therefore, our results showed good hepatic function of treated animals for the aforementioned reasons (Arüjo et al., 2005).

In general, all concentration levels of biochemical and haematological parameters evaluated in the present study were within the normal ranges (Barry et al., 1995; Feldams et al., 1997).

Acute toxicity of the aqueous extract of *B. sumatrana* leaves in rats

Animals were treated with single oral doses of the aqueous extract (AE-1) (500, 1000 and 5000 mg/kg body weight, respectively). In this test, no sign of toxicity such as alteration of the locomotion activity and gastro-intestinal disturbances were observed. Rats received all tested oral doses significantly gained body weight compared to negative control groups. According to Pieme et al. (2006), the growth response effect could be considered as a result of increased food and water intake. On Day 21, one death (6.66%) was noted in the third group receiving 1000 mg/kg bw of the extract and on Day 22, 3 deaths (20%) were recorded in the fourth group having received 5000 mg/kg body weight of the extract. This last percentage of mortality is weaker than 50%. According to Kennedy et al. (1986), substances that present LD_{50} higher than 5 g/kg body weight via oral route, may be considered as practically non-toxic. Therefore, it may be suggested that the acute toxicity of *B. sumatrana* aqueous leaves extract is practically null via oral route. Therefore, the LD_{50} of the extract was estimated to be greater than 5000 mg/kg body weight. In addition, histopathological examination of vital organs of treated animals did not show any abnormality compared to untreated groups indicating that their state was well maintained at the administered oral dose.

On the other hand, the acute toxicity of leaves ethanol extract of *Brucea javanica* Merr. collected in Indonesia on mice was previously reported (Marissa et al., 2012). Results from this study indicated that the oral administration of the leaves ethanol extract at oral doses of 562.5, 1125, 2250 and 4500 mg/kg body weight, respectively, were unable to induce acute toxic effects in mice. But at the highest oral dose of 4500 mg/kg body weight, 26% mortality occurred after 14 days, and its DL_{50} was determined to be 1003.65 mg/kg body weight. This DL_{50} determined by these authors seems not to be correct because not only 26% of death observed at the highest oral dose of 4500 mg/kg bw was weaker than 50% of death, but also not percentage death was reported after the administration of 1125 and 2250 mg/kg bw, respectively, suggesting that these oral doses did not induce mortality of animals. Taking account of these important observations, the DL_{50} of the administered extract in this previous study must be greater than 4500 mg/kg bw and not 1003.65 mg/kg bw as reported. Interestingly, in this same investigation, it was reported that vital organs and body average weights of treated animals did not show any difference compared to control groups. In addition, gross examination of the vital organs revealed no pathologic abnormality compared to control groups on the microscopic observation. These finding were in good agreement with our observations for the aqueous leaves extract tested in the present study. From these results of this study, these authors concluded that the extract can be considered to be slightly toxic since the damage caused by leaves ethanol extract is minor and not permanent considering the administered oral dose (Marissa et al., 2012).

The chemical composition of *B. sumatrana* leaves

Some plant parts of *B. javanica* growing in Asian regions were chemically previously investigated. Triterpenoids and quassinoids were isolated from the combined plant materials leaves, twigs and inflorescences. Flavonoids were also detected (Ismail et al., 2012) or isolated from the leaves (Dong et al., 2013). Results from our phytochemical screening conducted on *B. sumatrana* leaves collected in Mai-Ndombe, DR Congo, revealed the presence of alkaloids, steroids, terpenoids, flavonoids and tannins in the leaves. Anthraquinones, anthocyanins and coumarins were not detected in our experimental conditions. The presence mainly of alkaloids, flavonoids, steroids and terpenoids may largely contribute to the observed antiprotozoal activity because more chemicals belonging to these phytochemical groups present in other medicinal plant species had previously been reported to exhibit antiprotozoal activity at different extents (Wright et al., 1994; Camacho et al., 1998; Christensen and Kharazmi, 2001; Hoet et al., 2004: Bero et al., 2009; Bero and Quetin-Leclercq, 2011). Particularly, different terpenes belonging to the quassinoid groups mainly isolated from the seeds of *B. javanica* growing in Asian regions are known as active principles for various evaluated biological activities already mentioned earlier.

Conclusion

The present investigation has described for the first time the antiprotozoal and cytotoxic activities, and acute toxicity of extracts, fractions and sub-fractions from *B. sumatrana* leaves from RD Congo on a large spectrum of protozoa. The reported results showed that all samples possessed interesting *in vitro* antiprotozoal activity at different extents. The aqueous extract (AE-1), which is the used traditional preparation, was found to be non-toxic and did not affect the concentration levels of evaluated biochemical and hematological parameters, and can be considered as a sign of no appearance of pathologic abnormality. The reported results can partly justify and support the use of this plant part of *B. sumatrana* as raw material for the preparation of traditional remedy for the treatment of parasitic diseases such as malaria, sleeping sickness, leishmaniosis and in some extents American trypanosomiasis named Chagas disease, with no apparent toxic effects in patients. Further studies are in progress on the most active fractions, sub-fractions and the total alkaloids extract, leading to the isolation and structural elucidation of active constituents.

REFERENCES

Alen Y, Nkajima S, Nitoda T, Baba N, Kanzaki H, Kawazu K (2000). Antinematodal activity of some tropical rainforest plants against the pinewood nematode, *Bursaphelenchus*. Zeit. Naturf. 55:295-299.

Ameyaw Y, Owusu-Ansah SI (1998). Morphological studies of two plant species in Ethnomedicine. J. Herbs Spices Med. Plants 5:60-85.

Arüjo B.J.A., Sant'Ana D.M.G., Molinari SI (2005). Hematologic and biochemic parameters of rats subjected to hypoprotic and hyperprotic diet. Unuarama 8:139-140.

Barry SL (1995). Animal clinical pathology. In: Michael JD, Manfred AH (Eds), CRC Handbook of Toxicology. CRC Press, Inc., USA. pp. 517-537.

Bawm BS, Matsuura H, Elkhateeb A,. Nabeta K, Subeki, Nonaka N, Oku Y, Katakura K (2008). *In Vitro* Antitrypanosomal activities of quassinoid compounds from the fruits of a medicinal plant, *Brucea javanica*. Vet. Parasitol. 4:288-294.

Bero J, Frédérich M, Quetin-Leclercq J (2009). Antimalarial compounds isolated from plants used in traditional medicine. J. Pharm. Pharmacol. 61:1401-1433.

Bero J, Quetin-Leclercq J (2011).Natural products published in 2009 from plants traditionally used to treat malaria. Planta Med. 77:631-640.

Biruniya AL (1993). Recueil des plantes utilisées en médecine traditionnelle Zaïroise. Rev. Méd. Pharm. 9:101-115.

Camacho MDR (1998) Natural Products as sources of antiprotozoal drugs. Curr. Opin. Antiinfect. Investig. Drugs, 2, 47-62.

Camacho MDR, Phillipson, JD, Croft, SL, Solis, PN, Marshall, SJ, Ghazanfar SA (2003). Screening of plant extracts for antiprotozoal and cytotoxic activities. J. Ethnopharmacol. 89:185-191.

Christensen SB, Kharazmi A (2001). Antimalarial natural products. In: Trigali C (Ed.), Bioactive Compounds from Natural Sources. Isolation, Characterization and Biological Properties. Taylor and Francis, NY. pp. 379-342.

Crook MA (2006). Clinical Chemistry and Metabolic Medicine, 7th Edition. Hoker Arnold, London. 426 pp.

Dong SH, Liu YZ, Dongl, Xu CH, Yue JM (2013). Chemical constituents from *Brucea javanica*. Phytochemistry 85:175-174.

Eden DO, Usoh LF (2009). Biochemical changes in Wistar rats and oral doses of Mistletoe (*Loranthus micranthus*) Am. J. Pharm. Toxicol. 4: 94-97.

Feldams BV, Zinkj JG, Jain NC (1997). Scam's Veterinary Hematology, 5th Edition. Les Febiger, Philadelphia. pp. 1210-1218.

Harborne JB (1998). Phytochemical Methods. A guide to modern techniques of plants analysis. Chapman & Hall, London.

Hoet S, Opperdoes F, Brun R, Adjakijé V, Quetin-Leclercq J (2004). *In vitro* antitrypanosomal activity of ethnopharmacologically selected Beninese plants. J. Ethnopharmacol. 91:37-42.

Ismail N, Abdullah H, Janie S, Jamafullail MSS, Ratando B, Seidal V (2012). BP6M rich in flavonoids from the leaves of *Bruceajavanica* shown relatively potent cytotoxic activity in several cancer cell lines. VMT 11th International Annual Symposium in Sustainability Science and Management, Terengaan, Malaysia.

Kennedy GL, Ferems BL, Brugers BA(1986). Estimation of acute toxicity in rats by determination of the approximative lethal dose rather the LD_{50}. J. Appl. Toxicol. 4:145-148.

Kuypers K, Cos P, Ortega-Barria E, Vanden Berghe D, Maes L (2006). Bioassays for some parasitic protozoa, screening concepts and standard *in vitro* and *in vivo* laboratory model. In: MP, Gupta, SS, Handa, K and Vanish, (Eds.), Biological Screening of Plant Constituents. International Centre for Science and High Technology, Trieste. pp. 7-18.

Lee KH, ImakuraY, Seinida Y, Wu RY, Hall IH, Huang HC(1979). Antitumor agents, 33.Isolation and structural elucidation of bruceolide A and B from *Brucea javanica*. J. Org. Chem. 44:2180-2185.

Lima LB, Vasconcelo CFB, Maranha, HMI, Leite VR, Ferreira FA, Andrade BA, Arüjo EI, Xavier HE, Lafayette SSI, Vanderley AA (2009). Acute and subacute toxicity of *Schinus terebinthifolius* bark extract. J. Ethnopharmacol. 126:468-475.

Luka CD, Mohammed A (2012). Evaluation of the antidiabetic property of the aqueous extract of *Mangifera indica* leaf in normal and alloxan induced diabetic rats. J. Nat. Prod. Plants Res. 2:239-249.

Makler MT, Ries JM, Williams JA, Bancroft JE, Piper RC, Gibbins B, Hinrichs DJ (1993). Parasite lactate dehydrogenase as an assay for *Plasmodium falciparum* drug sensitivity. Am. J. Trop. Med. Hyg. 48:739-741,

Marissa A, Indah DD, Banjarnahoor SD., Mrgawati, Tri Yuliani (2012). Acute toxicity of *Brucea javanica* Merril leaves extract on mice. J. Trop. Life Sci. 2:29-31.

Mitscher LA., Park YH, Clark D, Clark III GW (1978). Antimicrobial agents from higher plants. An investigation of *Hunnemannia fumariaefolia* pseudoalcoholates of sanguinarine and chelerythrine. J. Nat. Prod. 41:145-150.

Musuyu Muganza D (2006). Contribution à la revue des plantes médicinales des Nkundaau Sud-Ouest du Parc National de Salonga. Mémoire DEA. Département de Biologie, Faculté des Sciences, Université de Kinshasa, Kinshasa, République Démocratique du Congo.

Neuwinger HD (2002). African Traditional Medicine. A Dictionary of Plant Uses and Application. Medipharm Scientific Publishers, Stuttgart. pp. 318, 379, 42-422.

Ngoma B, Bikengeli M (1993). Therapeutic Application of *Brucea sumatrana* Roxb. (Simaroubaceae). Al-Birunya 9:101-108.

Okoli CO, Ibiam AF, Ezike AC, Akali PA, Ekoye TC (2010). Evaluation of potientials of *Phyllanthus niruri* in alloxan diabetic rats. Afr. J. Biotechnol. 9:248-259.

O'Neill MJ, Bray DH, Boardman P, Phillip son JD, Warhurst DC (1985). Plants as sources of antimalarial drugs. Part. 1. *In vitro* test method for the evaluation of crude extracts from plants. Planta Med. 5:394-398.

O'Neill MJ, Bray DH, Boardman P, Chan KI, Phillipson, JD, Warhurst D, Peters W (1987). Plants as a source of antimalarial drugs Part 4: Activity of *Brucea javanica* fruits against chloroquine-resistant *Plasmodium falciparum in vitro* and against *Plasmodium bergheiberghei*. J. Nat. Prod. 50:41-48.

Pavanand K, Nutakul W, Dechatiwongse T, Yoshi-Hira K, Yongvanitchit K., Scovill JP, Flippen-Anderson LL, Gilardi R, George C, Kanchanapee P, Webster HK (1986). *In Vitro* Antimalarial Activity of *Brucea javanica* against Multidrug Resistant *Plasmodium falciparum*. Planta Med. 52:108-111.

Pieme CA, Penlap VN, Nkegdum A, Taziebou CL, Tekuvu EM, Eto FX, Ngongan J (2006). Evaluation of acute and subacutetoxicity of aqueous ethanolic extract of leaves of *Sennaalata* (L.) Roxb (Cesalpiniaceae). Afr. J. Biotechnol. 5:283-289.

Subeki H, Matssura K, Tabahashi K, Nabeta K, Ya-Masaki M, Maede Y, Katakura K (2007). Screening of Indonesian medicinal plant extracts for antibabesial activity and isolation of new quassinoids from *Brucea javanica*. J. Nat. Prod. 70:1654-1657.

Sawangjaroen N, Sawangjaroen, K (2005). The effect of extracts from anti-diarrheic Thai medicinal plants on the *in vitro* growth of the intestinal protozoa parasite *Blastocytis hominis*. J. Ethnopharmacol. 98:67-72.

The Organization Economic Co-operation and Development (OECD) (2001). The OECD Guidelines for the Testing Chemical 420 acute oral toxicity. OECD, Paris. pp. 1-14.

Tshodi EM, Mbenza PA, Nsaka LS, Kikweta MC, Bakana PD, TonaLG, Kambu KO, Cimanga KR, Matheussen A, Cos P, Apers S, Pieters L, Maes L, Vlietinck AJ (2012). *In vitro* antiprotozoal and cytotoxic activity of the aqueous extract, the 80% methanol extract and its fractions from the seeds of *Brucea sumatrana* Roxb. (Simaroubaceae) growing in Democratic Republic of Congo. Chin. Med. 3:65-71.

Vasudevan MM, Sreekumari S (2005). Textbook of Biochemistry (For Medical Students), 4th Edition, Jaygne Brothers Medical Publishers (P) Ltd. New Delhi, India. pp. 502-503.

Wasan MM, Najaph S, Wong T, Kwong M (2001). Assessing plasma lipid levels body weight and hepatic and renal toxicity following chronic and administration of water soluble physkand compound FM-VP4 to gerbih. J. Pharm. Sci. 4:228-234

Wright CW, O'Neill MJ, Phillipson JD, Warhurst DC (1988). Use of microdilution to assess *in vitro* antiamoebic activities of *Brucea javanica* fruits, *Simarouba amara*, stem and a number of quassinoids. Antimicrob. Agents Chemother. 22:1725-1729.

Wright CW, Anderson MM, Allen D, Phillipson JD, Kirby GC, Warhurst DC, Chang HR.(1993). Quassinoids exhibit greater selectivity against *Plasmodium falciparum* than against *Entamoeba histolytica*, *Giardia intestinalis* and *Toxoplasma gondii in vitro*. J. Eukaryot. Microbiol. 40:244-246.

Wright CW, Allen D, Cai Y, Chen Z, Phillipson JD, Kirby GC, Warhurst DC, Tits M, Angensot L (1994). Selectivity antiprotozoal activity of some alkaloids. Phytother. Res.8:149-152.

14

Analysis of bioactive chemical compounds of *Aspergillus niger* by using gas chromatography-mass spectrometry and fourier-transform infrared spectroscopy

Imad Hadi Hameed*, Lena Fadhil Hamza and Sabreen A. Kamal

Department of Molecular Biology, Babylon University, Hilla City, Iraq.

Bioactives are chemical compounds often referred to as secondary metabolites. Thirty five bioactive compounds were identified in the methanolic extract of *Aspergillus niger*. The identification of bioactive chemical compounds is based on the peak area, retention time molecular weight and molecular formula. Gas chromatography-mass spectrometry (GC-MS) analysis of *Aspergillus niger* revealed the existence of the 6-Acetyl-ß-d-mannose, 4-[Dichloromethyl]-2-[[2-[1-methyl-2-pyrrolidinyl]ethyl]amino-6-trichloro, 2-Furan-carboxaldehyde,5-methyl, 2,2,2-Trifluoro-N-[2-(1-hydroxy-2,2,6,6-tetramethyl-piperidin-4-yl), 2,4-Dihydroxy-2,5-dimethyl-3(2H)-furan-3-one, HEPES (4-(2-hydroxyethyl)-1-piperazineethanesulfonic acid), Tetraacetyl-d-xylonic nitrile, Eicosanoic acid, phenylmethyl ester, Dodecanoic acid, 3-hydroxy, Desulphosinigrin, Glycyl-dl-serine, 2,5-Dimethyl-4-hydroxy-3(2H)-furanone, 2,5-Furandicarboxaldehyde, 2H-Oxecin-2-one,3,4,7,8,9,10- hexahydro-4-hydroxy-10-methyl, 6-Acetyl-ß-d-mannose, DL-Leucine, N-glycyl, 4H-Pyran-4-one,2,3-dihydro-3,5-dihydroxy-6-methyl, l-Gala-l-ido-octonic lactone, 2H-Pyran,tetrahydro-2-(12-pentadecynyloxy), 5-Hydroxymethylfurfural, Strychane,1-acetyl-20α-hydroxy-16-methylene, α-D-Glucopyranoside, O-α-D-glucopyranosyl-(1.fwdarw.3)ß-D-fru, Boroxin, tris(2,3-dimethylbut-2-yl), 16-Nitrobicyclo[10.4.0]hexadecane-1-ol-13-one, 3-[3-Bromophenyl]-7-chloro-3,4-dihydro-10-hydroxy-1,9(2H,10H)-a, Uric acid, 1,2,4-Trioxolane-2-octanoic acid ,5-octyl-,methyl ester, Tetraacetyl-d-xylonic nitrile, 1,2-Cyclopentanedicarboxylic acid, 4-(1,1-dimethylethyl)-,dimethyl, 2-Bromotetradecanoic acid, i-Propyl 11,12-methylene-octadecanoate, 1H-2,8a-Methanocyclopenta[a]cyclopropa [e]cyclodecan-11-one, and Octadecanoic acid. The FTIR analysis of *A. niger* proved the presence of aromatic rings, alkenes, aliphatic fluoro compounds, tetiary amine, C-N stretch, aromatic nitro compounds, ammonium ions and organic nitrate which shows major peaks at 696.30, 744.52, 821.68, 844.82, 900.76, 931.62, 1026.13, 1145.72, 1207.44, 1234.44, 1261.45, 1315.45, 1359.82, 1377.17, 1413.82, 1452.40, 1631.78, 1741.72, 2924.09, 3118.90, 3217.27 and 3271.27. *Datura stramonium* was very active against *A. niger*. Methanolic extract of bioactive compounds of *A. niger* were assayed for *in vitro* antibacterial activity against *Pseudomonas aerogenosa, Escherichia coli, Proteus mirabilis, Staphylococcus aureus* and *Klebsiella pneumonia* by using the diffusion method in agar. The zones of inhibition were compared with different standard antibiotics. The diameters of inhibition zones ranged from 0.46±0.1 to 6.52±0.61 mm for all treatments.

Key words: *Aspergillus niger*, bioactive compounds, gas chromatography-mass spectrometry, fourier-transform infrared spectroscopy.

INTRODUCTION

Aspergillus spp are ubiquitous opportunistic moulds that cause both allergic and invasive syndromes. The genus comprises approximately 180 species, of which 33 have been associated with human disease (Segal et al., 1998; Perfect et al., 2001). *Aspergillus niger* is the third most common species associated with invasive pulmonary aspergillosis (Bellini et al., 2003; Anupama et al., 2007). *A. niger* has a great economical and biotechnological interest and is extensively used for production of extracellular enzymes and organic acids such as citric acid (Baker, 2006; Perrone et al., 2007; Mogensen et al., 2010). It also produces fumonisin B2 (FB2) along with OTA. 9, 19, 27. Fumonisins are suspected to cause human and animal toxicoses, and are regarded as carcinogenic (Susca et al., 2010; Chacko et al., 2012; Gebreselema et al., 2013). A culture yielding *Aspergillus* spp, in addition to enabling a diagnosis of invasive aspergillosis, may further define therapeutic options via susceptibility testing or the isolation of a species possessing inherent antifungal resistance; examples of the latter include *Aspergillus terreus* and *Aspergillus nidulans*, which are both resistant to amphotericin B (Walsh, 2004). The main disadvantage of culture is that it is relatively slow (the process takes days), is relatively insensitive, and requires specialized expertise for species determination.

In common with other pathogenic fungi, the ability to grow at 37°C distinguishes *Aspergillus* spp from other nonpathogenic environmental moulds. *Aspergillus* spp can be recovered on most routine solid and liquid microbiological media (example, blood agar, chocolate agar, brain heart infusion broth). A fungal-specific medium example, sabouraud dextrose agar should be included at the time of initial specimen set-up in clinical scenarios in which *Aspergillus* spp (or other moulds) are considered possible pathogens, because of superior yield (Horvath and Dummer, 1995). The addition of antibiotics example, chloramphenicol and gentamicin to the medium is required for the recovery of *Aspergillus* spp from specimens obtained from nonsterile sites, since they prevent bacterial overgrowth. Cycloheximide, a eukaryotic protein synthesis inhibitor, is frequently added to fungal media to inhibit the overgrowth of cultures by non-pathogenic environmental moulds; however, on occasion, cycloheximide may inhibit the growth of *Aspergillus* spp. The aim of this study were analysis of the secondary metabolites and the evaluation of antibacterial and antifungal activity .

MATERIALS AND METHODS

Collection and growth condition

A. niger was isolated from dried fruit and the pure colonies were selected, isolated and maintained in potato dextrose agar slants (Usha and Masilamani, 2013). After the species were identified by the identification key, spores were grown in a liquid culture of potato dextrose broth (PDB) and incubated at 25°C in a shaker for 16 days at 130 rpm.

Production, extraction and determination of metabolites

The metabolites were determined and extracted for gas chromatography (GC) analysis using the method of Siddiquee et al. (2012) with some modifications. The extraction was performed by adding 25 ml methanol to 100 ml liquid culture in an Erlenmeyer flask after the infiltration of the culture. The mixture was incubated at 4°C for 10 min, and then shook for 10 min at 130 rpm. Metabolites was separated from the liquid culture and evaporated to dryness with a rotary evaporator at 45°C. The residue was dissolved in 1 ml methanol, filtered through a 0.2 µm syringe filter, and stored at 4°C for 24 h before being used for gas chromatography–mass spectrometry (GC-MS) (Imad et al., 2014a). The identification of the components was based on comparison of their mass spectra with those of NIST mass spectral library as well as on comparison of their retention indices either with those of authentic compounds or with literature values.

GC-MS analysis

Bioactive compound were examined for the chemical composition using GC-MS (Agilent 789N) equipped with a DB-5MS column (30 m×0.25 mm i.d., 0.25 um film thickness, J&W Scientific, Folsom, CA). The oven temperature was programmed as for the previous analysis (Imad et al., 2015a; Muhanned et al., 2015). Helium was used as the carrier gas at the rate of 1.0 ml/min. Effluent of the GC column was introduced directly into the source of the MS via a transfer line (250°C). Ionization voltage was 70 eV and ion source temperature was 230°C. Scan range was 41 to 450 amu. The constituents were identified after being compared with available data in the GC-MS library in the literatures (Imad et al., 2015b; Mohammed et al., 2013).

Fourier transform infrared spectrophotometer (FTIR)

The powdered sample of the *A. niger* specimen was treated for fourier transform infrared spectroscopy (Shimadzu, IR Affinity 1, Japan). The sample was run at infrared region between 400 nm and 4000 nm.

Determination of antibacterial activity of crude fraction of *A. niger* compounds

The test pathogens (*E. coli, Pseudomonas aeruginosa, Klebsiella pneumoniae* and *Staphylococcus aureus)* were swabbed in Muller Hinton agar plates. 90µl of fungal extracts was loaded on the bored wells. The wells were bored in 0.5cm in diameter. The plates were incubated at 37°C for 24 h and examined. After the incubation the diameter of inhibition zones around the discs was measured.

*Corresponding author. E-mail: imad_dna@yahoo.com.

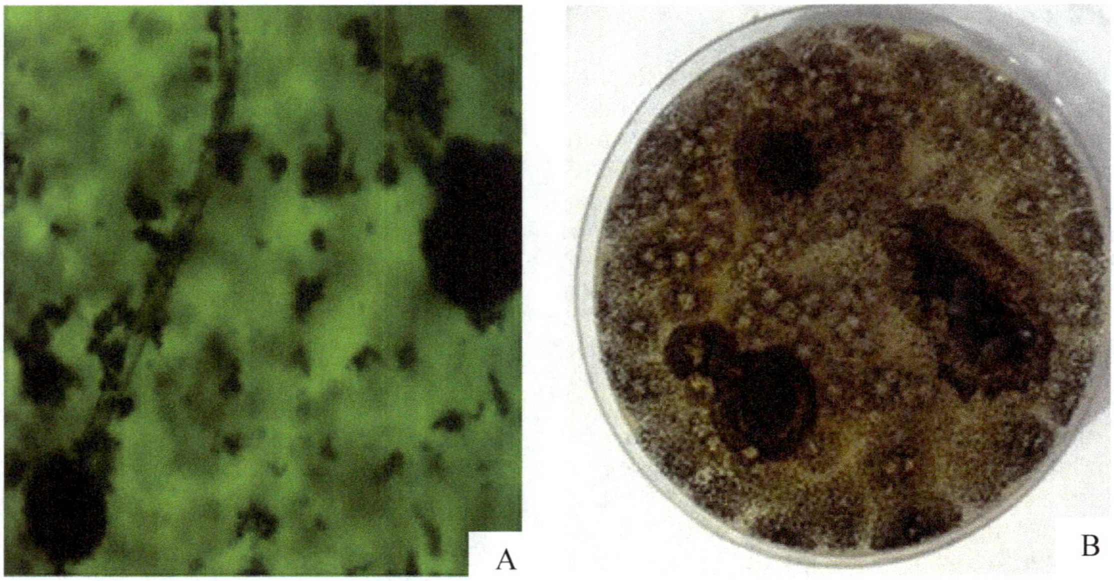

Figure 1. Morphological characterization of *Aspergillus niger*. (B) Microscopic observation (A) colony.

Determination of antifungal activity

A. niger isolate was suspended in potato dextrose broth and diluted to approximately 105 colony forming unit (CFU) per ml. They were "flood inoculated onto the surface of Potato dextrose agar and then dried. Standard agar well diffusion method was followed (Perez et al., 1990; Perez et al., 1999; Erdemogllu et al., 2003; Bagamboula et al., 2004). Five-millimeter diameter wells were cut from the agar using a sterile cork-borer, and 25 µl of the samples solutions (*Nerium olender, Ricinus communis, Datura stramonium*, *Linum usitatissimum*, *Anastatica hierochuntica* and *Gramineae poaceae*) were delivered into the wells. The plates were incubated for 48 h at room temperature (Huda et al., 2015a; Ameera et al., 2015; Imad et al., 2015c). Antimicrobial activity was evaluated by measuring the zone of inhibition against the test microorganisms. Methanol was used as solvent control. Amphotericin B and fluconazole were used as reference antifungal agent (Anesini and Perez, 1993; Rukayadi et al., 2006; Huda et al., 2015b). The tests were carried out in triplicate. The antifungal activity was evaluated by measuring the inhibition-zone diameter observed after 48 h of incubation.

Statistical analysis

Data were analyzed using analysis of variance (ANOVA), and differences among the means were determined for significance at $P < 0.05$ using Duncan's multiple range test (by statistical package for the social sciences (SPSS) software) Version 9.1 (Imad et al., 2014b).

RESULTS AND DISCUSSION

Isolation of fungi from dried fruit

The fungi were isolated from dried fruit by serial dilution method. Based on morphological, characteristics of fungi was isolated in selective media of potato dextrose agar media. Morphological, Microscopical and microscopical characteristics of fungal strains were determined using specific media light and compound microscope Figure 1.

Production and Identification of secondary metabolites from the methanolic crude extract of *A. niger* by gas chromatography and mass spectrometry and fourier-transform infrared spectroscopy

The 400 ml of fermentation broth (PDA broth) which contain 200 µl of the standardized fugal suspensions were used to inoculate the flasks and incubated at 37°C on a shaker at 90 rpm for 7 days. After fermentation, the secondary metabolites were produced by isolated microorganisms.

Gas chromatography and mass spectroscopy analysis of compounds was carried out in methanolic extract of *A. niger*, as shown in Table 1. The GC-MS chromatogram of the seventeen peaks of the compounds detected was shown in Figure 2. Chromatogram GC-MS analysis of the methanol extract of *A. niger* showed the presence of twenty major peaks and the components corresponding to the peaks were determined as follows. The First set up peak were determined to be 6-Acetyl-ß-d-mannose (Figure 3). The second peak indicated to be 4-[Dichloromethyl]-2-[[2-[1-methyl-2-pyrrolidinyl]ethylamino-6-trichloro (Figure 4). The next peaks considered to be 2-Furan-carboxaldehyde, 5-methyl, 2,2,2-Trifluoro-N-[2-(1-hydroxy-2,2,6,6-tetramethyl-piperidin-4-yl), 2,4-Dihydroxy-2,5-dimethyl-3(2H)-furan-3-one, HEPES, Tetraacetyl-d-xylonic nitrile, eicosanoic acid, phenylmethyl ester, dodecanoic acid , 3-hydroxy, Desulphosinigrin,

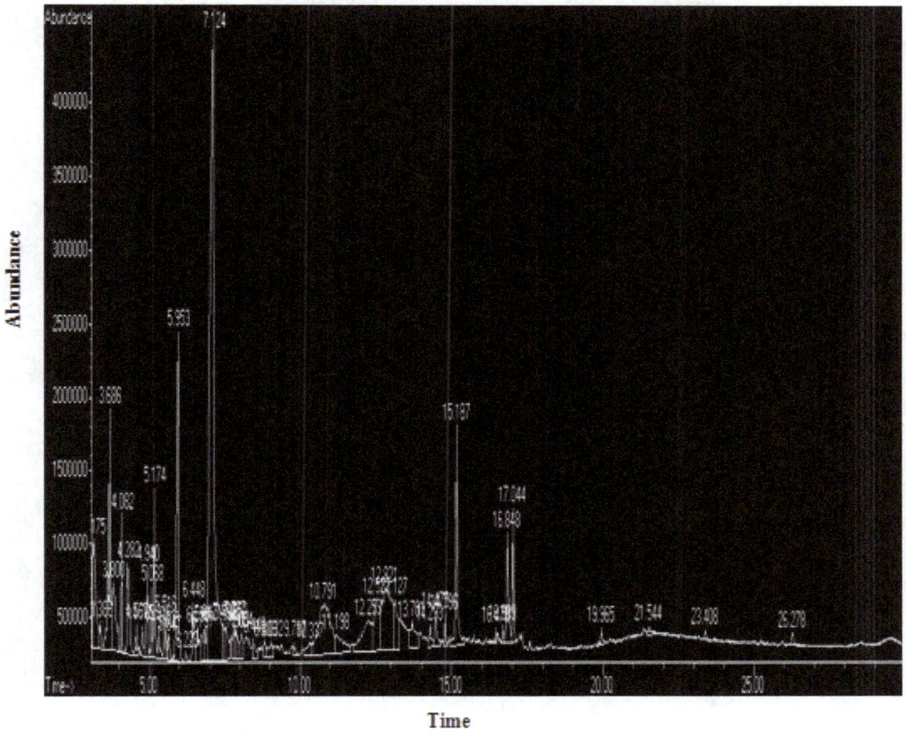

Figure 2. GC-MS chromatogram of methanolic extract of *A. niger.*

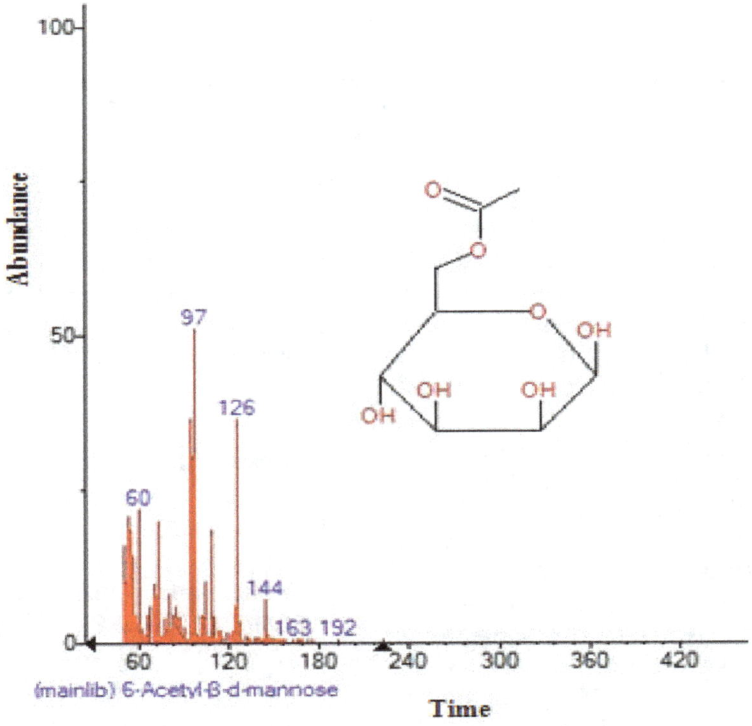

Figure 3. Mass spectrum of 6-Acetyl-ß-d-mannose with Retention Time (RT)= 3.201.

Glycyl-dl-serine, 2,5-Dimethyl-4 -hydroxy-3(2H)-furanone, 2,5-Furandicarboxaldehyde, 2H-oxecine-2-one, 3,4,7,8,9

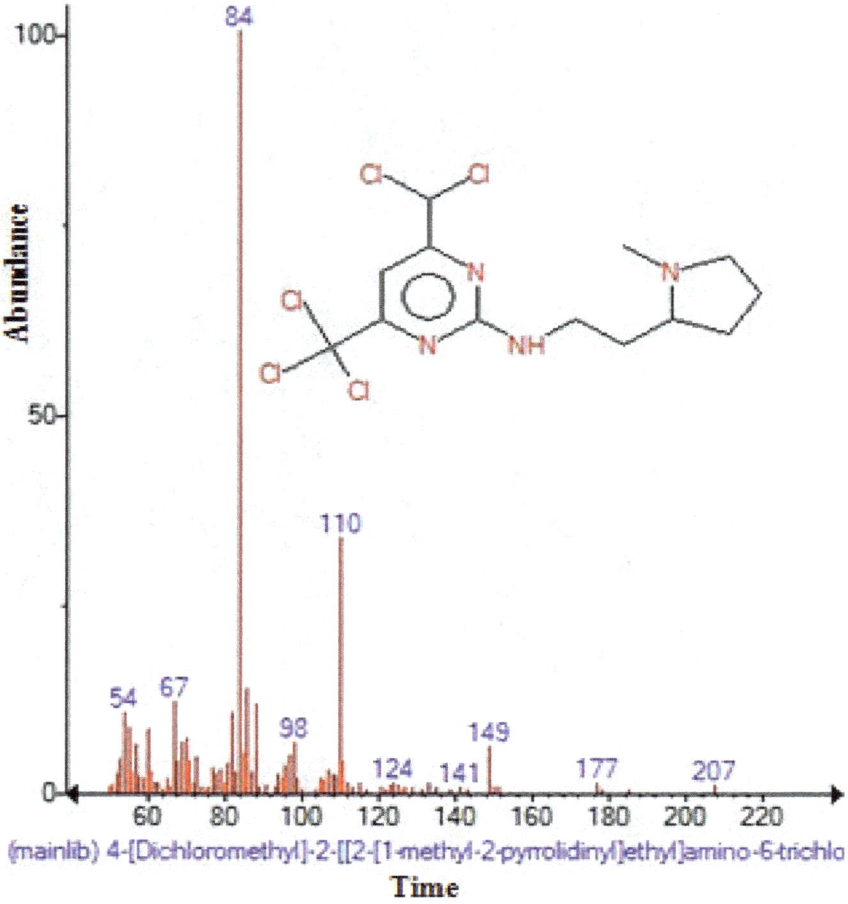

Figure 4. Mass spectrum of 4-[Dichloromethyl]-2-[[2-[1-methyl-2-pyrrolidinyl]ethyl]amino-6-trichloro with Retention Time (RT)= 3.613.

10-hexahydro-4-hydroxy-10-methyl, 6-Acetyl-ß-d-mannose, DL-Leucine, N-glycyl, 4H-Pyran-4-one,2,3-dihydro-3,5-dihydroxy-6-methyl, l-Gala-l-ido-octonic lactone, 2H-Pyran,tetrahydro-2-(12-pentadecynyloxy), 5-Hydroxymethylfurfural, Strychane,1-acetyl-20α-hydroxy-16-methylene, α-D-Glucopyranoside, O-α-D-glucopyranosyl-(1.fwdarw.3)ß-D-fru, Boroxin, tris (2,3-dimethylbut-2-yl), 16-Nitrobicyclo[10.4.0]hexadecane-1-ol-13-one, 3-[3-Bromophenyl]-7-chloro-3,4-dihydro-10-hydroxy-1,9(2H,10H)-a, Uric acid, 1,2,4-Trioxolane-2-octanoic acid ,5-octyl-,methyl ester, Tetraacetyl-d-xylonic nitrile, 1,2-Cyclopentanedicarboxylic acid ,4-(1,1-dimethylethyl)-,dimethyl, 2-Bromotetradecanoic acid, i-Propyl 11,12-methylene-octadecanoate, 1H-2,8a-Metha-nocyclopenta[a]cyclopropa[e]cyclodecan-11-one and Octadecanoic acid (Figures 5 to 34). Many compounds are identified in the present study. Some of them are biological compounds with antimicrobial activities.

Fourier-transform infrared analysis of dry methanolic extract of *A. niger* proved the presence of aromatic rings, alkenes, aliphatic fluoro compounds, alcohols, ethers, carboxlic acids, esters, nitro compounds, aldehydes, ketones, alkanes, hydrogen bonded alcohols and phenols compounds shows major peaks at 894.97, 927.76, 1024.20, 1236.37, 1317.38, 1608.63, 2306.86, 2850.79, 2922.16, 3184.48, 3277.06 and 3292.49, respectively. (Table 2 and Figure 35).

Antibacterial activity

Four clinical pathogens selected for antibacterial activity namely, *k. pneumoniae, P. aeroginosa, E. coli, S. aeureus.* and maximum zone formation against *k. pneumonia* (Table 3 and Figure 36).

Antifungal activity

Each extract plant showed notable antifungal activities against *A. niger* (Figure 37). In agar well diffusion method the selected medicinal plants (*N. olender, R. communis, D. stramonium*, *L. usitatissimum*, *A. hierochuntica* and *G.*

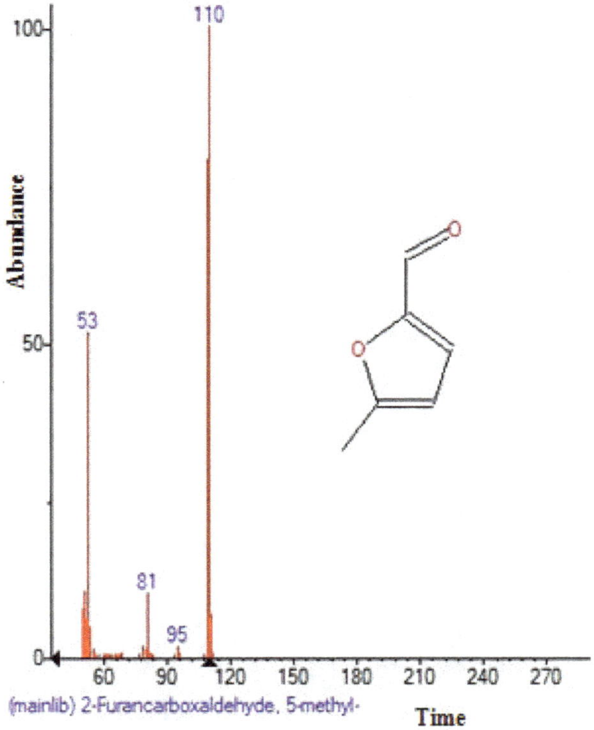

Figure 5. Mass spectrum of 2-Furancarboxaldehyde,5-methyl with Retention Time (RT)= 3.722.

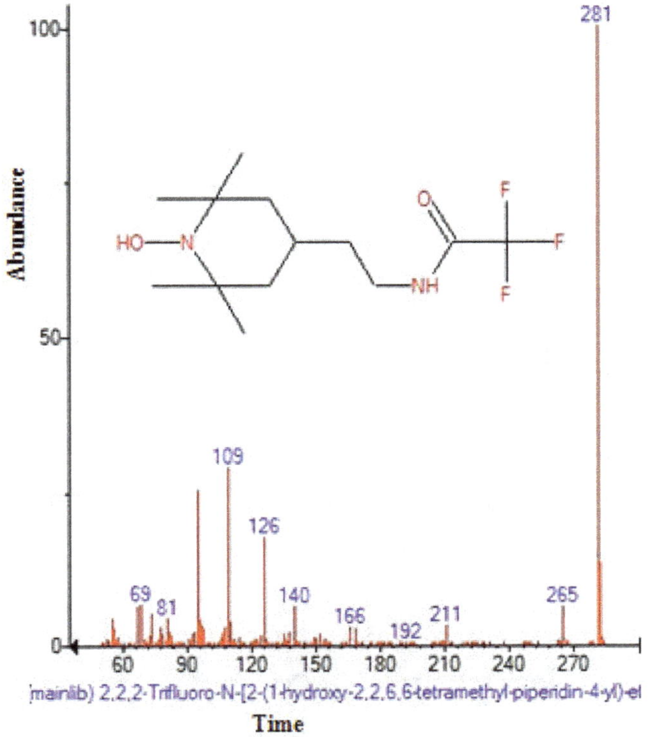

Figure 6. Mass spectrum of 2,2,2-Trifluoro-N-[2-(1-hydroxy-2,2,6,6-tetramethyl-piperidin-4-yl)-el with Retention Time (RT)= 3.779.

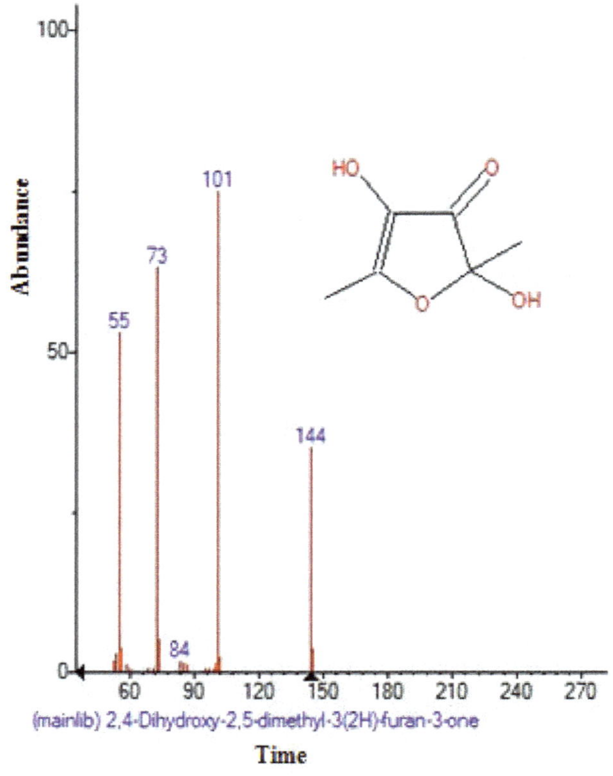

Figure 7. Mass spectrum of 2,4-Dihydroxy-2,5-dimethyl-3(2H)-furan-3-one with Retention Time (RT)= 4.076.

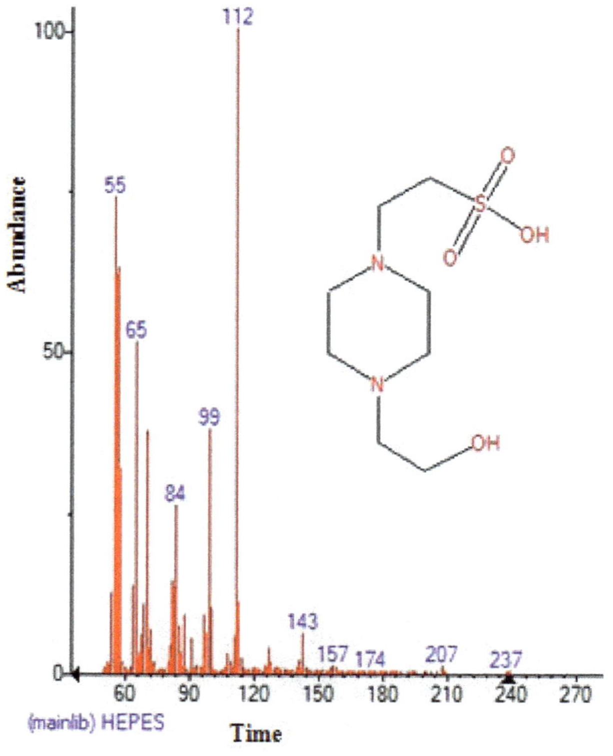

Figure 8. Mass spectrum of 2 HEPES with Retention Time (RT)= 4.271.

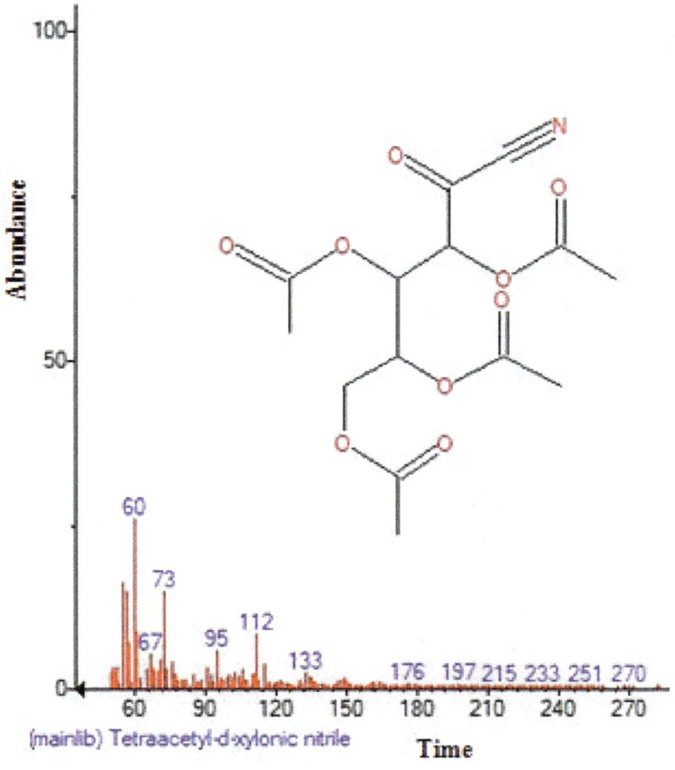

Figure 9. Mass spectrum of Tetraacetyl-d-xylonic nitrile with Retention Time (RT)= 4.465.

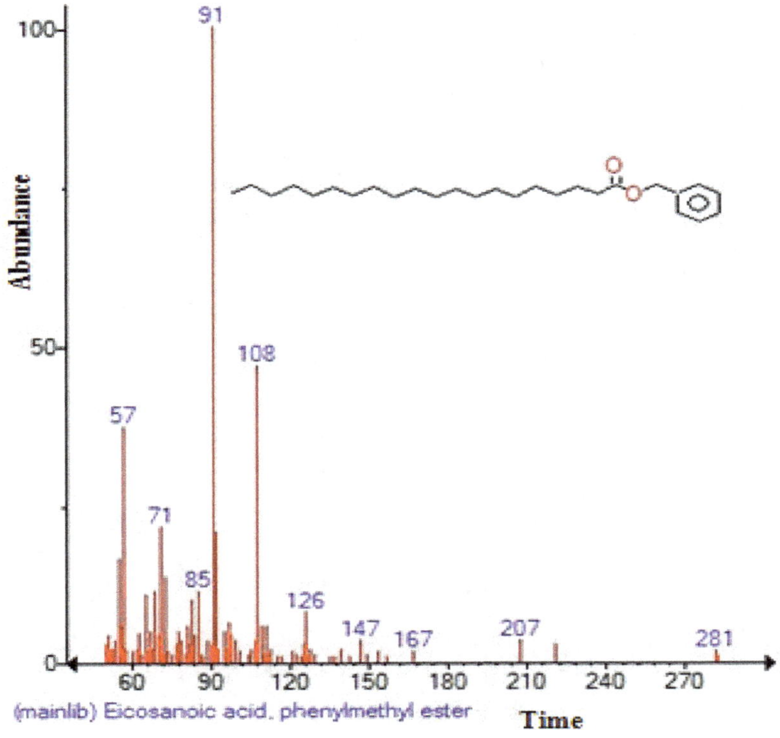

Figure 10. Mass spectrum of eicosanoic acid , phenylmethyl ester with retention time (RT)= 4.546.

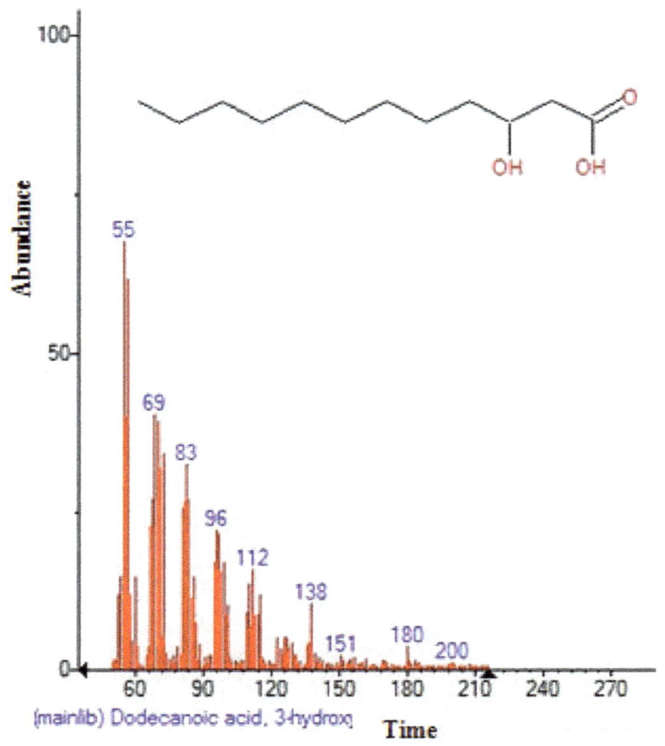

Figure 11. Mass spectrum of dodecanoic acid , 3-hydroxy with retention time (RT)= 4.574.

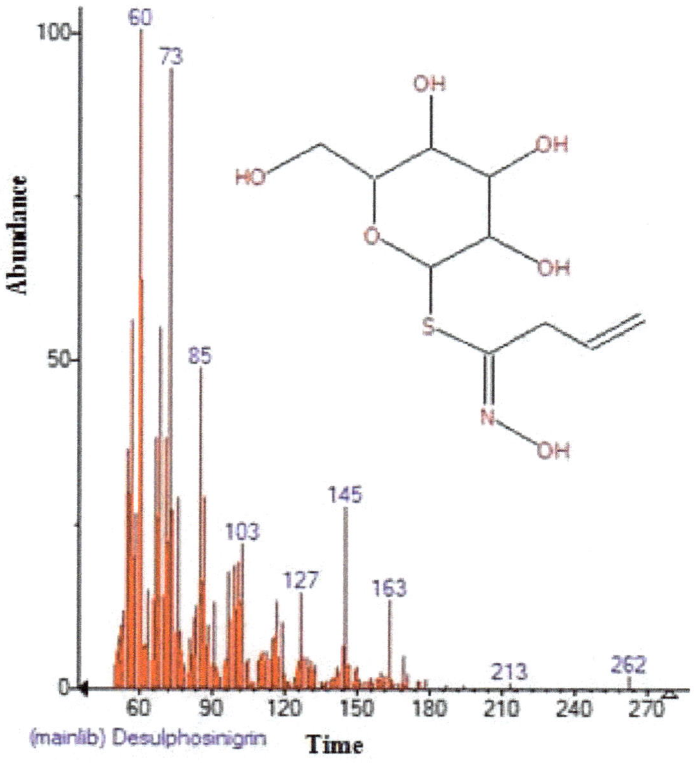

Figure 12. Mass spectrum of desulphosinigrin with retention time (RT)= 4.654.

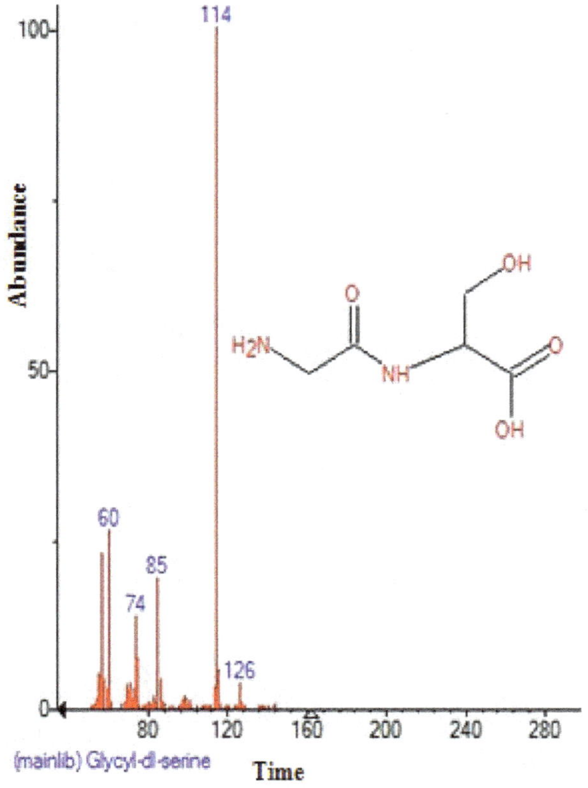

Figure 13. Mass spectrum of Glycyl-dl-serine with retention time (RT)= 4.763.

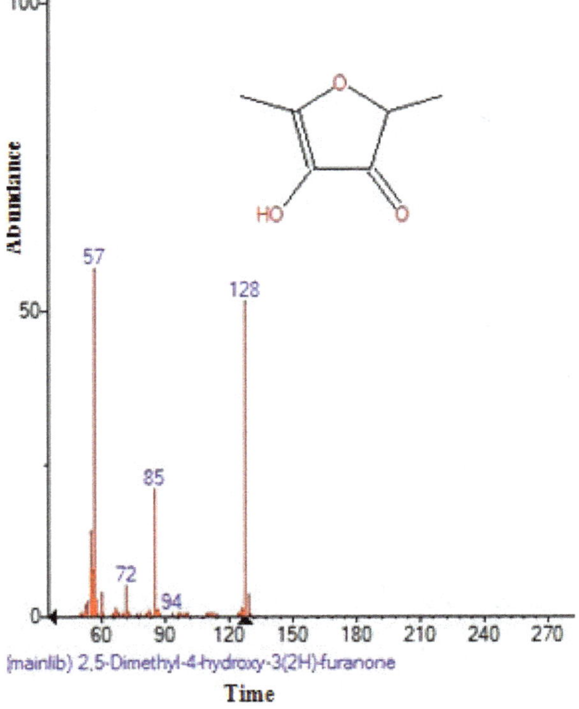

Figure 14. Mass spectrum of 2,5-Dimethyl-4-hydroxy-3(2H)-furanone with retention time (RT)= 4.929.

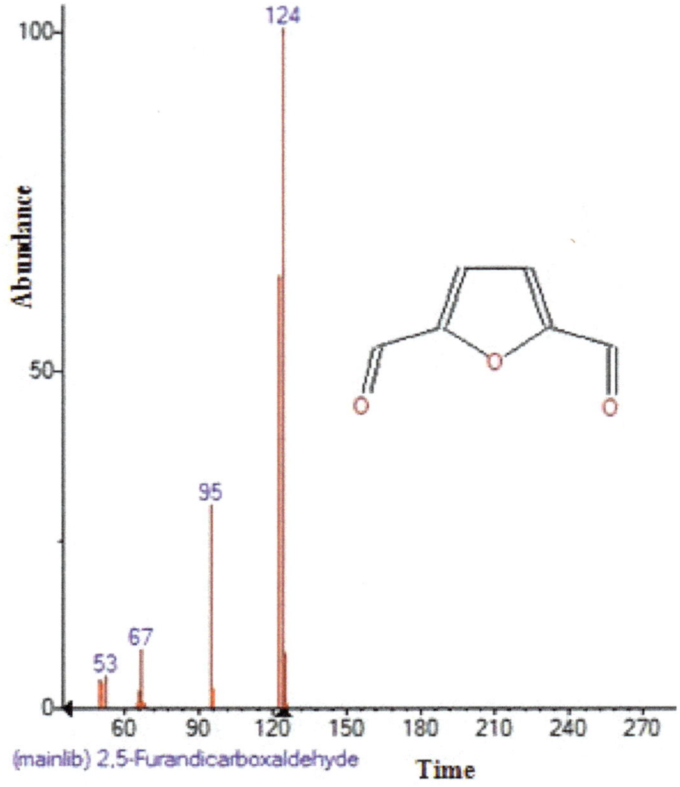

Figure 15. Mass spectrum of 2,5-Furandicarboxaldehyde with retention time (RT)= 5.066.

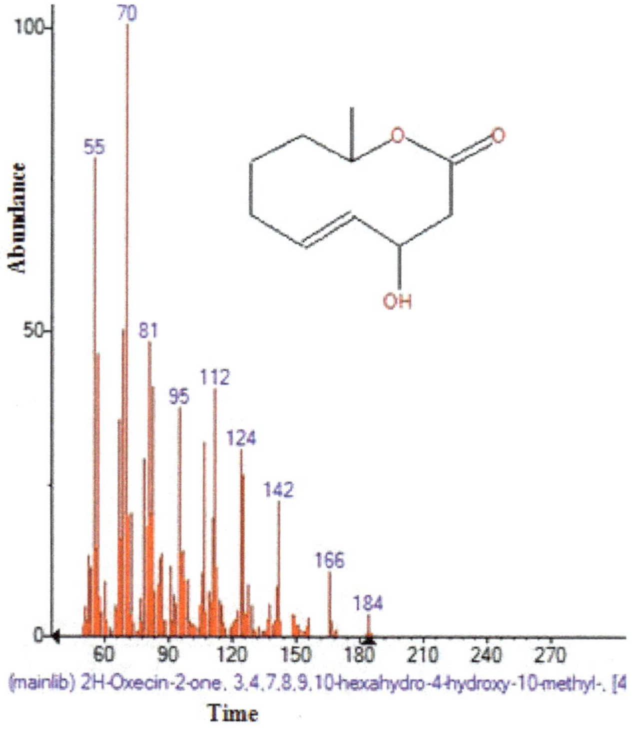

Figure 16. Mass spectrum of 2H-Oxecin-2-one,3,4,7,8,9,10-hexahydro-4-hydroxy-10-methyl-,[4 with retention time (RT)= 5.261.

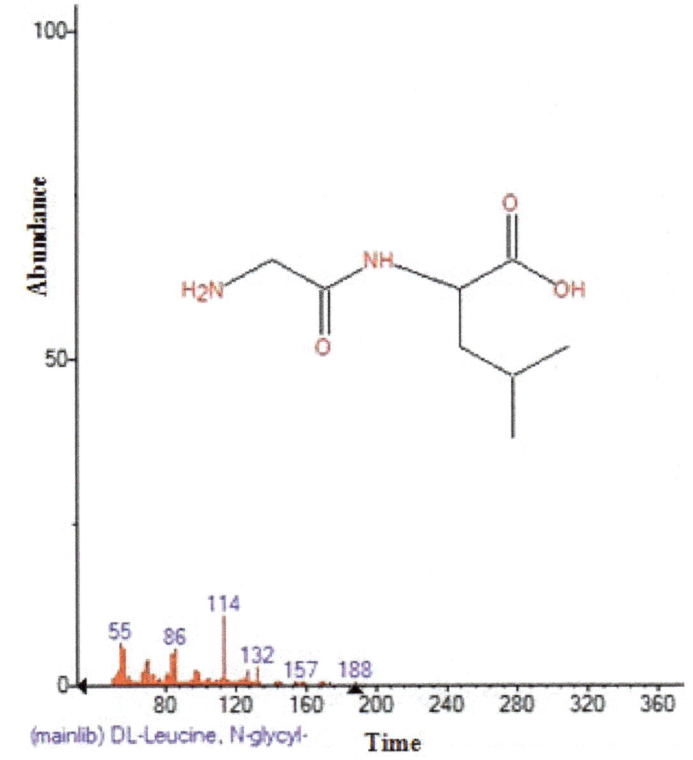

Figure 17. Mass spectrum of DL-Leucine , N-glycyl with retention time (RT)= 5.616.

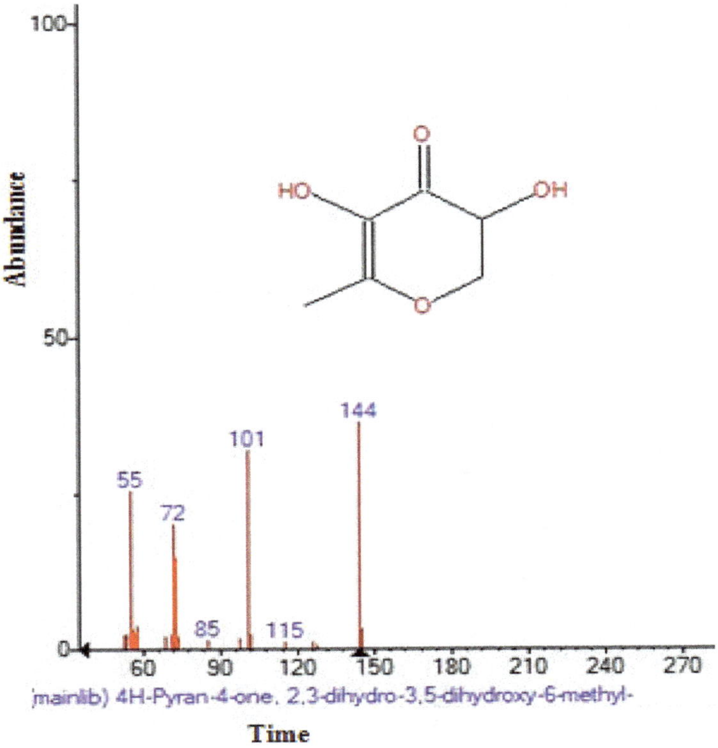

Figure 18. Mass spectrum of 4H-Pyran-4-one,2,3-dihydro-3,5-dihydroxy-6-methyl with retention time (RT)= 5.942.

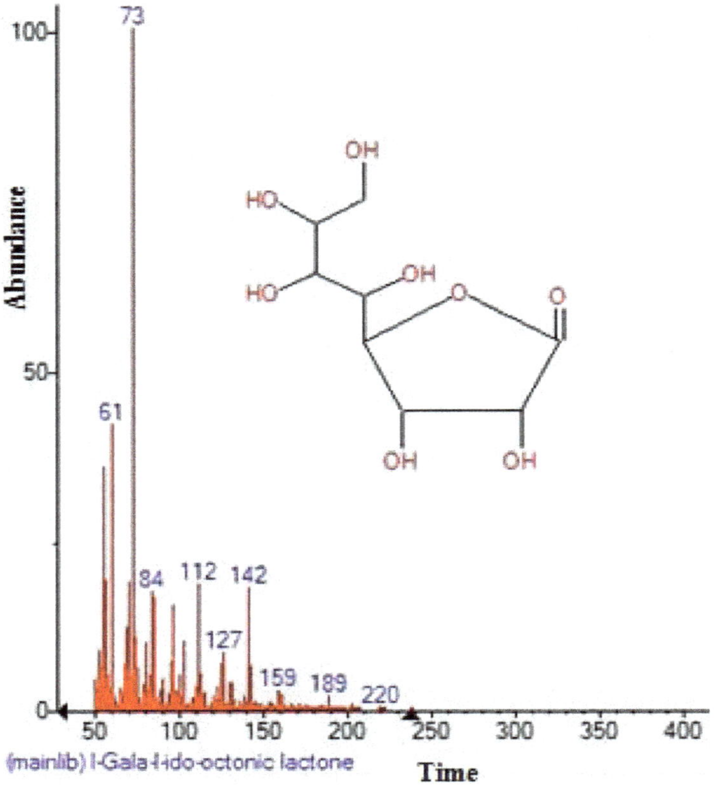

Figure 19. Mass spectrum of l-Gala-l-ido-octonic lactone with retention time (RT)= 6.577.

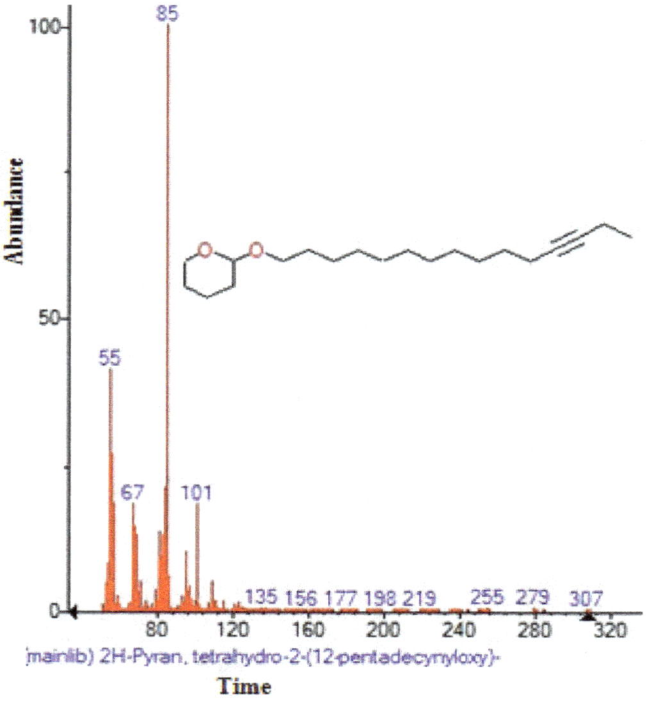

Figure 20. Mass spectrum of 2H-Pyran,tetrahydro-2-(12-pentadecynyloxy) with retention time (RT)= 6.737.

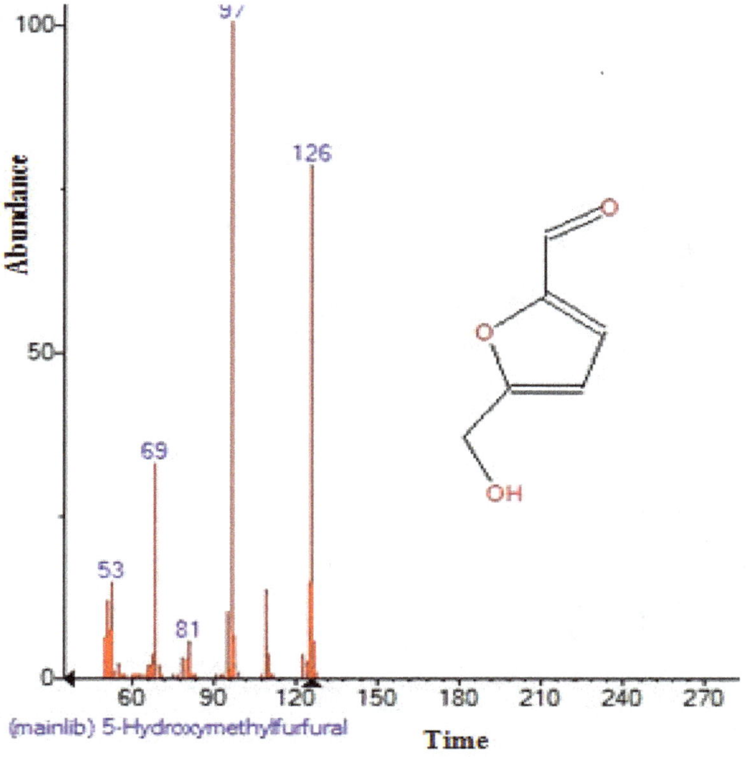

Figure 21. Mass spectrum of 5-Hydroxymethylfurfural with retention time (RT)= 7.120.

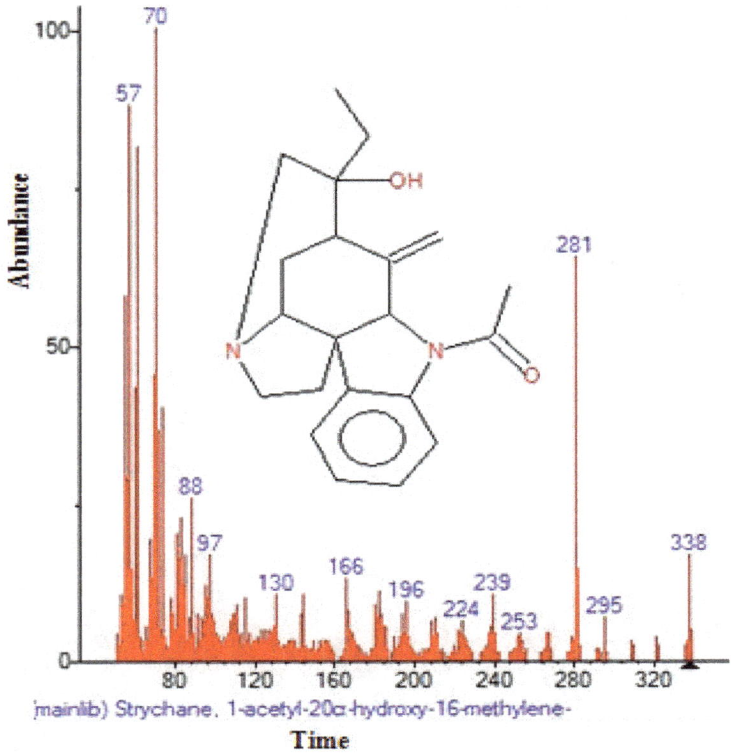

Figure 22. Mass spectrum of Strychane,1-acetyl-20α-hydroxy-16-methylene with retention time (RT)= 8.053.

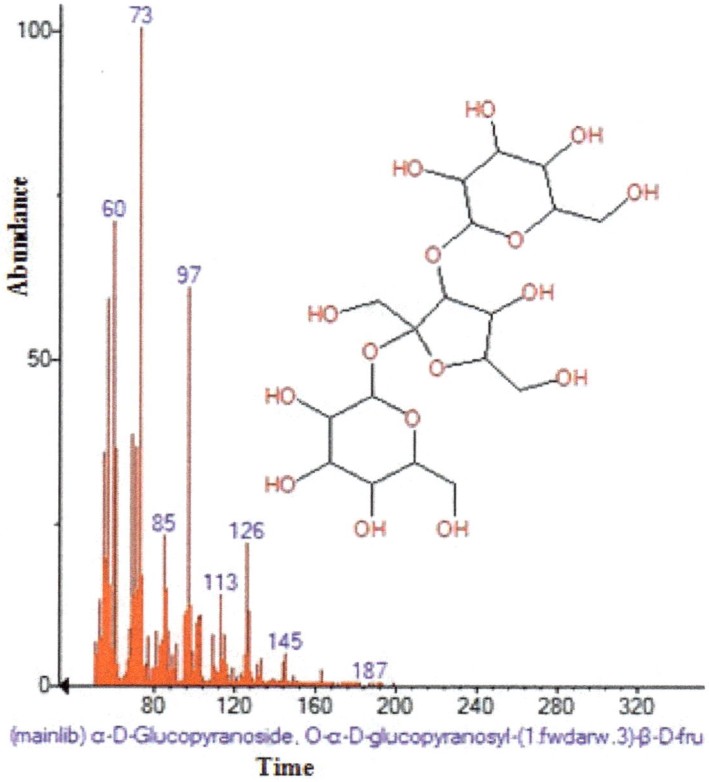

Figure 23. Mass spectrum of α-D-Glucopyranoside ,O-α-D-glucopyranosyl-(1.fwdarw.3)ß-D-fru with retention time (RT)= 7.836.

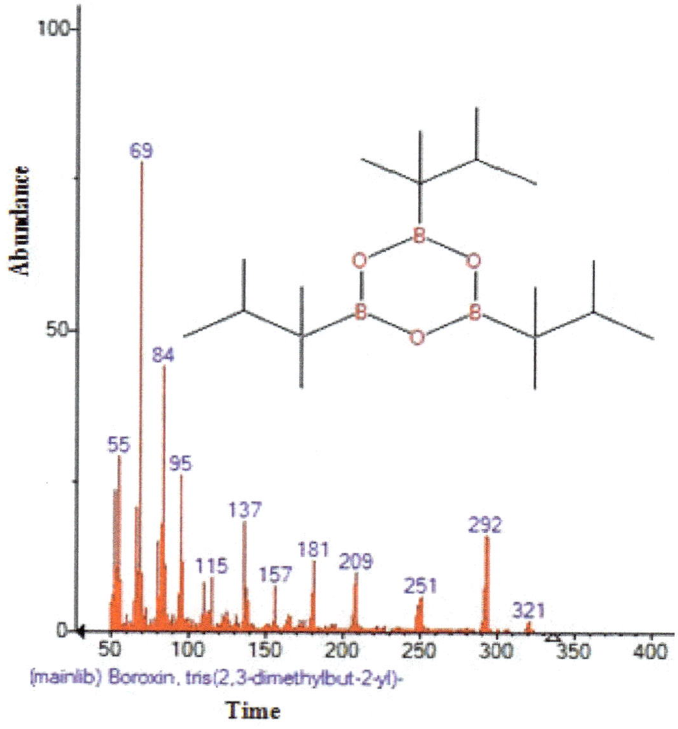

Figure 24. Mass spectrum of Boroxin , tris(2,3-dimethylbut-2-yl) with retention time (RT)= 8.442.

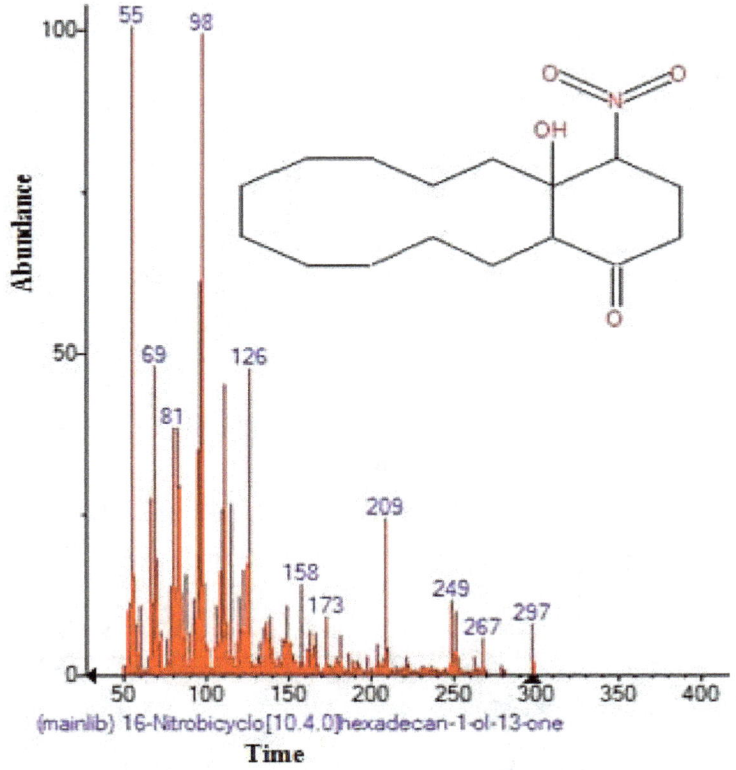

Figure 25. Mass spectrum of 16-Nitrobicyclo[10.4.0]hexadecane-1-ol-13-one with retention time (RT)= 8.797.

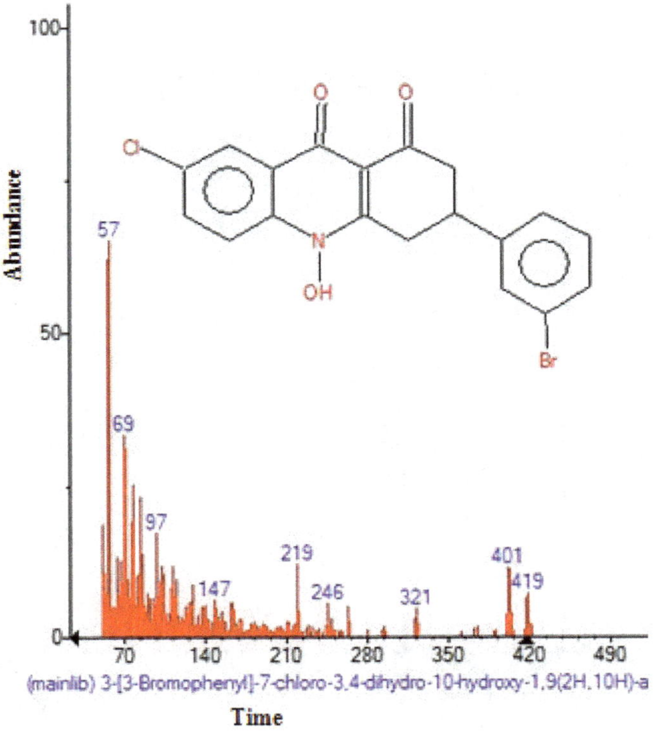

Figure 26. Mass spectrum of 3-[3-Bromophenyl]-7-chloro-3,4-dihydro-10-hydroxy-1,9(2H,10H)-a with retention time (RT)= 9.043.

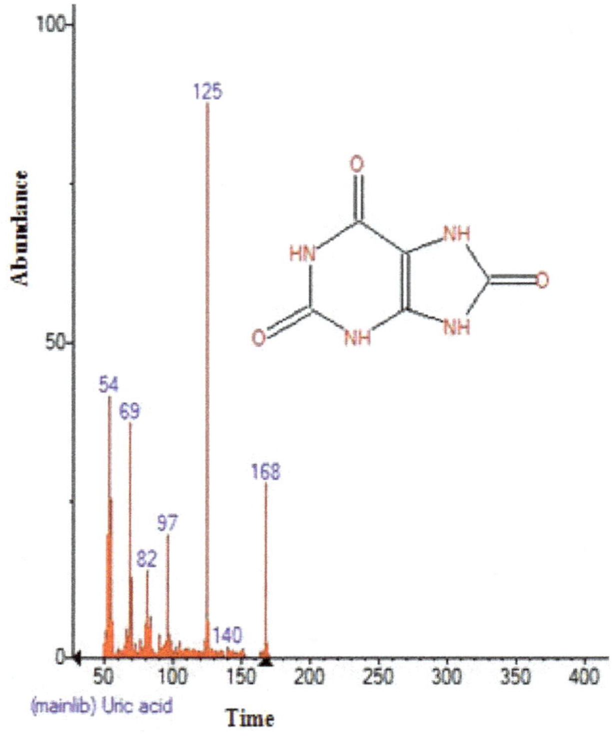

Figure 27. Mass spectrum of uric acid with retention time (RT)= 9.672.

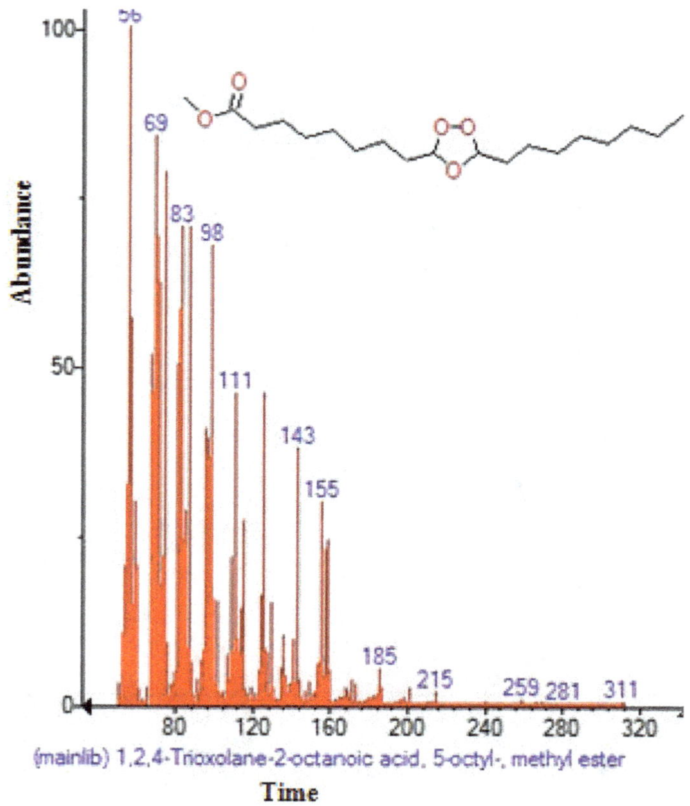

Figure 28. Mass spectrum of 1,2,4-Trioxolane-2-octanoic acid ,5-octyl-,methyl ester with retention time (RT)= 11.320.

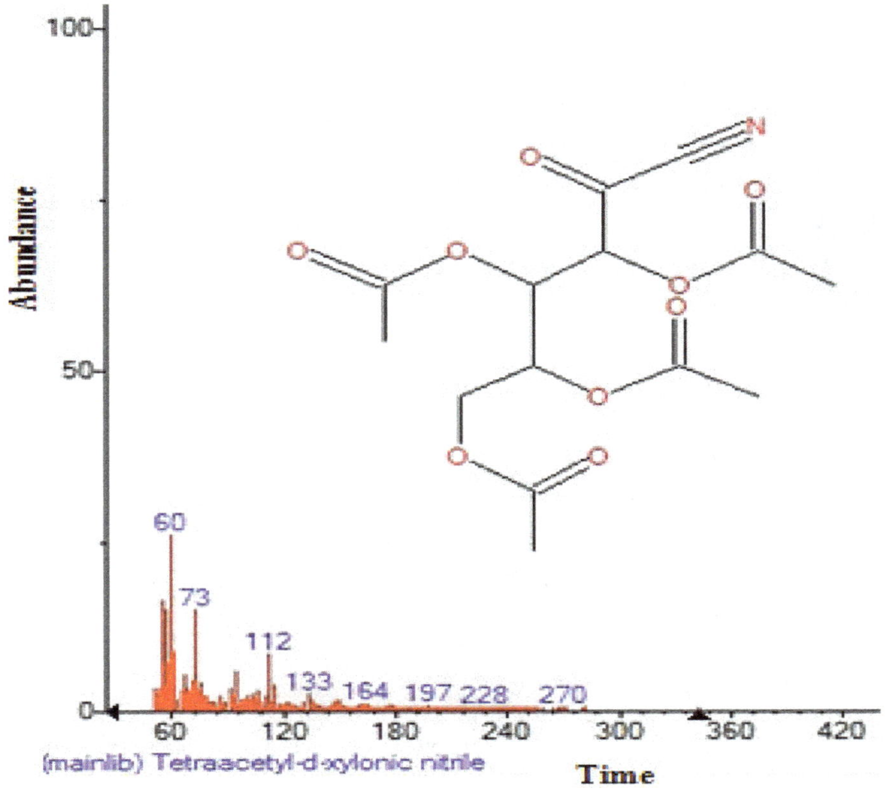

Figure 29. Mass spectrum of Tetraacetyl-d-xylonic nitrile with retention time (RT)= 12.276.

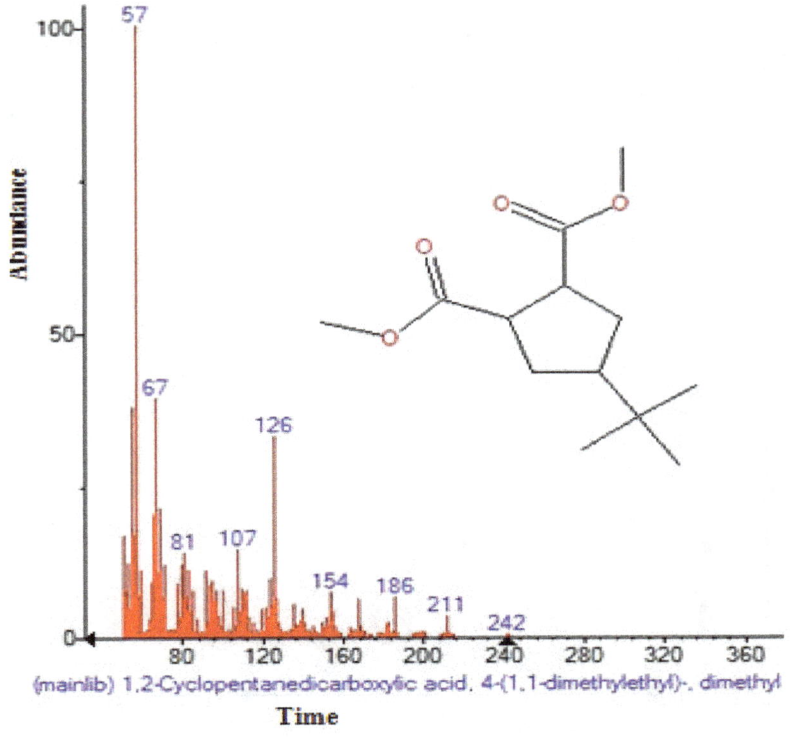

Figure 30. Mass spectrum of 1,2-Cyclopentanedicarboxylic acid ,4-(1,1-dimethylethyl)-,dimethyl with retention time (RT)= 13.975.

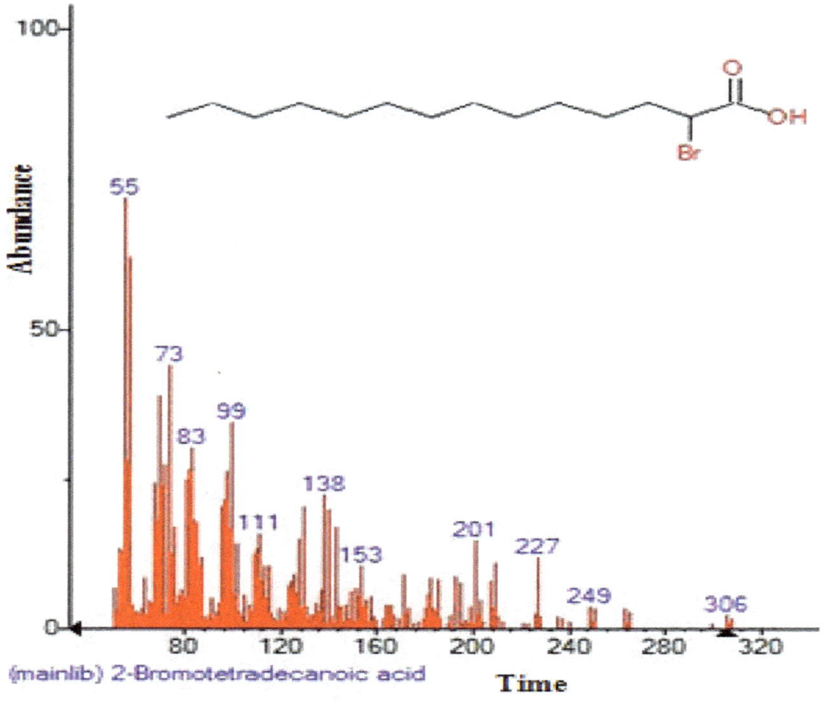

Figure 31. Mass spectrum of 2-Bromotetradecanoic acid with retention time (RT)= 14.771.

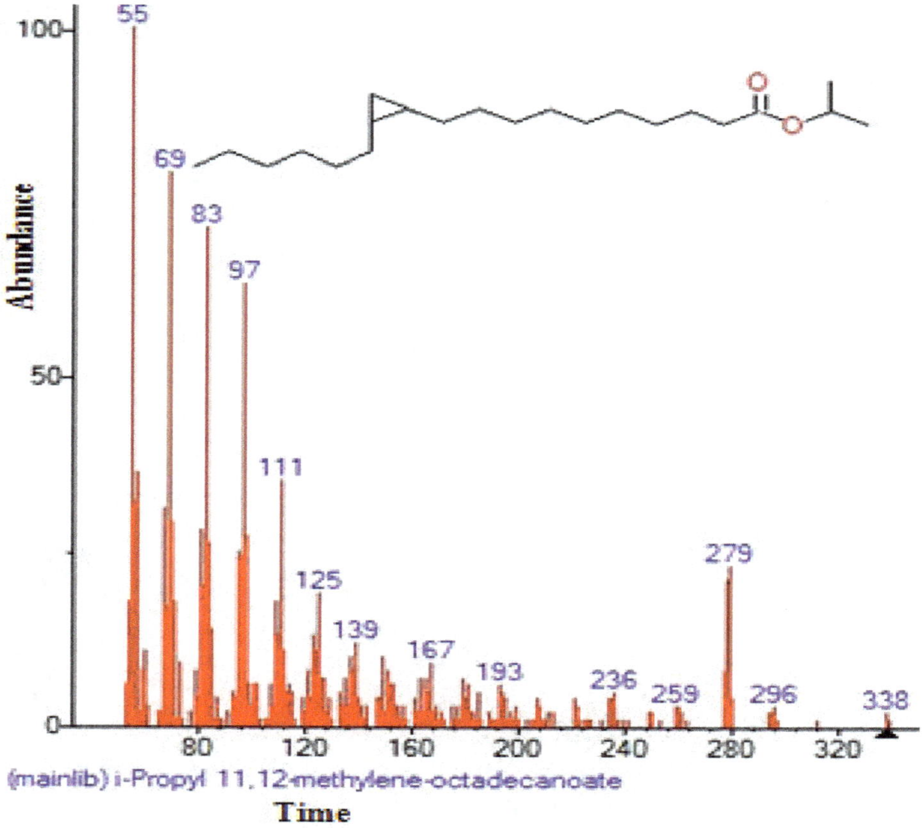

Figure 32. Mass spectrum of i-Propyl 11,12-methylene-octadecanoate with retention time (RT)= 15.022.

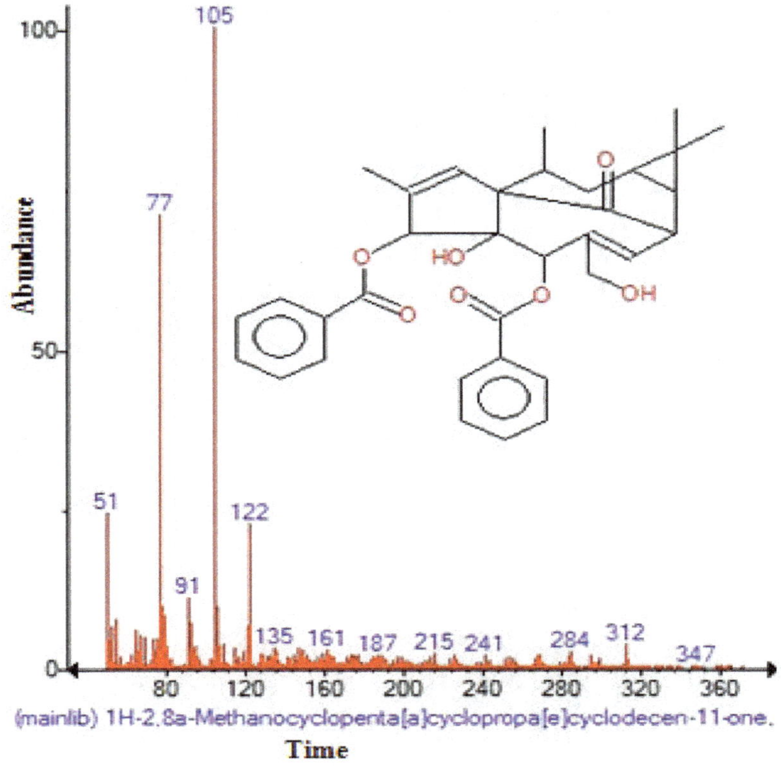

Figure 33. Mass spectrum of 1H-2,8a-Methanocyclopenta[a]cyclopropa[e]cyclodecan-11-one with retention time (RT)= 17.214.

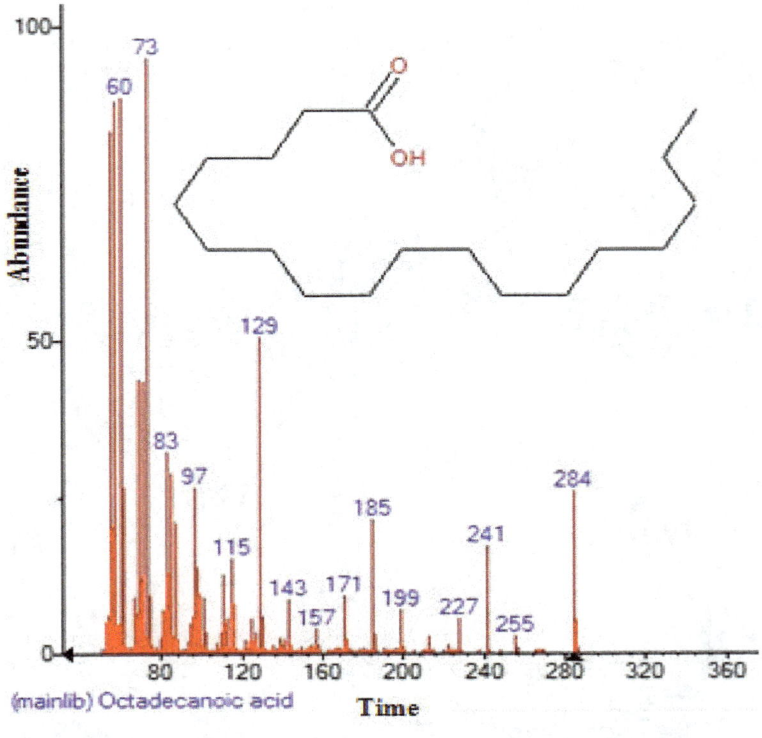

Figure 34. Mass spectrum of octadecanoic acid with retention time (RT) = 17.048.

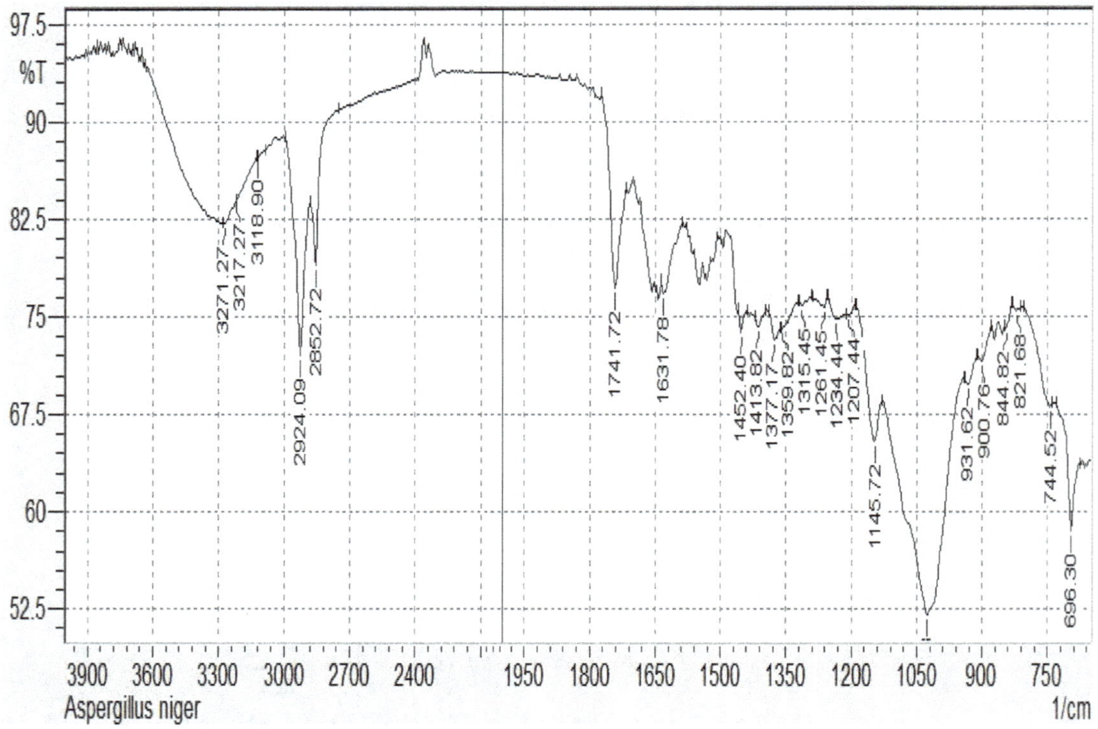

Figure 35. Fourier-transform infrared spectroscopy peak values of *A. niger*

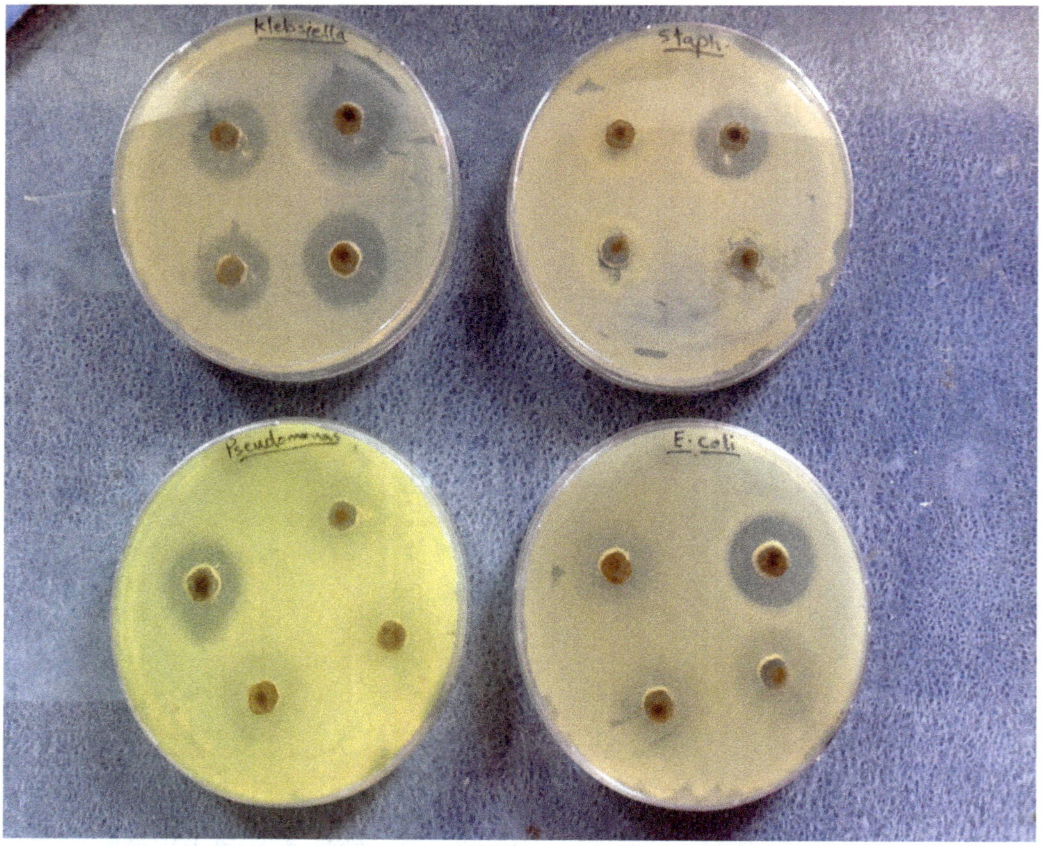

Figure 36. Antimicrobial activity of *A. niger.*

Table 1. Major bioactive chemical compounds identified in methanolic extract of *Aspergillus niger*.

S/N	Phytochemical compound	RT (min)	Formula	Molecular weight	Exact mass	Chemical structure	MS Fragment- ions
1	6-Acetyl-ß-d-mannose	3.201	$C_6H_{14}O_7$	222	222.073953	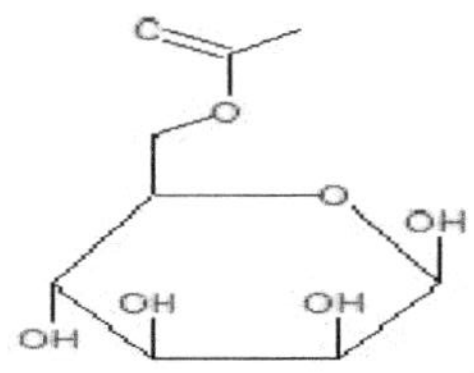	60, 97, 126, 144, 163, 192
2	4-[Dichloromethyl]-2-[[2-[1-methyl-2-pyrrolidinyl]ethyl]amino-6-trichloro	3.613	$C_{13}H_{17}Cl_5N_4$	403	403.989586	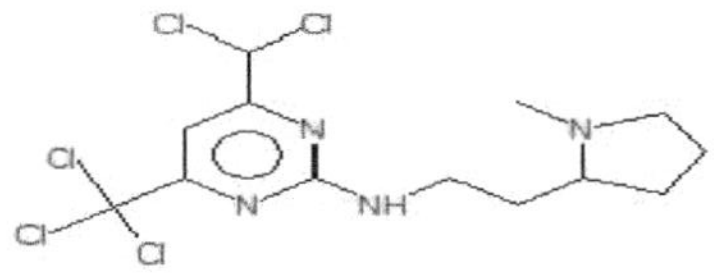	54, 67, 84, 98, 110, 124, 141, 149, 177, 207
3	2-Furancarboxaldehyde,5-methyl	3.722	$C_6H_6O_2$	110	110.0367794	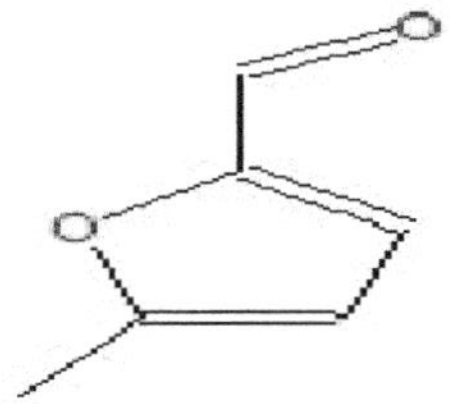	53, 81, 95, 110
4	2,2,2-Trifluoro-N-[2-(1-hydroxy-2,2,6,6-tetramethyl-piperidin-4-yl)	3.779	$C_{13}H_{23}F_3N_2O_2$	296	296.171164	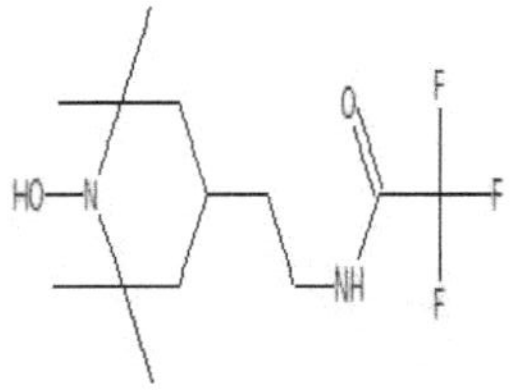	69, 81, 109, 126, 140, 166, 192, 211, 265, 281

poaceae) were effective against *A. niger* (Table 4). *D. stramonium* was very highly active against *A. niger*. *A. niger* was found to be sensitive to all test medicinal plants, and mostly comparable to the standard reference antifungal drug amphotericin B and fluconazole to some extent.

CONCLUSION

The results of this study showed that *A. niger*

Table 1. Contd.

5	2,4-Dihydroxy-2,5-dimethyl-3(2H)-furan-3-one	4.076	$C_6H_8O_4$	144	144.042258	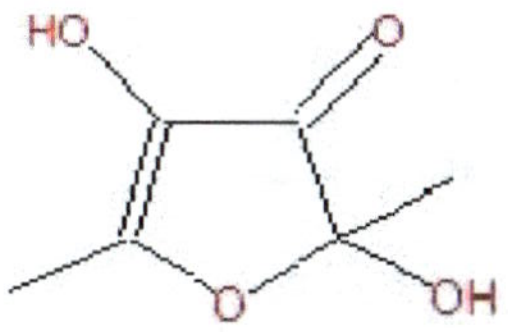	55, 73, 84, 101,144
6	HEPES	4.271	$C_8H_{18}N_2O_4S$	238	238.098728	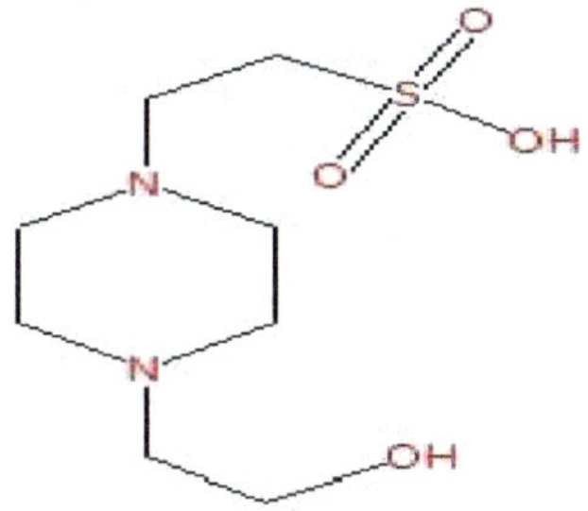	55, 65, 84, 99, 112, 143, 157, 174, 207, 237
7.	Tetraacetyl-d-xylonic nitrile	4.465	$C_{14}H_{17}NO_9$	343	343.090332	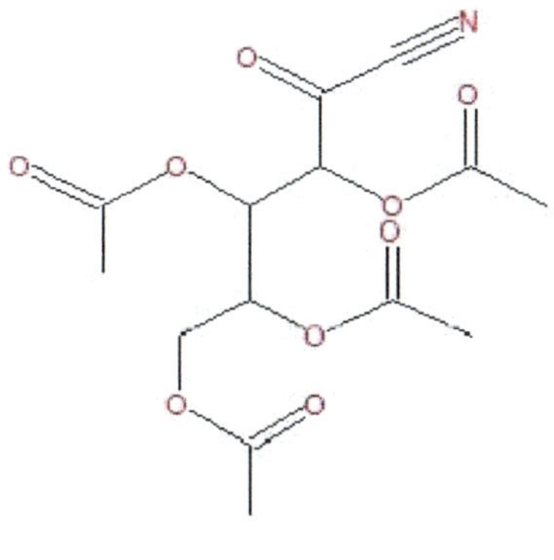	60, 67, 73, 95, 112, 133, 176, 197, 215, 233, 251, 270
8	Eicosanoic acid , phenylmethyl ester	4.546	$C_{27}H_{46}O_2$	402	402.349781	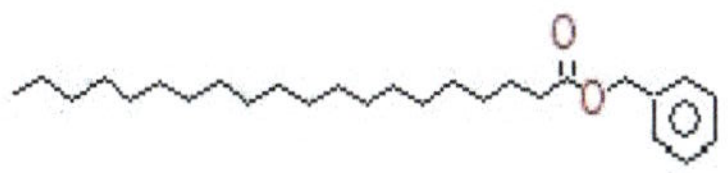	57, 71, 85, 91, 108, 126, 147, 167, 207, 281

Table 1. Contd.

9	Dodecanoic acid , 3-hydroxy	4.574	$C_{12}H_{24}O_3$	216	216.125445	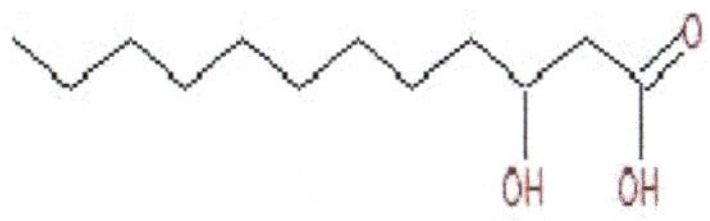	55, 69, 83, 96, 112, 138, 151, 180, 200
10	Desulphosinigrin	4.654	$C_{10}H_{17}NO_6S$	279	279.077658	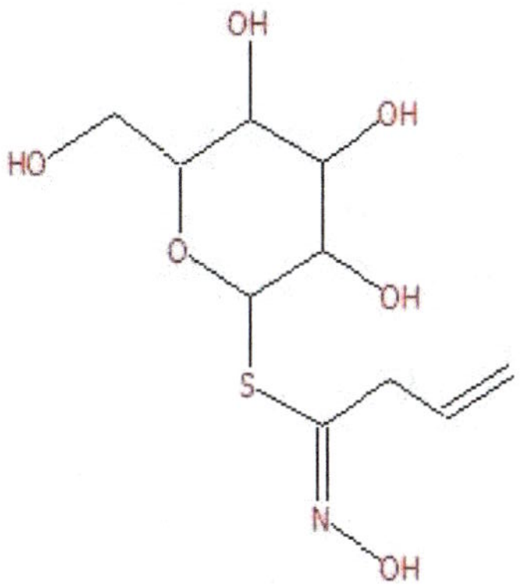	60, 73, 85, 103, 127, 145, 163, 213, 262
11	Glycyl-dl-serine	4.763	$C_5H_{10}N_2O_4$	162	162064056	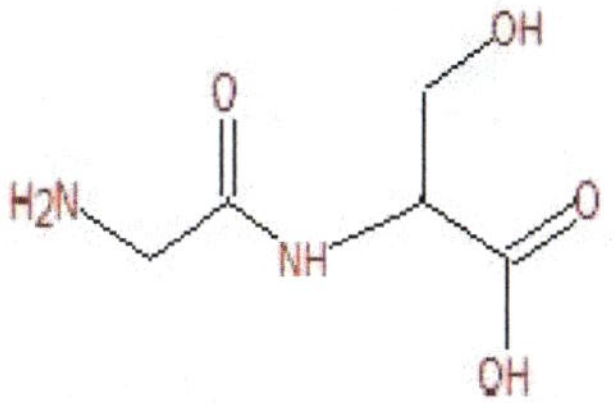	60, 74, 85, 114, 126
12	2,5-Dimethyl-4-hydroxy-3(2H)-furanone	4.929	$C_6H_8O_3$	128	128.047344	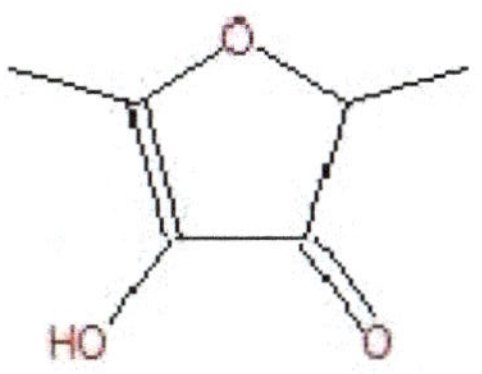	57, 72, 85, 94,128

Table 1. Contd.

13	2,5-Furandicarboxaldehyde	5.066	$C_6H_4O_3$	124	124.016044	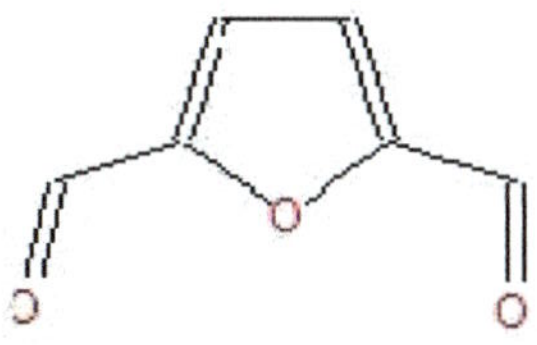	53, 67, 95, 124
14	2H-Oxecin-2-one,3,4,7,8,9,10- hexahydro-4-hydroxy-10-methyl-,[4	5.261	$C_{10}H_{16}O_3$	184	184.109944	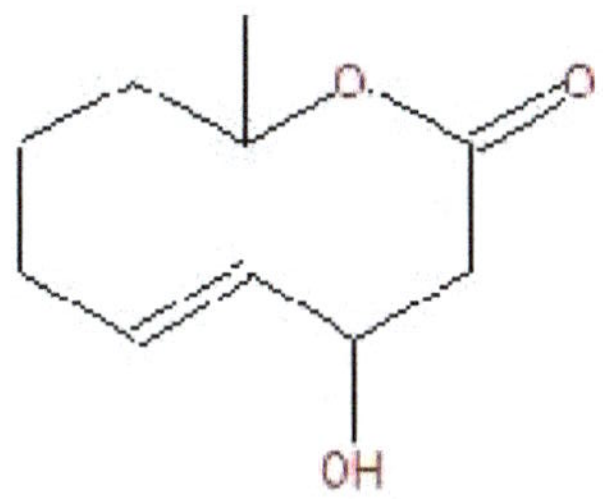	55, 70, 81, 95, 112, 124, 142, 166, 184
16	DL-Leucine , N-glycyl	5.616	$C_8H_{16}N_2O_3$	188	188.116093	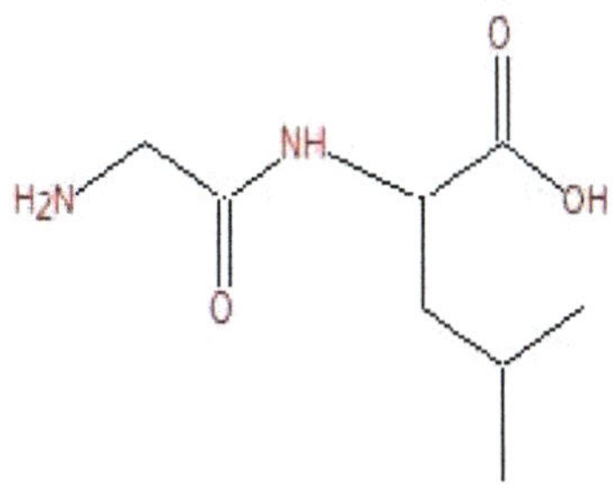	55, 86, 114, 132, 157, 188
18	4H-Pyran-4-one,2,3-dihydro-3,5-dihydroxy-6-methyl	5.942	$C_6H_8O_4$	144	144.042258	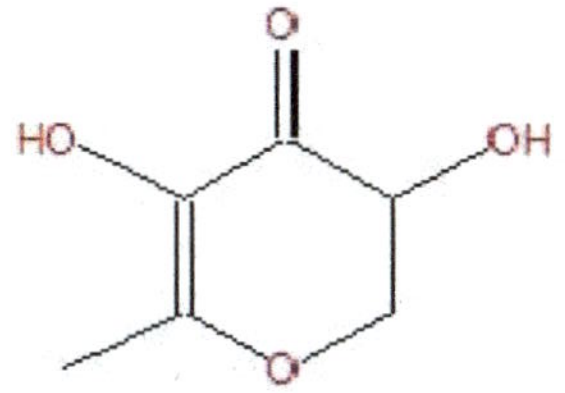	55, 72, 85, 101, 115, 144

Table 1. Contd.

19	l-Gala-l-ido-octonic lactone	6.577	$C_8H_{14}O_8$	238	238.068868	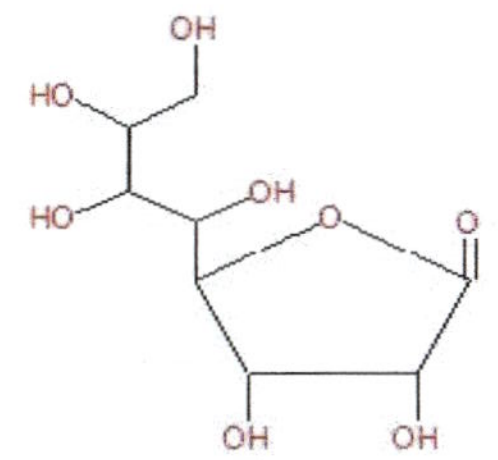	61, 73, 84,112, 127, 142, 159, 189, 220
20	2H-Pyran,tetrahydro-2-(12-pentadecynyloxy)	6.737	$C_{20}H_{36}O_2$	308	308.27153	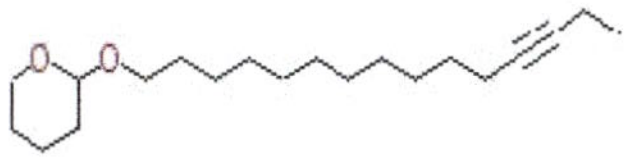	55, 67, 85, 101, 135, 156, 177, 198, 219, 255, 279, 307
21	5-Hydroxymethylfurfural	7.120	$C_6H_6O_3$	126	126.031694	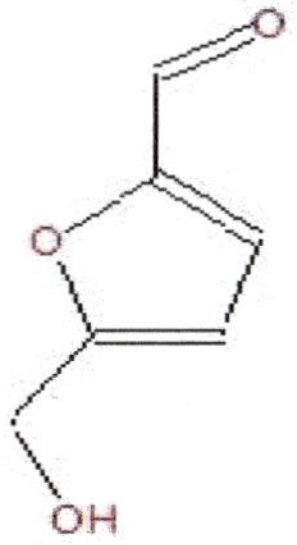	53, 69, 81, 97, 126
22	Strychane,1-acetyl-20α-hydroxy-16-methylene	8.053	$C_{21}H_{26}N_2O_2$	338	338.199429	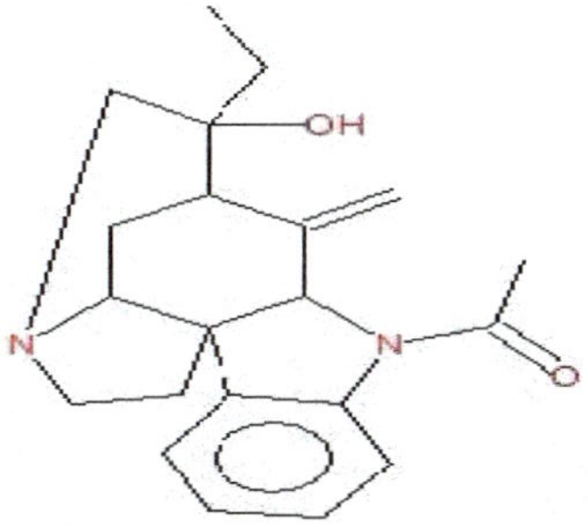	57, 70, 88, 97, 130, 166, 196, 224, 239, 253, 281, 295, 338

Table 1. Contd.

23	α-D-Glucopyranoside ,O-α-D-glucopyranosyl-(1.fwdarw.3)ß-D-fru	7.836	$C_{18}H_{32}O_{16}$	504	504.169035	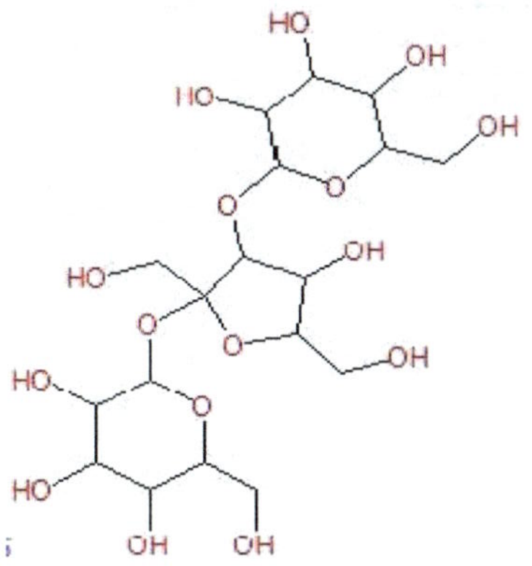	60, 73, 85, 97,113, 126, 145, 187
24	Boroxin , tris(2,3-dimethylbut-2-yl)	8.442	$C_{18}H_{39}B_3O_3$	336	336.317837	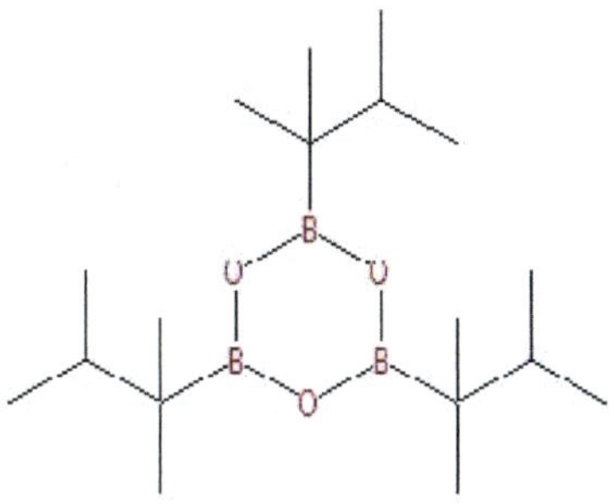	55, 69, 84, 95, 115, 137, 157, 181, 209, 251, 292, 321
25	16-Nitrobicyclo[10.4.0]hexadecane-1-ol-13-one	8.797	$C_{16}H_{27}NO_4$	297	297.194008	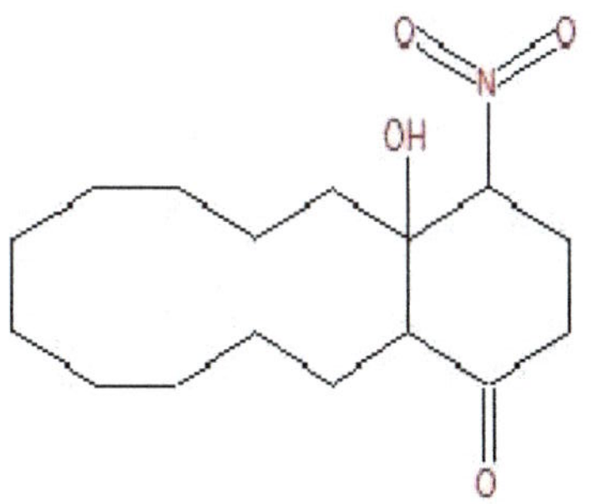	55, 69, 81, 98, 126, 158, 173, 209, 249, 267, 297

Table 1. Cont'd.

26	3-[3-Bromophenyl]-7-chloro-3,4-dihydro-10-hydroxy-1,9(2H,10H)-a	9.043	$C_{19}H_{13}BrClNO_3$	416	416.976732	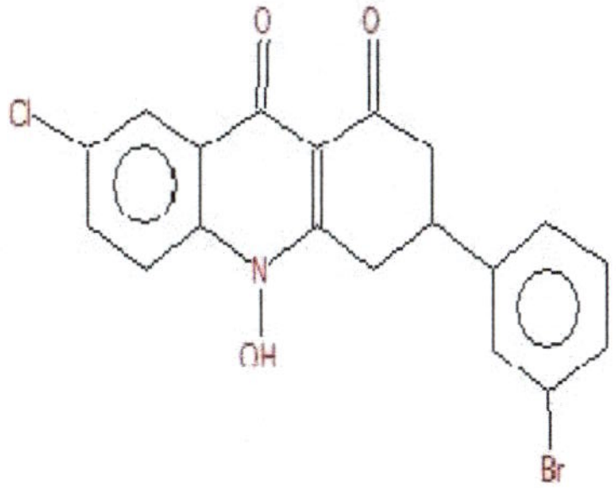	57, 69, 97, 147, 219, 246, 321, 401, 419
27	Uric acid	9.672	$C_5H_4N_4O_3$	168	168.02834	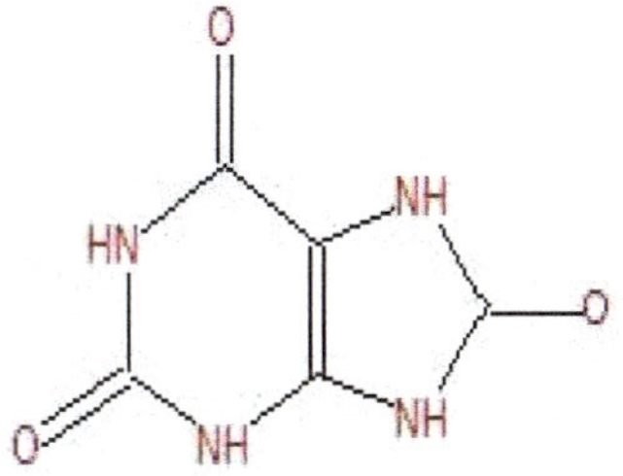	54, 69, 82, 97, 125, 140, 168
28	1,2,4-Trioxolane-2-octanoic acid ,5-octyl-,methyl ester	11.320	$C_{19}H_{36}O_5$	344	344.256275	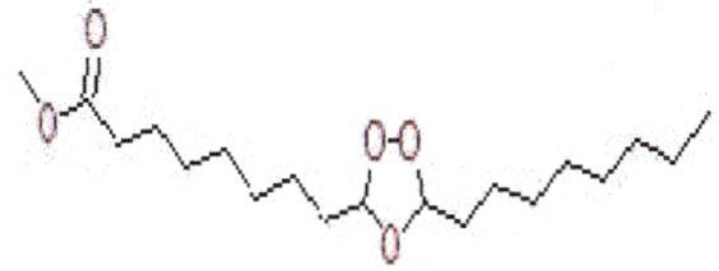	56, 69, 83, 98, 111, 143, 155, 185, 215, 259, 281, 311
29	Tetraacetyl-d-xylonic nitrile	12.276	$C_{14}H_{17}NO_9$	343	343.090332	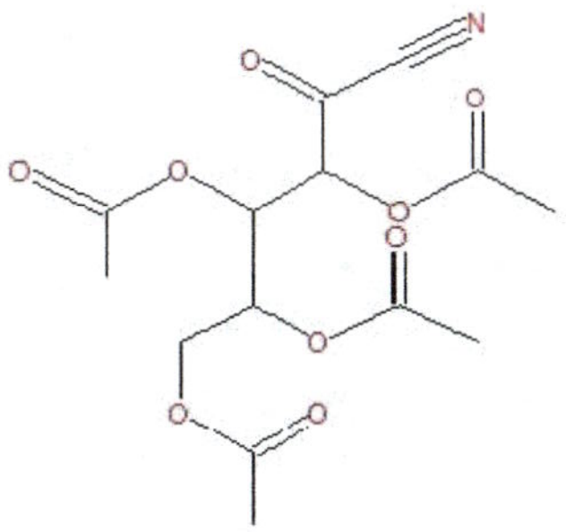	60, 73, 112, 133, 164, 197, 228, 270

Table 1. Cont'd.

30	1,2-Cyclopentanedicarboxylic acid ,4-(1,1-dimethylethyl)-,dimethyl	13.975	$C_{13}H_{22}O_4$	242	242.151809	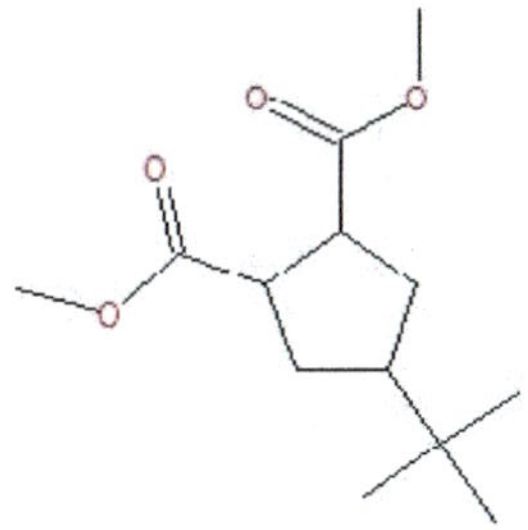	57, 67, 81, 107, 126, 154, 186, 211, 242
31	2-Bromotetradecanoic acid	14.771	$C_{14}H_{27}BrO_2$	306	306.119442	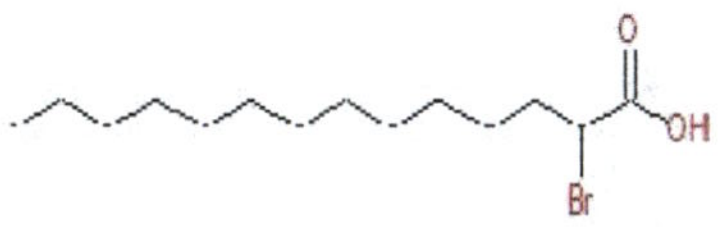	55, 73, 83, 99, 111, 138, 153, 201, 227, 249, 306
32	16-Nitrobicyclo[10.4.0]hexadecane-i-1-ol-13-one	14.908	$C_{16}H_{27}NO_4$	297	297.194008	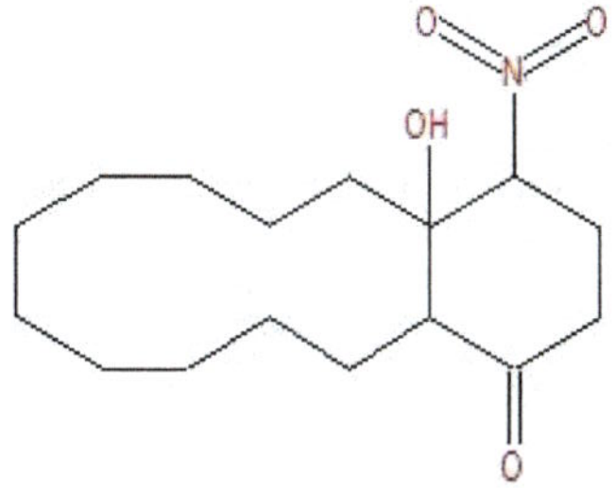	55, 69, 81, 98, 126, 158, 173, 209, 221, 249, 267, 297
33	i-Propyl 11,12-methylene-octadecanoate	15.022	$C_{22}H_{42}O_2$	338	338.318481	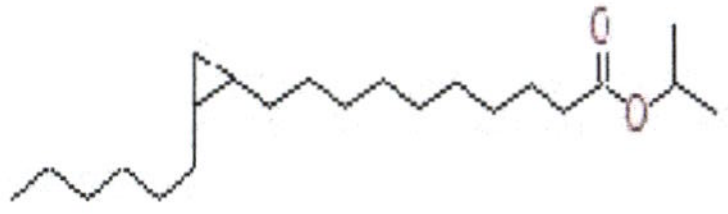	55, 69, 83, 97, 111, 125, 139, 167, 193, 236, 259, 279, 296, 338
34	1H-2,8a-Methanocyclopenta[a]cyclopropa[e]cyclodecan-11-one	17.214	$C_{34}H_{36}O_7$	556	556.246105	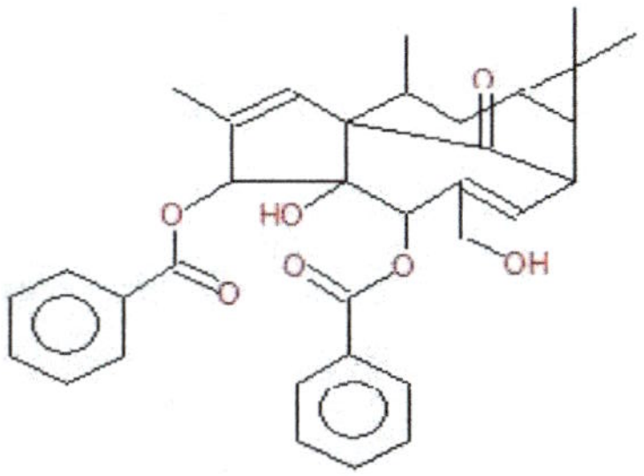	51, 77, 91, 105, 122, 135, 161, 187, 215, 241, 284, 312, 347

Table 1. Cont'd.

35	Octadecanoic acid	17.048	$C_{18}H_{36}O_2$	284	284.27153	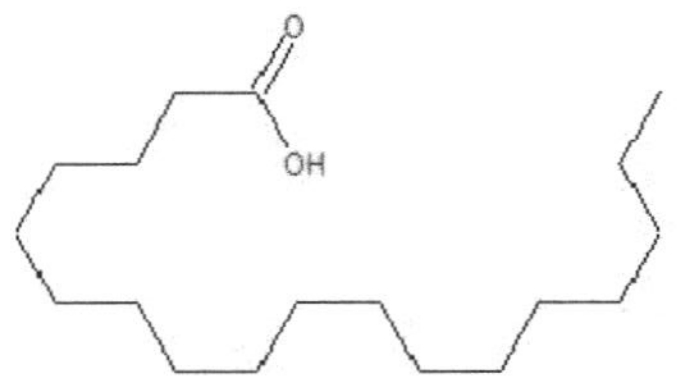	60, 73, 83, 97, 115, 129, 143, 157, 171, 185, 199, 227, 241 ,255, 284

Table 2. Fourier-transorm infrared spectroscopy peak values of *A. niger.*

S/N	Peak (Wave number cm-^{l})	Intensity	Bond	Functional group assignment	Group frequency
1	696.30	58.479	C-H	Aromatic rings	690-900
2	744.52	68.028	C-H	Alkenes	675-995
3	821.68	75.498	C-H	Alkenes	675-995
4	844.82	74.141	C-H	Alkenes	675-995
5	900.76	71.557	C-H	Alkenes	675-995
6	931.62	69.887	C-H	Alkenes	675-995
7	1026.13	52.098	C-F stretch	Aliphatic fluoro compounds	1000-10150
8	1145.72	65.416	C-F stretch	Aliphatic fluoro compounds	1000-10150
9	1207.44	75.125	C-H	Tetiary amine, C-N stretch	1150-1207
10	1234.44	74.798	-	Unknown	-
11	1261.45	75.761	-	Unknown	-
12	1315.45	75.890	-	Aromatic nitro compounds	1310-1390
13	1359.82	74.081	-	Aromatic nitro compounds	1310-1390
14	1377.17	73.205	-	Aromatic nitro compounds	1310-1390
15	1413.82	74.198	-	Ammonium ions	1390-1430
16	1452.40	73.841	-CH3	Methyl-CH. asym	1430-1470
17	1631.78	76.752	-	Organic nitrate	1620-1640
18	1741.72	77.128	-	Unknow	-
19	2852.72	78.925	-	Methylene-CH. asym	2840-2860
20	2924.09	72.033	-	Methylene-CH. asym	2915-2935
21	3118.90	87.299	-	Unknown	-
22	3217.27	83.936	O-H	Normal polymeric O-H stretch	3200-3400
23	3271.27	82.140	O-H	Normal polymeric O-H stretch	3200-3400

Table 3. Zone of inhibition (mm) of test bacterial strains to *A. niger* bioactive compounds and standard antibiotics.

Fungal products Antibiotics	Bacteria				
	Klebsiella pneumonia	***Pseudomonas eurogenosa***	***Staphylococcus aureus***	***Proteus mirabilis***	***Escherichia coli***
Fungal products	6.52±0.61	4.71±0.52	6.16±0.42	5.51±0.62	6.30±0.43
Rifambin	1.12±0.1	1.10±0.1	1.21±0.5	0.60±0.1	0.81±0.2
Streptomycin	1.25±0.3	1.11±0.3	1.30±0.5	1.73±0.2	1.34±0.6
Kanamycin	0.82±0.3	0.53±0.4	0.60±0.2	0.46±0.1	0.92±0.1
Cefotoxime	1.29±0.5	1.50±0.1	1.27±0.1	1.22±0.6	1.25±0.3

Table 4. Zone of inhibition (mm) of test different bioactive compounds and standard antibiotics of plants to *A. niger*.

S/N	Plant	Zone of inhibition (mm)
1	*Nerium olender* (Alkaloids)	4.19±0.25
2	*Ricinus communis* (Alkaloids)	4.70
3	*Datura stramonium* (Alkaloids)	7.81±0.61
4	*Linum usitatissimum* (Crude)	7.60±0.50
5	*Anastatica hierochuntica* (Crude)	3.52±0.09
6	*Gramineae poaceae* (Crude)	7.50±0.13
7	Amphotericin B	5.0±0.20
8	Fluconazol	13.0±0.00
9	Control	0.00

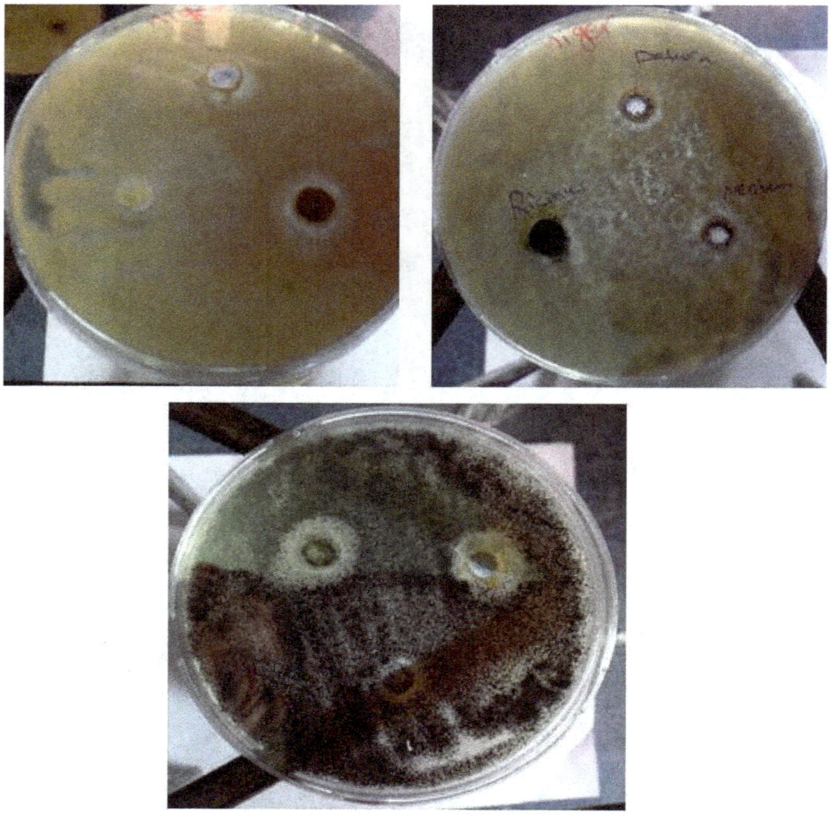

Figure 37. Antifungal activity of extract plant on *A. niger*.

produce many important secondary metabolites with high biological activities. Based on the significance of employing bioactive compounds in pharmacy to produce drugs for the treatment of many diseases, the purification of compounds produced by *A. niger* can be useful.

ACKNOWLEDGEMENTS

The author's sincere thanks go to Dr. Ali Al-Marzuqi for providing them with the opportunity to work on this study. They also would like to thank Zainab Al-Habubi from the Department of Biology for her guidance and help in the laboratory work.

REFERENCES

Ameera OH, Imad HH, Huda J, Muhanned AK (2015). Determination of Alkaloid Compounds of *Ricinus communis* by gas chromatography-mass spectroscopy (GC-MS). J. Med. Plant. Res. 9(10):349-359.

Anesini C, Perez C (1993). Screening of plants used in Argentine folk medicine for antimicrobial activity. J. Ethnopharmacol. 39:119-128.

Anupama M, Narayana KJ, Vijayalakshmi M (2007). Screening of streptomyces perpuofucus for antimicrobial metabolites. Res. J. Microbiol. 2:992-994.

Baker SE (2006). *Aspergillus niger* genomics: past, present and into the future. Med. Mycol. 44:17–21.

Bellini C, Antonini P, Ermanni S (2003). Malignant otitis externa due to *Aspergillus niger*. Scand. J. Infect. Dis. 35(4):284-288.

Chacko S, Vijay S, Ernest D (2012). A comparative study on selected marine actinomycetes from pulicat, Muttukadu, and Ennore estuaries. Asian Pac. J. Trop. Biomed. 2(3):S1827-S1834.

Gebreselema G, Feleke M, Samuel S, Nagappan R (2013). Isolation and characterization of potencial antibiotic producing actinomycetes from water and sediments of lake Tana, Ethiopia. Asian Pac. J. Trop. Biomed. 3(6):426-435.

Horvath JA, Dummer S (1996). The use of respiratory-tract cultures in the diagnosis of invasive pulmonary aspergillosis. Am. J. Med. 100:171-178.

Huda J, Ameera OH, Imad HH, Muhanned AK (2015a). Characterization of alkaloid constitution and evaluation of antimicrobial activity of *Solanum nigrum* by using (GC-MS). J. Pharmacogn. Phytother. 7(4):56-72.

Huda J, Imad HH, Muhanned AK (2015b). Analysis of alkaloid phytochemical compounds in the ethanolic extract of *Datura stramonium* and evaluation of antimicrobial activity. Afr. J. Biotechnol. 14(19):1668-1674.

Imad H, Ameer I, Mohammed A, Cheah Y, Aamera J (2014a). Haplotypes and variable position detection in the mitochondrial DNA coding region encompassing nucleotide positions 10,716–11,184. Mitochondrial DNA 26(4):544-9.

Imad H, Mohammed A, Aamera J, Ameer I, Cheah Y (2014b). Haplotype data of mitochondrial DNA coding region encompassing nucleotide positions 11,719–12,184 and evaluate the importance of these positions for forensic genetic purposes in Iraq. Mitochondrial DNA 4:1-4.

Imad HH, Huda J, Muhanned AK, Ameera OH (2015c). Alkaloid constitution of *Nerium oleander* by using gas chromatography- mass specroscopy (GC-MS). J. Med. Plant. Res. 9(9):326-334.

Imad HH, Israa A, Hawraa J (2015a). Gas chromatography mass spectrum and fouriertransform infrared spectroscopy analysis of methanolic extract of *Rosmarinus oficinalis* leaves. J. Pharmacogn. Phytother. 7(6):90-106.

Imad HH, Mohammed AJ, Muhanned AK (2015b). Forensic analysis of mitochondrial DNA hypervariable region HVII (encompassing nucleotide positions 37 to 340) and HVIII (encompassing nucleotide positions 438-574) and evaluate the importance of these variable positions for forensic genetic purposes. Afr. J. Biotechnol. 14(5):365-375.

Mogensen JM, Frisvad JC, Thrane U, Nielsen KF (2010). Production of fumonisin B2 and B4 by Aspergillus niger on grapes and raisins. J Agric. Food Chem. 58:954-8.

Mohammed A, Imad H (2013). Autosomal STR: From locus information to next generation sequencing technology. Res. J. Biotechnol. 8(10):92-105.

Muhanned AK, Ameer IA, Imad HH, Mohammed AJ (2015). A New Polymorphic Positions Discovered in Mitochondrial DNA Hypervariable Region HVIII From Central and North-Central of Iraq. Mitochondrial DNA 23:1-5.

Perfect JR, Cox GM, Lee JY (2001). The impact of culture isolation of Aspergillus species: a hospital-based survey of aspergillosis. Clin. Infect Dis. 33:1824-1833.

Perrone G, Susca A, Cozzi G, Ehrlich K, Varga J, Frisvad JC (2007). Biodiversity of Aspergillus species in some important agricultural products. Stud. Mycol. 59:53-66.

Rukayadi Y, Yong D, Hwang JK (2006). In vitro anticandidal activity of xanthorrhizol isolated from Curcuma xanthorrhiza Roxb. J. Antimicrob. Chemother. 57:1231-1234.

Segal BH, DeCarlo ES, Kwon-Chung KJ, Malech HL, Gallin JI, Holland SM (1998). *Aspergillus nidulans* infection in chronic granulomatous disease. Medicine (Baltimore) 77:345-54.

Susca A, Proctor RH, Mule G, Stea G, Ritieni A, Logrieco A (2010). Correlation of mycotoxin fumonisin B2 production and presence of the fumonisin biosynthetic gene fum8 in Aspergillus niger from grape. J. Agric. Food Chem. 58:9266-7922.

Usha NS, Masilamani SM (2013). Bioactive compound produced by streptomycin strain. Int. J. Pharm. Pharm. Sci. 5(1):0975-14.

Walsh TJ (2004). Detection of galactomannan antigenemia by enzyme immunoassay for the diagnosis of invasive aspergillosis: variables that affect performance. J. Infect. Dis. 190:641-49.

Hepatoprotective effects of the decoction and macerated leaves of *Rhamnus alaternus* L. on rats exposed to carbon tetrachloride

Abdelkrim Berroukche*, Khaled Kahloula, Miloud Slimani, Imane Denai and Kheira Ammour

Laboratory of Biochemistry, Biology Department, Faculty of Sciences, Dr. Tahar Moulay University, Saida 20000, Algeria.

The plant of *Ramnus alaternus* L. (Rhamnaceae) has been object of many therapeutic indications for traditional medicine. Many studies have showed a hepatoprotective activity of *R. alaternus* L. The objective of this study was to compare the hepatoprotective activities of decoction and macerated *R. Alaternus* L. leaves extracts on rats initially exposed to carbon tetrachloride CCl_4 (1 ml/kg). The macerated leaves (250 mg/kg body weight) showed a highly significant hepatoprotective activity ($p < 0.01$) expressed by a significant decrease in enzymatic biochemical markers such as total bilirubin, alkaline phosphatase (ALP) and transaminases (GOT and GPT). Mean serum biochemical marker levels were 4.5 ± 0.9 mg/dL, 143 ± 3.7, 43.5 ± 9.2 and 32.2 ± 5.1 U/L, respectively. These results illustrate the dominance of the hepatoprotective pharmacological activity of macerated *R. alaternus* L. leaves.

Key words: Rhamnaceae, traditional medicine, hepatoprotective activity, biochemical markers, alcaline phosphatase.

INTRODUCTION

Liver diseases have a multifactorial etiology including infectious factor. High mortality rate has been correlated with two types of liver diseases namely, jaundice and hepatitis. (Pang et al., 1992). Hepatitis, has been associated with the drinking of contaminated water and poor hygiene (WHO, 2005). Jaundice which is common in children has been characterized by yellow skin because of an excess of bilirubin (Sourabie et al., 2012). Hepatoprotective effects of drugs and plant extracts have been studied by using carbon tetrachloride (CCl_4) induced hepatotoxicity in animal models (Suja et al., 2002). Studies have shown toxicity of CCl_4 which leads to free radicals in tissues such as liver, kidney, heart, lung, testis, brain and blood (Kumar et al., 2005; Khan and Ahmed, 2009). Research in herbal medicine has been an alternative therapy for liver disease (Pramyothin et al., 2005). Plant drugs have been known for their role in the management of hepatic diseases.

*Corresponding author. E-mail: kerroum1967@yahoo.fr.

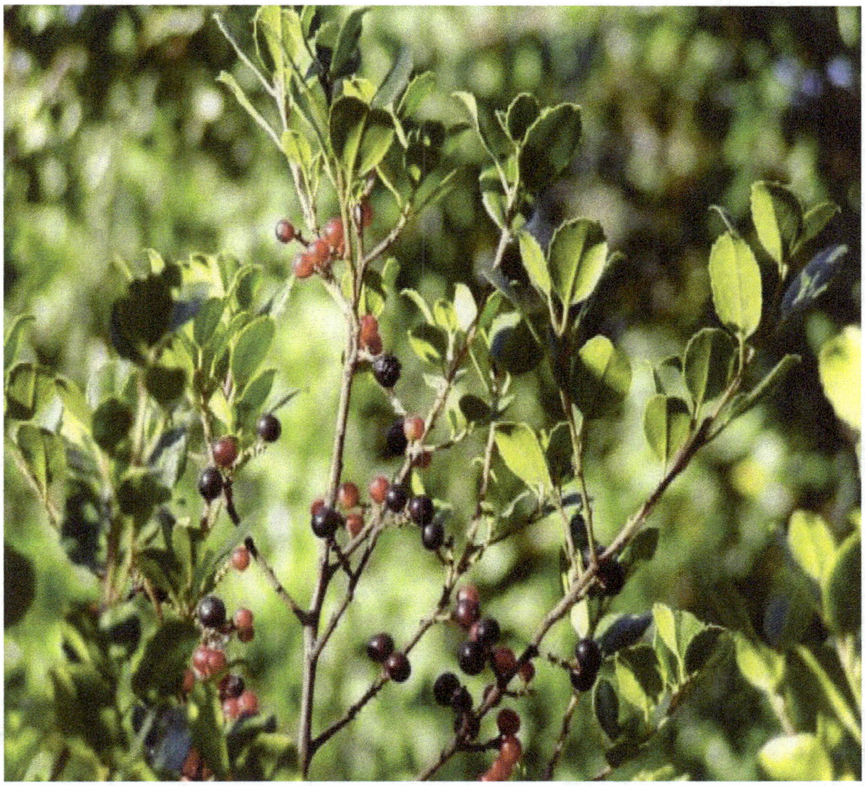

Figure 1. The shrub of *Rhamnus alaternus* L.
Source: Rameau et al. (2008).

Medicinal plants have been an important source of bioactive molecules, used in the food industry, cosmetics and pharmacy.

These molecules include coumarins, alkaloids, phenolic acids, tannins, flavonoids and terpenes (Bahorun et al., 1996). Polyphenols have therapeutic virtues, mainly against cancer and cardiovascular disease. These molecules are involved in the protection of plants against microbial attacks (Bruneton, 1999). Different medicinal plants species such as *Tinospora bakis*, *Cochlospermum tinctoria*, *Nauclea latifolia* and *Argemone mexicana*, have been used in traditional medicine for the therapy of jaundice (Sourabie et al., 2012). Through a rich literature on the phototherapy, it has been found that *Rhamnus alaternus* L. known by populations of different areas of Algeria for its therapeutic activities against jaundice (Figure 1). Important works on the chemistry of *R. alaternus* L. have been carried out and significant pharmacological properties have been reported by studies in Algeria and Tunisia (Ben Ammar et al., 2008; Chemli et al., 2006). Therapeutic properties of this species have been demonstrated *in vitro* because of their active compounds (Ben Ammar et al., 2008). The present study aimed to compare the hepatoprotective effects of the decoction and macerated leaves of *R. alaternus* L. on rats exposed to CCl_4.

MATERIALS AND METHODS

Description of plant

Leaves of *R. alaternus* have been collected during the month of October, 2013 in rural areas of Mohammedia, located in North-West of Algeria (Figure 2). *R. alatenus* L. is a sun-loving plant, growing in Mediterranean areas. It is a shrub of 5 m high with non spiny leaves and fruits (Chemli et al., 2006; Rameau et al., 2008). The leaves are oval or lance-shaped with slightly toothed edges, buckthorn, short-stalked, thick and leathery. The fruits appear in late fall. There are small red and black berries, grouped in compact clusters. Identification of the plant was made by M. Terras, researcher and team member of Laboratory of water sources and environment Biology Department at the University of Saida (Algeria). Dried leaves have been transformed into powder using an electric mill (Moulinex model D5001). Powders have been used to prepare aqueous decoction and macerated extract of the leaves.

Preparation of extract

To prepare an aqueous decoction, two hundred fifty grams (250 g) of powder leaves of *R. alaternus* have been used in a flask containing 1000 ml of distilled water. Decoction has been maintained under continuous reflux for 2 h at 80°C (Belhattab et al.,

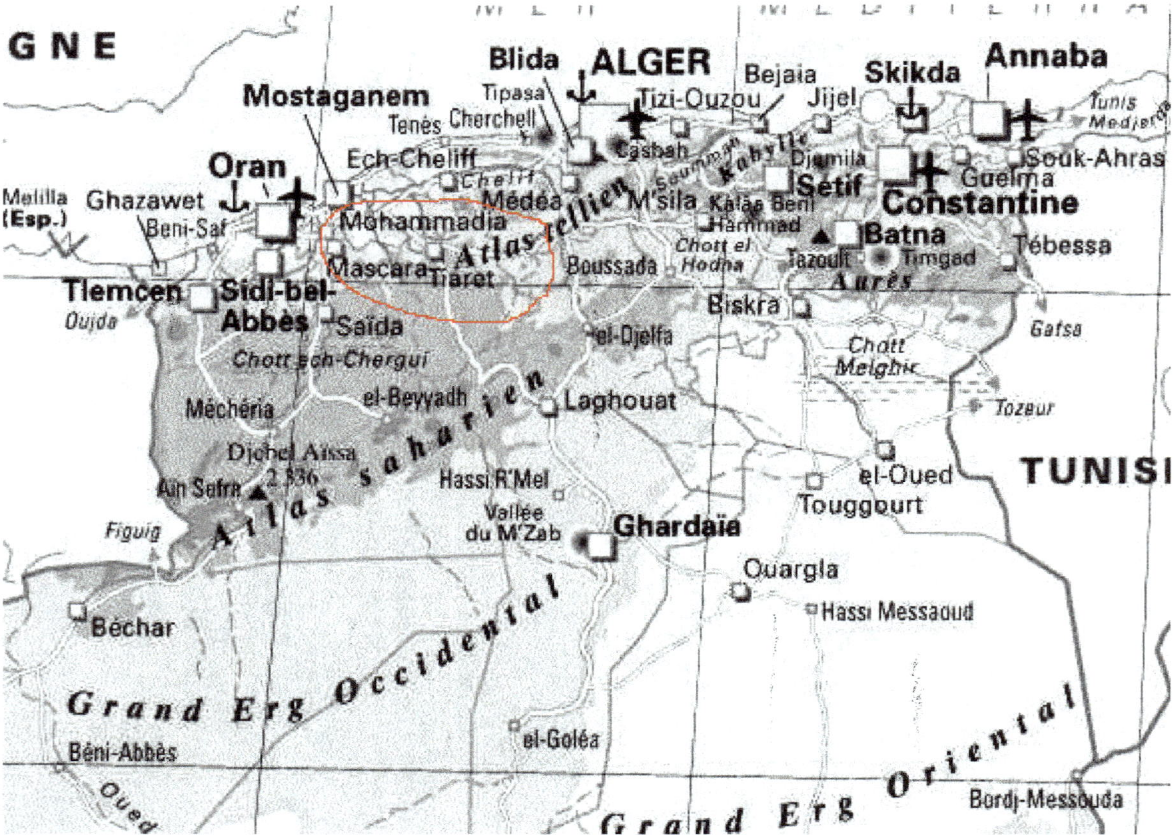

Figure 2. Geographical map of Mohammedia, located in North- West of Algeria. (Diagram tourism development of the department of Mascara, 2015).

2004). Decoction has been filtered through a funnel containing cotton wool and then centrifuged at 2500 rpm for 5 min. Aqueous macerated extract of the leaves was obtained in the same conditions as the decoction with the only difference that it has made macerated extract (cold extraction) without any heating process of the test portion (250 g).

Preparation of animals

Forty (40) male adult Wistar rats, 2 months old and weighing about (180 to 200 g) from the central animal house of the Department of Biology of Saida University, were used in this study. They were kept under standard environmental conditions at 25°C with 12:12 h light-dark cycle in ventilated plastic cages. The rats were fed with standard feed livestock and water ad libitum. The animals were divided into 4 groups (10 rats per group) as follow:

Group 1: served as normal controls (NC) and rats received a tap water daily for 7 days orally.
Group 2: served as toxic control and the rats were injected intraperitoneal with carbon tetrachloride (CCl_4) (1 ml/kg body weight) daily for the same period (7 days).
Group 3: (CCl_4 + decoction of *R. alaternus* leaves): the rats were injected intraperitoneal with CCl_4 (1 ml/kg body weight) and treated orally with the decoction of *R. alaternus* leaves (250 mg/kg body weight) daily for the same period.
Group 4: (CCl_4 + macerated *R. alaternus* leaves): the rats were injected intraperitoneal with CCl_4 (1 ml/kg body weight) and treated orally with the macerated *R. alaternus* leaves (250 mg/kg body weight) daily for the same period (Sourabie et al., 2012).

Biochemical study

At the end of the experiments, all animals were sacrificed and the blood from each animal was taken into haemolysis tubes (5 mL). The blood samples were centrifuged at 2500 rpm for 10 to 15 min and the sera isolated were used for estimation of the serum biochemical markers of liver; as serum glutamic oxaloacetic transaminase (GOT), serum glutamic pyruvic transaminase (GPT), alkaline phosphatase (ALP) and total bilirubin.

Histopathology

The animals were dissected to isolate liver tissues. After draining the blood, liver samples were excised, washed with normal saline and processed separately for histological observations. Initially, the materials were fixed in 10% buffered neutral formalin for 48 h and then with bovine solution for 6 h. Paraffin sections were taken at 5 mm thickness, processed in alcohol-xylene series and were stained

Table 1. Effects of decoction and macerated *Rhamnus alatenus* leaves on serum hepatic parameters in groups of control rats and exposed to CCl_4.

Groups of rats (n = 40)	Total bilirubin (mg/dL)	ALP (U/L)	SGOT (U/L)	SGPT (U/L)
Group 1 (NC)				
Mean ± SD	1.49 ± 0.03	130.25 ± 4.4	26.5 ± 4	26 ± 4.6
Min-Max	1.41 - 1.56	120 - 139	17 - 36	19 - 39
Mean CI (95%)	1.47 - 1.50	128.09 - 132.4	24.53 - 28.46	17 - 28.2
Group 2 (CCl_4)				
Mean ± SD	**11.0 ± 0.94	**185.5 ± 5.95	**88.25 ± 6.96	**69.25 ± 2.92
Min-Max	9.88 - 13.74	169 - 197	69 - 99	66 - 78
Mean CI (95%)	10.53 - 11.46	182.58 - 188.41	84.83 - 91.66	67.81 - 70.68
Group 3 (CCl_4 + D)				
Mean ± SD	10.00 ± 1.07	161.5 ± 8.7	49 ± 1.08	61.5 ± 3.77
Min - Max	7.13 - 12.04	145 - 186	46 - 51	55 - 69
Mean CI (95%)	9.47 - 10.52	157.23 - 165.76	48 - 57	59.65 - 63.34
Group 4 (CCl_4 + M)				
Mean ± SD	4.51 ± 0.45	135.25 ± 0.85	30.75 ± 3.54	34.5 ± 2.21
Min - Max	3.33 - 5.33	133 - 137	22 - 37	29 - 39
Mean CI (95%)	4.28 ± 4.73	134.83 - 135.66	29.01 - 32.48	33.47 - 35.58

NC: Normal control; D: Decoction, M: Maceration; SD: Standard deviation; Min: Minimum; Max: Maximum; CI: Confidence interval; ALP: Alkaline phosphatase; GOT: Glutamic oxaloacetic transaminase; GPT: Glutamic pyruvic transaminase; P**: Highly significant (< 0.001).

with alum haematoxylin and eosin (Galighter et Koyloff, 1971). The sections were examined microscopically for histopathological changes.

Statistical analysis

Data are expressed as mean ± SD, with a value of $p < 0.05$ considered statistically significant. Statistical evaluation was performed by one way analysis of variance (ANOVA) followed by the Tukey's t-test for multiple comparisons. All analysis was made with the statistical software Sigmaplot (version 11.0).

RESULTS

As shown in Table 1 and Figure 3, body weight of rats exposed to CCl_4 (Group 2) was highly decreased significantly ($p^{**} < 0.01$) compared with normal control rats (Group 1). The median body weight in group of rats administered CCl_4 was lower (174.57 ± 5.2 g) compared to normal control rats (Group1) which showed a higher mean body weight (224.28 ± 6.6 g). Whereas the body weight of rats (Groups 3 and 4) has not showed a significant difference. Their mean body weights were 179.85 ± 1.68 and 196.28 ± 1.63 g, respectively.

The administration of carbon tetrachloride CCl_4 (1 ml/kg body weight) developed a significant increase in serum enzymatic markers ($p^{**} < 0.01$), especially serum transaminase (GOT and GPT) and alkaline phosphatase (ALP). Similarly, it was observed concomitantly, a significant increase in serum total bilirubin ($p^{**} < 0.01$) (Table 1). This phenomenon was particularly observed in rats of Group 2 which were administrated CCl_4, in comparison with the normal control rats of Group 1 as shown in Figures 4, 5, 6, 7.

The aqueous extracts (decoction and macerated) administered at the same dose (250 mg/kg) developed a significant decrease in serum enzymes (GOT and GPT) ($p^{**} < 0.01$) and a decrease in the serum total bilirubin concentration as compared to animals which were administered CCl_4 (Group 2) (Figures 4, 5, 6, 7). The effect of different treatments (decoction and macerated) on serum enzyme markers and serum total bilirubin is reported in Figures 4, 5, 6, 7. From the perspective of pharmacological activity, the decrease of biological parameters observed in the test Groups 3 and 4 is a clear sign and an illustration of the ability of these extracts to reduce the hepatotoxicity induced by the administration of toxic organochlorine (CCl_4, 1 ml/ kg B.W). Histopathologies of various groups are shown in Figure 8. In Group 1 (normal control rats), liver tissue section

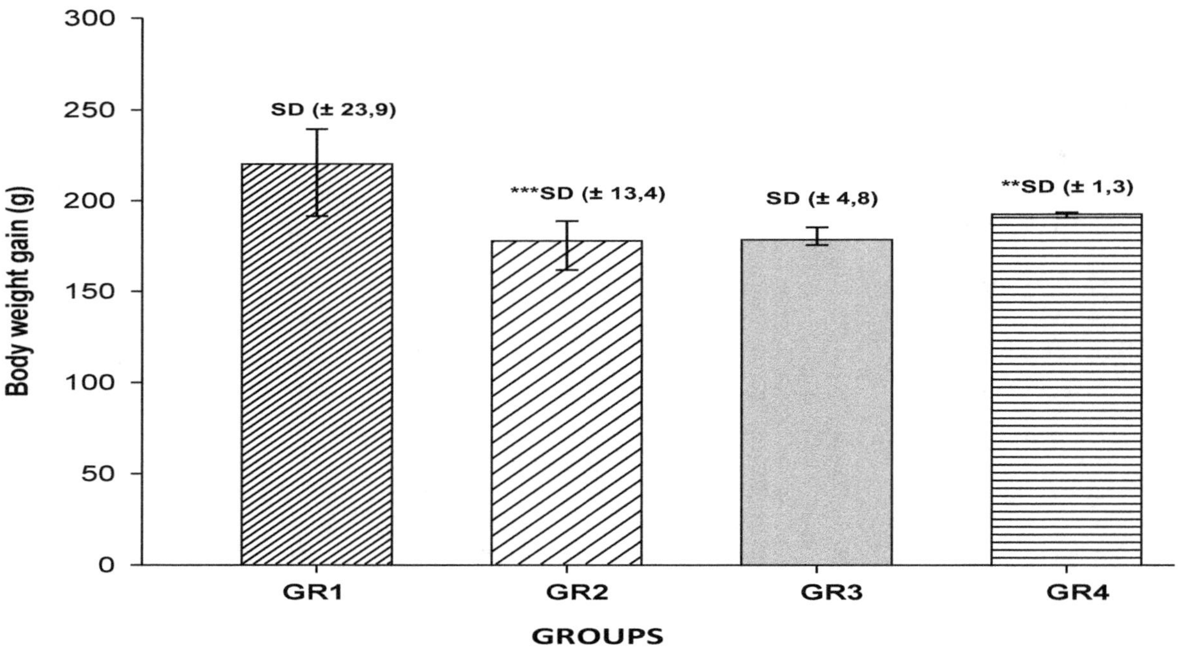

Figure 3. Variation of body weight in groups of animals. GR1 (NC): Group 1 of normal control rats; GR2 ($CC1_4$): Group 2 of treated rats with CCl_4; GR3 (CCl_4-D): Group 3 of treated rats with CCl_4 and decoction *Rhamnus alaternus* leaves; GR4 (CCl_4-M): Group 4 of treated rats with CCl_4 and macerated *Rhamnus alaternus* leaves; SD: standard deviation; ** ($p < 0.01$): statistically significant difference between the groups of animals.

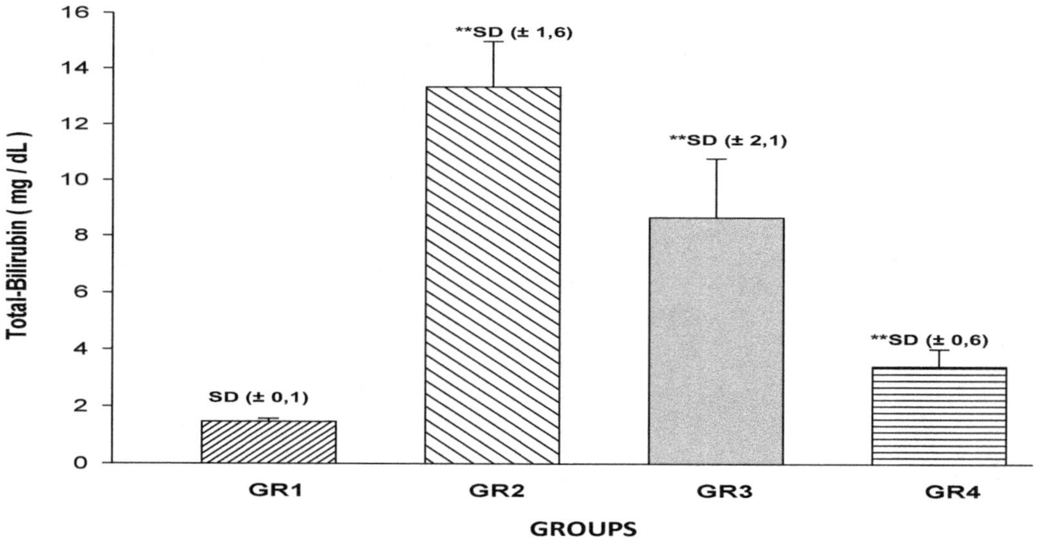

Figure 4. Effects of decoction and macerated *Rhamnus alatenus* leaves on serum total-bilirubine in groups of animals exposed to CCl_4.

(Figure 8A) shows a normal architecture of liver cells. Hepatocyte, hepatic sinusoids, portal tract, shows normal size and Shape. The nuclei are round and are uniform with little variation in size.

In Group 2 (Rats treated with CCl_4), liver tissue section (Figure 8B) shows extreme degeneration of hepatic

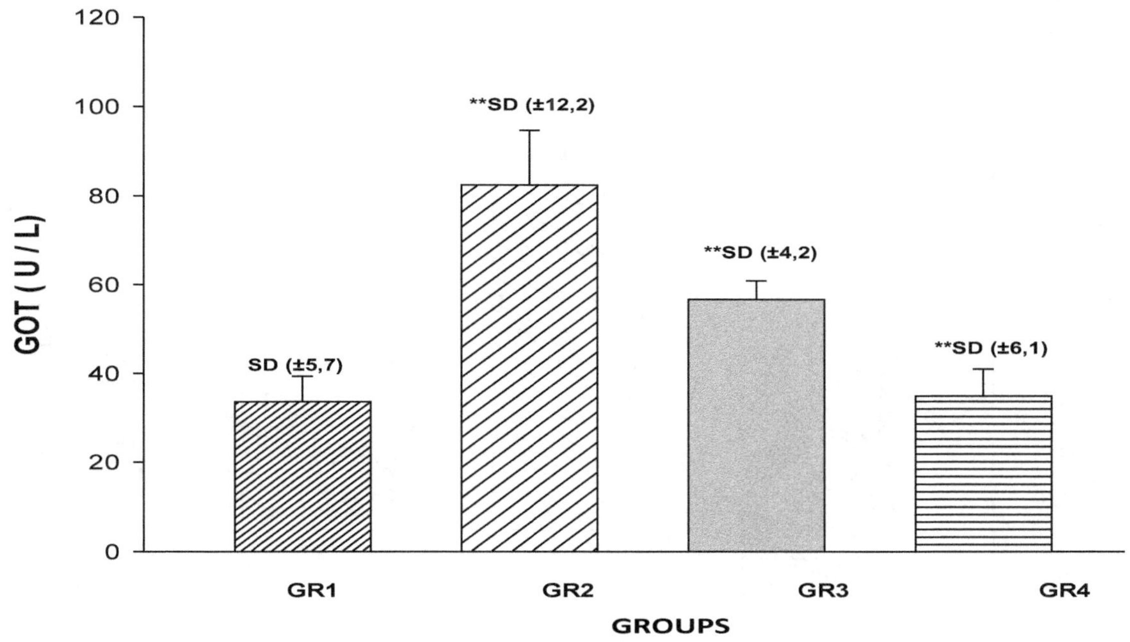

Figure 5. Effects of decoction and macerated *Rhamnus alatenus* leaves on serum glutamic oxaloacetic transaminase (GOT) in groups of animals exposed to CCl_4.

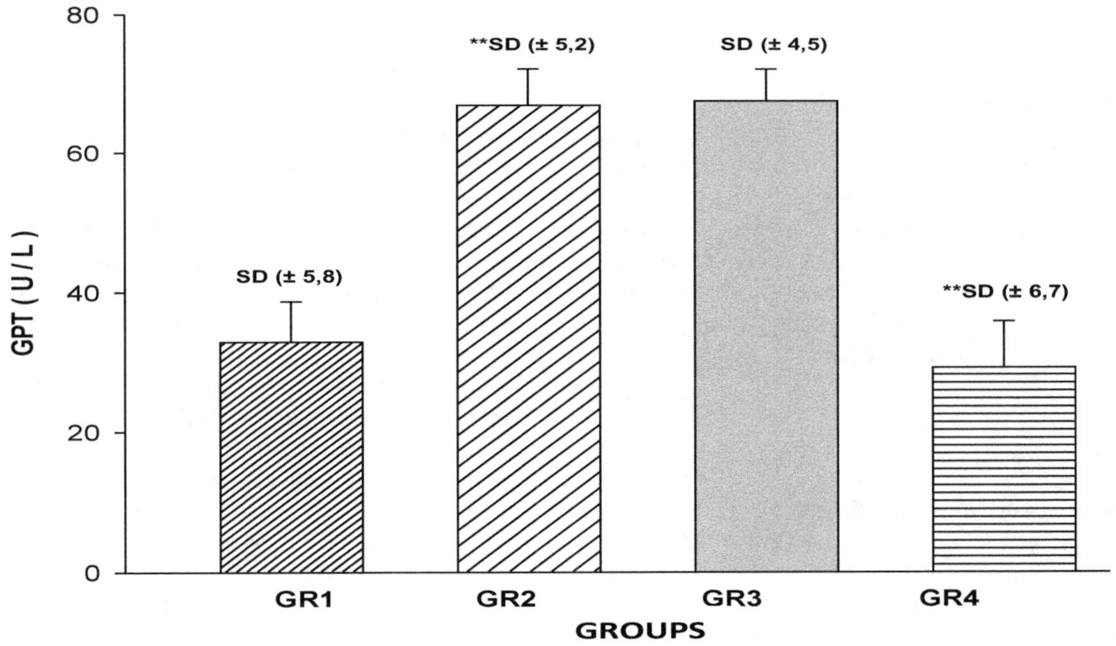

Figure 6. Effects of decoction and macerated *Rhamnus alatenus* leaves on serum glutamic pyruvic transaminase (GPT) in groups of animals exposed to CCl_4.

architecture by necrosis, foci of haemorrhage, fatty changes and vein crowding. Hepatocyte are arranged like disks and shows a typical proliferation. In Group 3 (Rats treated with CCl_4 and decoction of *R. alaternus* leaves),

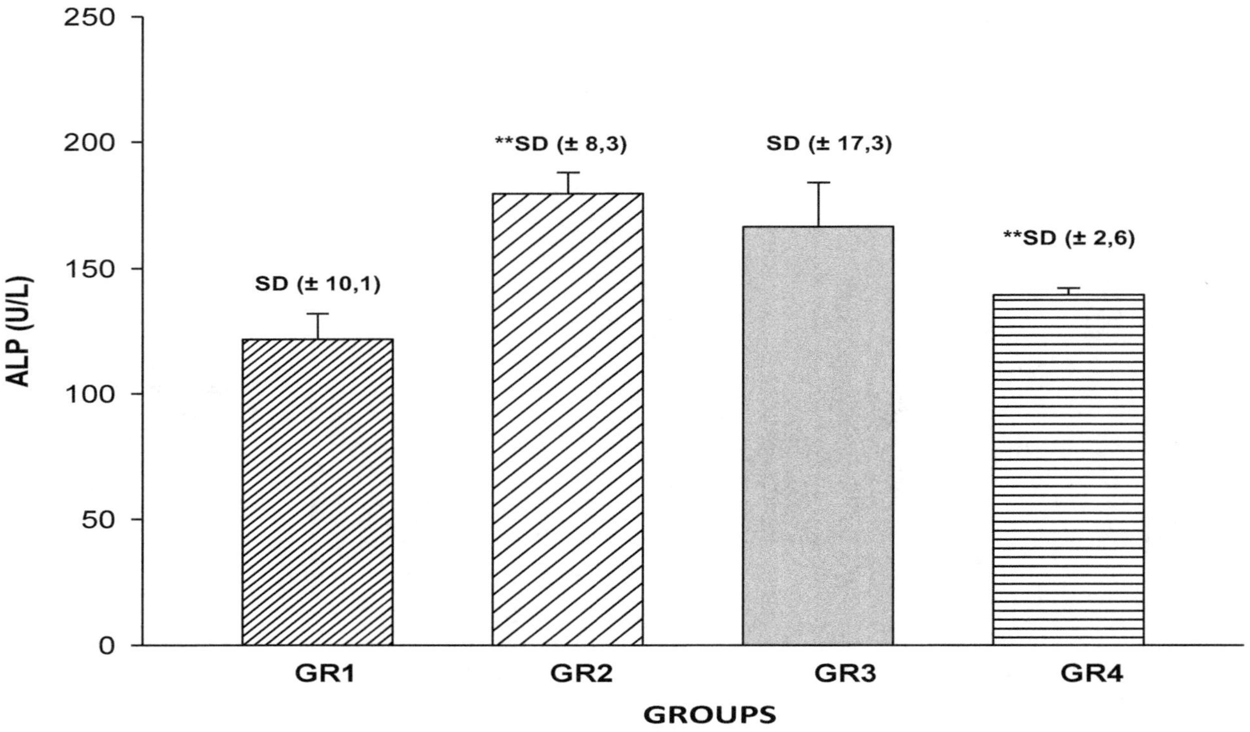

Figure 7. Effects of decoction and macerated *R. alatenus* leaves on serum alkaline phosphatase (ALP) in groups of animals exposed to CCl_4.

liver tissue section (Figure 8C) shows mild degree of liver necrosis. Hepatocytes are compact. Hepatic sinusoids appear normal. The Hepatocytes are well arranged like clusters. In Group 4 (rats treated with CCl_4 and the macerated *R. alaternus* leaves), liver tissue section (Figure 8D) shows that hepatocytes were regenerative and showed no visible changes and prominent nuclei, reduced score of necrosis and no fatty changes. Thus, confirming the safety of the extract.

DISCUSSION

CCl_4 has been used in this present study for its liver toxicity and tropism for hepatocytes. Cell mechanism of CCl_4, has been previously described in different studies (Sarada et al., 2012; Letteron et al., 1990), showing alteration and necrosis of liver cells. Hepatic metabolism of CCl_4 has been initiated by transforming it into its primary metabolites (trichloromethyl and trichlorométhyl peroxyde) through the hepatic cytochrome P450 oxidase and main enzymatic system involved into redox reactions of xenobiotics in the liver. Trichloromethyl peroxide is highly reactive free radicals that will initiate a lipid peroxidation (Sourabie et al., 2012). Free radicals have caused an important flow of GOT and GPT from hepatocyte membranes into blood medium (Sourabie et al., 2012). Results of this present study showed that a dose of CCl_4 (250 ml/kg) have caused severe hepatocellular injury as indicated by the massive elevations of GPT, GOT, ALP and total bilirubin levels in rats intoxicated with CCl_4 (Group 2) when compared with normal control animals (Group 1).

Treated rats (Groups 3, 4) have preserved the integrity of liver cells and significantly decreased elevated enzymatic parameters (GOT, GPT and ALP) and total bilirubin levels. Dose (250 mg/kg) of aqueous extract *R. alaternus* leaves has been used in the present study based on some published studies demonstrating the hepatoprotective activity of this dose (Gopal et al., 2008). In this present study, decoction and specially macerated leaves treated groups (Groups 3 and 4) have exhibited lower levels of GPT, GOT, ALP and bilirubin as compared to CCl_4 treated group (Group 1). Reduction of these parameters is an indication of the stabilization of cell membranes as well as repair of hepatic tissue damage caused by CCl_4 (Lin et al., 2008). The stabilization of serum bilirubin, GPT, GOT, and ALP levels by decoction and macerated plant leaves is a clear indication of the improvement of the functional status of

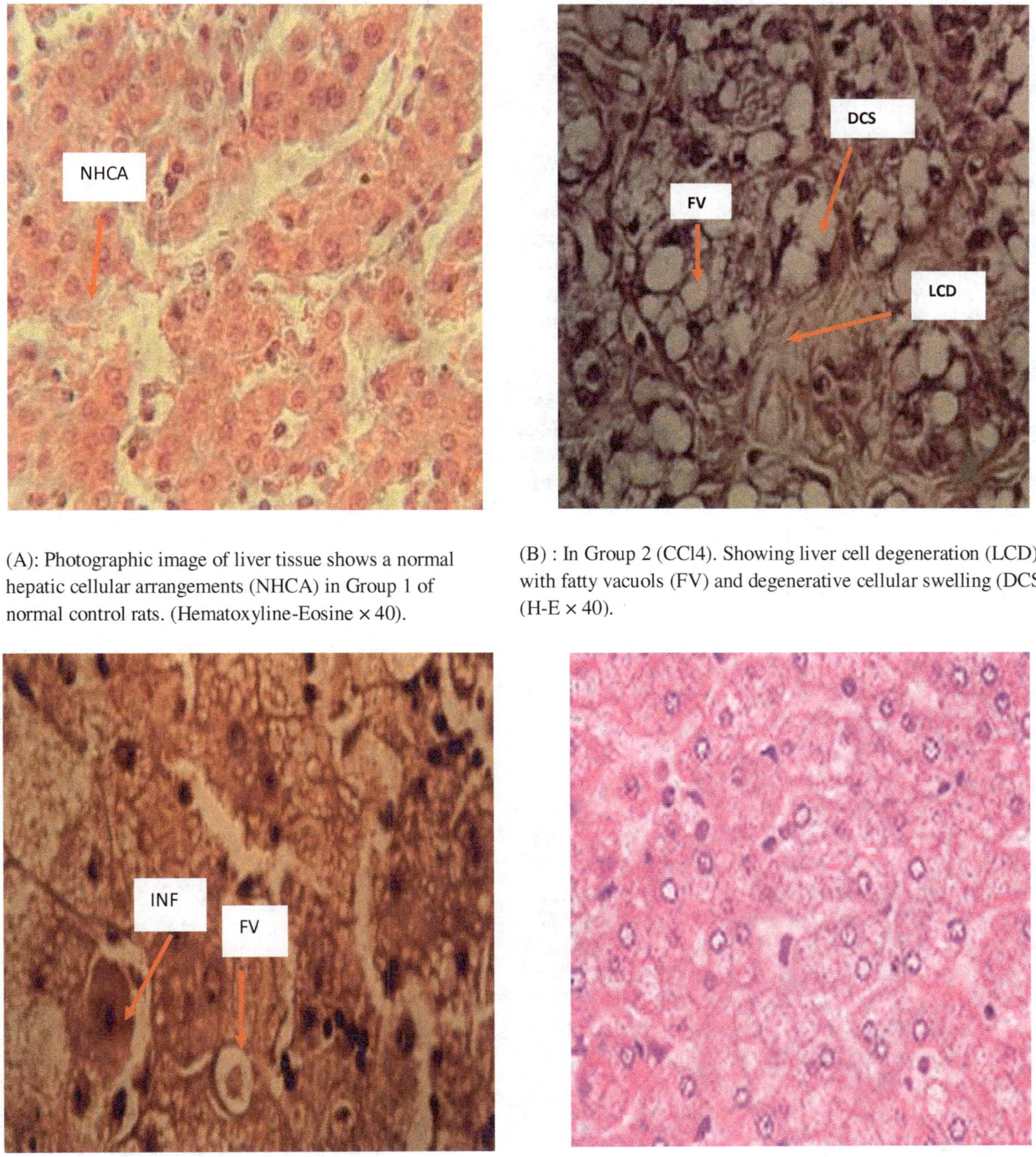

(A): Photographic image of liver tissue shows a normal hepatic cellular arrangements (NHCA) in Group 1 of normal control rats. (Hematoxyline-Eosine × 40).

(B) : In Group 2 (CCl4). Showing liver cell degeneration (LCD), with fatty vacuols (FV) and degenerative cellular swelling (DCS) (H-E × 40).

(C) : In Group 3 (CCl4 + decoction leaves). Less cellular necrosis associated with inflammation (INF) and low presence of fatty vacuoles (FV) (H-E × 40).

(D) : In Group 4 (CCl4 + macerated leaves). Absence of fatty vacuoles and inflammation and normal cell arrangements (H-E × 40).

Figure 8. Histopathologies of various groups.

the liver cells. This indicates the anti-lipid peroxidation of aqueous extract of *R. alaternus* leaves which acted against the damaging effects of free radicals produced by CCl_4.

Histopathological examination clearly reveals that the hepatic cells, central vein and portal triad are almost normal in decoction and macerated *R. alaternus* leaves treated group (250 mg/kg) in contrast to group which received CCl_4. Thus, decoction and macerated *R. alaternus* leaves can be considered to be an effective hepatoprotective agent as it ameliorated almost to normalcy the damage caused by CCl_4 to hepatic function. In literature, it has been suggested that administration of extract of *R. alaternus* increased enzymatic parameters (GOT, GPT and ALP) and total bilirubin level and it may be due to the presence of active constituents such as flavonoids and alkaloids (Ben Ammar et al., 2009). Studies have shown that phenolic compounds had an antioxidant activity as scavenging free radicals (Seyoum et al., 2006).

Phenolic compounds can also act as antioxidants by chelating metal ions, preventing radical formation and improving the antioxidant endogenous system (Al-Azzawie et al., 2006). These compounds are known to act as antioxidants not only because of their ability to donate hydrogen or electrons but also because they are stable radical intermediates. Probably the most important natural phenolics are flavonoids because of their broad spectrum of chemical and biological activities, including antioxidant and free radical scavenging properties (Kahkonen et al., 1999). In fact, flavonoids have been reported as antioxidants, scavengers of a wide range of reactive oxygen species and inhibitors of lipid peroxidation (Williams et al., 2004).

CONCLUSION

Both decoction and macerated *R. alaternus* L. leaves have exhibited a potent hepato-ameliorating and antioxidant effects in rats exposed to CCl_4. But hepato-ameliorating and antioxidant effects of macerated *R. alaternus* L. leaves were found to be better than those of decoction plant leaves. In two cases, the hepatoprorective qualities of aqueous extract of *R. alaternus* L. leaves need to be addressed by isolating and characterizing the active principle(s) responsible for hepatoprotective activity.

ABBREVIATIONS

(NC): Normal control; **(GOT):** Glutamic oxaloacetic transaminase; **(GPT):** Glutamic pyruvic transaminase; **(ALP):** Alkaline phosphatase; **(SD):** Standard deviation; **(ANOVA):** analysis of variance.

Authors' contributions

All authors read and approved the final manuscript.

ACKNOWLEDGEMENT

Our thanks to Dr. M. Terras, member of the Laboratory of Water Resources and Environment of the Saida University and Dr. S. Amara. We also thank technicians of THE Para medical team of Laboratory of Biology Analysis led by Dr. Z. Haddi.

REFERENCES

Al-Azzawie HF, Mohamed-Saiel SA (2006). Hypoglycemic and antioxidant effect of oleuropein in alloxan-diabetic rabbits. Life Sci. 78:1371–1377.

Bahorun T, Gressier B, Trotin F, Brunet C, Dine T, Luyckx M, Vasseur J, Cazin *M*, Cazin JC, Pinkas M (1996). Oxygen species scavenging activity of phenolic extracts from hawthorn fresh plant organs and pharmaceutical preparations. Arznei. Forschung 46:1086-1089.

Belhattab R, Larous L, Kalantzakis G, Bouskou D, Exarchou V (2004). Antifungal properties of *Origanum glandulosum* Desf. extracts. Food, Agric. Environ. 2:63-69

Ben Ammar R, Ben Sghaeir M, Boubaker J, Bhouri W, Naffeti A, Skandrani I, Bouhlel I, Kilani S, Ghedira K, Chekir-Ghedira L (2008). Antioxidant activity and inhibition of aflatoxin B1-, nifuroxaside-, and sodium azide-induced mutagenicity by extracts from *Rhamnus alaternus* L. Chim. Biol. Interact. 174:1-10.

Ben Ammar R, Bhouri W, Ben Sghaier M, Boubaker J, Skandrani I, Neffati A, Bouhlel I, Kilani S, Mariotte AM, Chekir-Ghedira L, Dijoux-Franca MG, Ghedira K (2009). Antioxidant and free radical-scavenging properties of three flavonoids isolated from the leaves of Rhamnus alaternus L. (Rhamnaceae): A structure-activity relationship study. Food Chem. 116: 258–264.

Bruneton J (1999). Pharmacognosy, phytochemistry, medicinal plants. Ed. International Medical. Technical Editions & Documentation, Cachan S1 : 647-673.

Chemli R, Dahmen M, Khaldi A (2006). Guides of medicinal and aromatic plants. pp. 13-116.

Diagram tourism development of the Wilaya of Mascara. In: Project selected tourist development plan. Report No. 3, CENEAP 2012. https://fr.scribd.com/doc/101586413/Report-mascara-Final-doc. Accessed 10 April 2015.

Galighter AE, Koyloff EN (1971). Essential of practical microtechnique. 2nd ed. Lea and Febiger: Philadelphia.

Gopal N, Sengottuvelu S (2008). Hepatoprotective activity of *Clerodendruminerme* against CCl_4 induced hepatic injury in rats. Fitoterapia 79:24-26.

Kahkonen MP, Hopia AI, Vuorela HJ, Rauha JP, Pihlaja K, Kujala TS, Heinonen M (1999). Antioxidant activity of plant extracts containing phenolic compounds. J. Agric. Food Chem. 47:3954–3962.

Khan MR, Ahmed D (2009). Protective effects *of Digera muricata (L.)* Mart. on testis against oxidative stress of carbon tetrachloride in rat. Food Chem. Toxicol. 47:1393-1399.

Kumar G, Banu GS, Pandian MR (2005). Evaluation of the antioxidant activity of *Trianthema portulacastrum L.* Ind. J. Pharmacol. 37:331–333.

Lettéron P, Labbe G, Degott C, Berson A, Fromenty B, Delaforge M, Larrey D, Pessayre D (1990). "Mechanism for the protective effects of silymarin against carbon tetrachloride-induced lipid peroxidation and hepatotoxicity in mice: evidence that silymarin acts both as an inhibitor of metabolic activation and as a chain-breaking antioxidant." Biochem. Pharmacol. 39(12):2027-2034.

Lin HM, Tseng HC, Wang CJ, Lin JJ, Lo CW, Chou FP (2008). Hepato-protective effects of *Solanum nigrum* Linn extract against CCl_4-induced oxidative damage in rats. Chem. Biol. Interact. 171:283-293.

Pang S, Xin X, Stpierre MV (1992). Determinants of Metabolic Disposition. Ann. Rev. Pharmacol. Toxicol. 32:625-626.

Pramyothin P, Chirdchupunsare H, Rungsipipat A, Chaichantipyuth C (2005). Hepatoprotective activity of *Thunbergia laurifolia* Linn extract in rats treated with ethanol: *In vitro* and *in-vivo* studies. J. Ethnopharmacol. 102:408-411.

Rameau D, Mansion G, Dumé C (2008). Flore forestière française, guide écologique illustré, région méditerranéenne, ministère de l'agriculture et de la pèche. P 2426.

Sarada K, Jothibai MR, Mohan VR (2012). Hepatoprotective and antioxidant activity of ethanol extracts of *Naringi crenulata* (Roxb) Nicolson against CCl_4 induced hepatotoxicity in rats. Int. J. Pharm. Sci. Res. 3:874-880.

Seyoum A, Asres K, El-Fiky FK (2006). Structure–radical scavenging activity relationships of flavonoids. Phytochemistry 67:2058–2070.

silymarin against carbon tetrachloride induced lipid peroxidation and hepatotoxicity in mice. Evidence that silymarin acts both as an inhibitor of metabolic activation and as a chainbreaking antioxidant. Biochem. Pharmacol. 39:2027-2034.

Sourabie TS, Nikiema JB, Guissou IP, Nacoulma OG (2012). Comparative study of anti-hepatotoxic effects of extracts of *Argemone mexicana* L. (Papaveraceae), a plant used in traditional treatment of jaundice in Burkina Faso. Int. J. Bio. Chem. Sci. 6: 1139-1147.

Suja SR, Latha PG, Pushpangadan P, Rajasekharan S (2002). Aphrodisiac property of *Helminthostachys zeylanica* in mice. J. Trop. Med. Plants 3:191-195.

WHO guidelines for the safe use of wastewater, excreta and greywater (2005). Volume VI: The use of excreta and greywater in agriculture. World Health Organization, PNUE.

Williams RJ, Spencer JP, Rice-Evans C (2004). Flavonoids: Antioxidants or signalling molecules? Free Rad. Biol. Med. 36:838-849.

Preliminary screening of anti-inflammatory effect of phytochemicals on chemotaxis of human neutrophils

Uthayashanker R. Ezekiel* and Rita M. Heuertz

Department of Biomedical Laboratory Science,Doisy College of Health Sciences,Saint Louis University, 3437 Caroline Street,Saint Louis, USA.

Neutrophils are leukocytes that are actively recruited to sites of tissue infection and/or injury by directed movement (chemotaxis). *In vitro* assessment of inhibition of neutrophil chemotaxis is a physiologic indicator of anti-inflammatory potential. To identify nontoxic, anti-inflammatory agents, plant-derived compounds (curcumin, resveratrol, rosmarinic acid and piperine) were assessed for effects on *in vitro* neutrophil movement. Effects were determined on directed migration (chemotaxis) towards the potent chemoattractant of bacterial cell wall origin, f-met-leu-phe (fMLP). Curcumin significantly inhibited neutrophil chemotaxis in a concentration-dependent manner with statistically significant inhibition at 50 and 100 μM. Similarly, resveratrol (25, 50, 100 μM) and rosmarinic acid (100 μM) significantly inhibited fMLP-induced chemotaxis in concentration-dependent manners. Piperine had no effect on neutrophil chemotaxis. These results indicate that curcumin, resveratrol and rosmarinic acid have the potential to elicit anti-inflammatory effects.

Key words: Neutrophils, phytochemicals, chemotaxis, inflammation.

INTRODUCTION

An important *in vivo* biological event is chemotaxis, which is directed cell movement towards a chemical or biological agent. Chemotaxis occurs in many cell types with examples being leukocyte influx into an inflammatory nidus, migration of endothelial cells for blood vessel formation during angiogenesis, development of an embryo and cancer cell metastasis. Chemotaxis is regularly assessed in immune cells where their mobilization and deployment to sites of inflammation are integral parts of the immune response (Kruger et al., 2015).

One immune cell type, the polymorphonuclear neutrophil (PMN), has been well studied for its chemotactic behavior relevant to its important role in innate immunity and inflammation (Headland and Norling, 2015). Recruitment of neutrophils to sites of inflammation or injury involves the following commonly recognized steps: tethering, rolling, adhesion, crawling and endothelial transmigration (Kolaczkowska and Kubes, 2013). Neutrophil chemotaxis is induced by chemoattractants such as chemokines (interleukin-8: IL-8), bacteria-derived agents (f-met-leu-phe: fMLP) and

*Corresponding author. E-mail: uezekiel@slu.edu.

vasculature-derived components (complement proteins such as C5a) (McNeely et al., 1993). Regardless of the cue, neutrophils in circulation first recognize chemotactic signals in the endothelium close to an inflammatory site, roll along the endothelium and extravasate into the tissue where they fight infections and interact with other cells of the immune system. Neutrophils are the first cells to arrive at an inflammatory site and they do that in massive numbers (Bardoel et al., 2014).

Therefore, assessment of neutrophil chemotaxis is an important early function in acute inflammation. Noteworthy is the fact that impaired recruitment or inappropriate or excessive activation of neutrophils can lead to disease states such as rheumatoid arthritis, inflammatory bowel disease and chronic obstructive pulmonary disease (den Broeder et al., 2003; Kaur and Singh, 2013; Larmonier et al., 2011). It is for this reason that neutrophils have become targets for pharmaceutical approaches to functional regulation. Constant concerns about an ever-expanding population of patients with inflammation-mediated diseases coupled with lack of nontoxic yet efficacious anti-inflammatory agents are sufficient reasons to continue the search for other therapeutic options and strategies. One alternative strategy is the use of plant compounds that have anti-inflammatory properties.

Reports indicate anti-inflammatory properties of rosmarinic acid (derived from rosemary), resveratrol (from skins of red grapes), curcumin (derived from turmeric) and piperine (derived from black pepper). Rosmarinic acid caused susbstantial reduction in inflammation in three different rat models of inflammation, local (carrageenin-induced paw edema) and systemic (liver ischemia/reperfusion injury, thermal injury) (Rocha et al., 2015). Additionally, it reduced inflammation (example, neutrophil infiltration) in LPS-challenged horses (Pearson et al., 2012) and reduced number of inflammatory cells in the airways of an experimental model of respiratory allergy (Costa et al., 2012). Resveratrol inhibited inflammation, with reduced neutrophil infiltration as a marker, in a rat cerebral ischemia/reperfusion model of stroke (Fang et al., 2015) and inhibited airway inflammation and hyperreactivity in mice (Zang et al., 2015). Curcumin, administered as oral doses, inhibited neutrophil infiltration into lavage fluid in mouse models of extrinsic (Hemophilus influenza-induced) and intrinsic (tumor-induced) airway inflammation (Moghaddam et al., 2009), and significantly inhibited neutrophil infiltration and inflammatory cytokine production in a murine model of asthma (Narumoto et al., 2012). Piperine inhibited inflammation in a rat periodontitis model (Dong et al., 2015) and reduced proinflammatory cytokine levels, infarct volume and neuronal loss in a rat model of stroke (Vaibhav et al., 2012).

Given the cited reports, plant-derived compounds with anti-inflammatory potential, specifically curcumin, resveratrol, rosmarinic acid and piperine, were selected for assessment of effects on chemotaxis of human neutrophil. These compounds were assessed by the leading front method of chemotaxis to determine their effects on fMLP-induced chemotaxis of human neutrophils (Kinane et al., 1989). Other reports document anti-inflammatory potential of each one of these plant compounds (Budhiraja and Dhingra, 2014; Hassan-Khabbar et al., 2010; Nonose et al., 2014; Sabina et al., 2011) as well as nontoxic host effects (Wang et al., 2015; McCrea et al., 2015).

MATERIALS AND METHODS

Isolation of human neutrophils

Heparinized venous blood was obtained from normal healthy, medication-free human donors after receiving informed consent following a protocol approved by the Saint Louis University Institutional Review Board. Neutrophils were isolated by dextran sedimentation and Ficoll-Hypaque density gradient centrifugation (Boyum, 1968). Contaminating erythrocytes were removed by hypotonic lysis. Cell purity was determined by differential counts of Wright-Giemsa stain (Sigma-Aldrich, St. Louis, MO) of cytospin preparations (routinely >95%) and neutrophil viability was determined by trypan blue (Sigma-Aldrich) exclusion (routinely >98%).

Phytochemical compounds

The phytochemicals, curcumin, resveratrol, rosmarinic acid and piperine were obtained commercially (Sigma-Aldrich). The compounds were solubilized in dimethylsulfoxide (DMSO: Sigma-Aldrich) at 100 mM stock concentrations and stored at -80°C. Phytochemicals used for chemotaxis were assessed at several concentrations (0.01, 0.1, 1, 10, 100 µM: concentrations were generated by diluting stock solutions in chemotaxis buffer (formulation described below)). The highest concentration (0.1%) of DMSO used for solubilization of plant-derived compounds was assessed in the assay as the vehicle control.

Leading front method of neutrophil chemotaxis

Appropriate concentrations of the bacteria-derived chemoattractant, f-met-leu-phe (fMLP: Sigma-Aldrich), was determined empirically by ascertaining concentration response curves of fMLP. Chemotaxis was measured using the leading front method of Zigmond and Hirsch (1973) as modified by Heuertz et al. (1999). Briefly, neutrophils were pretreated (10 min, 37°C) with plant-derived compounds in chemotaxis buffer consisting of Hanks' balanced salt solution (Sigma-Aldrich) containing N-2-hydroxyl-ethyl-piperazine-N'-2-ethanesulfonic acid (Hepes, 10 mM, pH 7.4: Sigma-Aldrich) and bovine serum albumin (1%: Sigma-Aldrich). Chemoattractant (fMLP) or buffer control (random neutrophil movement) was added to wells of the lower chamber in the chemotaxis assembly. A cellulose-nitrate filter (3 µm pore size: Sartorius Filters, Inc., Hayward, CA) was positioned on top of the lower chamber.

The 48-well chemotaxis apparatus (Neuroprobe, Cabin John, MD) was assembled and neutrophils (200,000 in 50 µl/well) were added to wells of the upper chamber. After set-up, the chemotaxis apparatus was incubated (35 min, 37°C) to allow time for the neutrophils to detect and react to the fMLP. After incubation, filters were removed from the chemotaxis assembly, fixed in isopropanol and stained with Harris acid hematoxylin (Sigma-

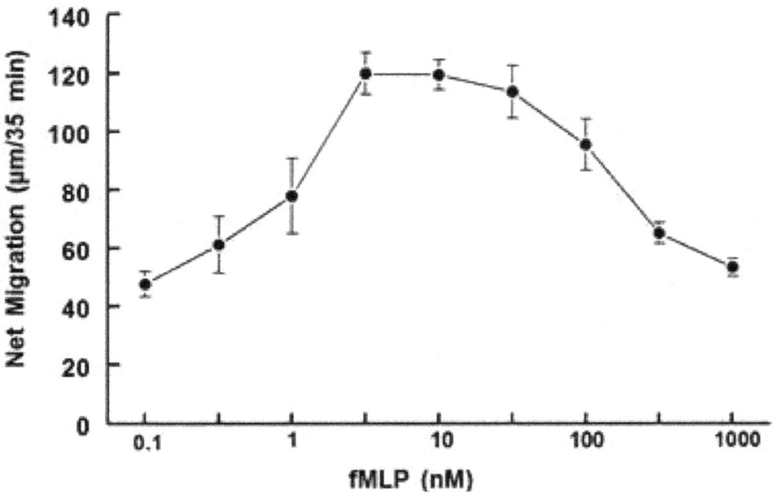

Figure 1. Concentration response curve of fMLP-induced chemotaxis by human neutrophils. The leading front method of chemotaxis was used. n=5.

Aldrich). Filters were viewed microscopically and neutrophil movement into the filter was quantified by identifying distance traveled by the leading two neutrophils, hence the reason the procedure is called the leading front assay. Net neutrophil migration into the filter was determined using the formula: (distance moved in response to treatment) minus (distance moved in response to buffer) = net migration of neutrophil movement in µm/35 min. A suboptimal concentration of fMLP was used for testing plant-derived compounds in order to determine whether inhibition or augmentation of neutrophil movement resulted.

Statistical analysis

All data were reported as the mean ± SEM. Comparisons of sample means were analyzed using repeated measures ANOVA followed by Dunnett multiple comparisons. Differences with $p < 0.05$ were considered significant.

RESULTS

fMLP concentration response curve

Results of the fMLP concentration response curve indicated that peak neutrophil movement was at 5 nM fMLP (Figure 1). Suboptimal concentrations were 0.5 and 1 nM fMLP. Declining neutrophil chemotaxis was evident at 50 to 1,000 nM fMLP.

Neutrophil chemotaxis after pretreatment with plant-derived compounds

The suboptimal concentration of 0.5 nM fMLP was used for assessment of effects of phytochemical-pretreatment on neutrophils. Several concentrations of phytochemicals (0, 0.01, 0.1, 1, 10, 100 uM) were assessed to determine their effects on neutrophil chemotaxis. Curcumin significantly inhibited fMLP-induced neutrophil chemotaxis in a concentration-dependent manner with statistically significant inhibition at 50 and 100 µM (Figure 2A) whereas vehicle (0.1% DMSO) had no effect on the chemotaxis (data not shown). Resveratrol inhibited fMLP-induced chemotaxis in a concentration-dependent manner with statistically significant inhibition at 25, 50 and 100 µM (Figure 2B). Rosmarinic acid inhibited fMLP-induced neutrophil chemotaxis in a concentration-dependent manner with statistically significant inhibition evident at 100 µM (Figure 2C). Piperine had no effect on fMLP-induced chemotaxis of neutrophils (Figure 2D). Trypan blue viability assays were performed in parallel with chemotaxis assays using the highest concentrations of all agents tested. None of the agents tested had any effect on PMN viability.

DISCUSSION

Neutrophils are actively recruited to sites of tissue infection and/or injury by directed movement (chemotaxis). *In vitro* assessment of inhibition of neutrophil chemotaxis is a physiologic indicator of anti-inflammatory potential (Antonicelli et al., 2004). The concentration response curve of fMLP showed suboptimal (0.5 and 1 nM fMLP), peak (5 nM fMLP) and declining (50 to 1,000 nM fMLP) neutrophil chemotaxis. Use of suboptimal concentrations allowed for interpretation of augmentation as well as inhibition outcomes. Declining chemotaxis at higher fMLP concentrations was not used due to the desensitization of neutrophil surface receptors to fMLP at those concentrations.

Plant-derived compounds (curcumin, resveratrol, rosmarinic acid, piperine) were assessed for effects on *in*

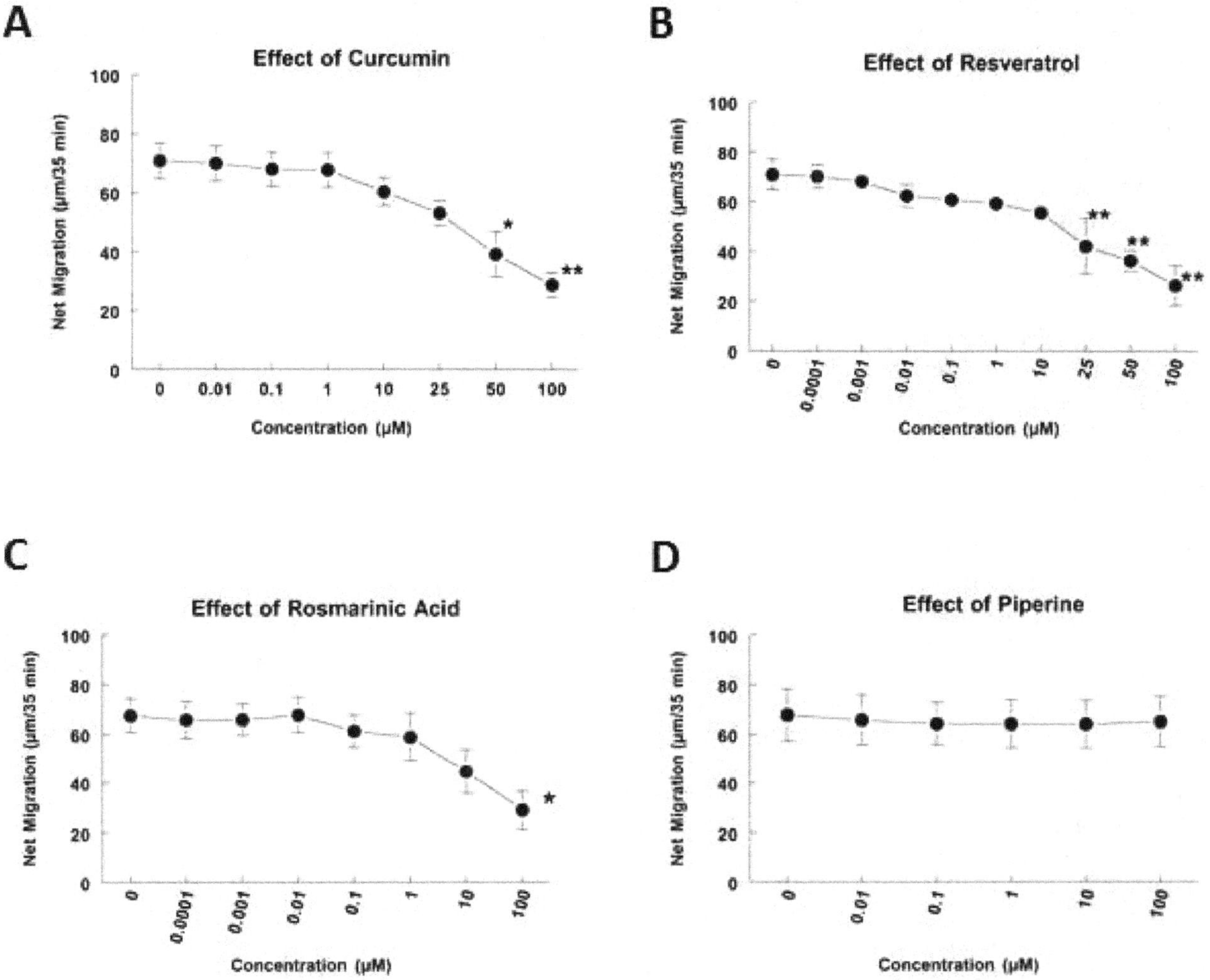

Figure 2. Effect of phytochemicals on fMLP-induced chemotaxis of human neutrophils. Cells were pretreated (10 minutes, 37°C) with indicated compounds and concentrations and then added to the chemotaxis unit for assessment of fMLP (0.5 nM)-induced chemotactic movement by the leading front method. A. Curcumin concentration response curve. n=6 at each concentration. B. Resveratrol concentration response curve. n= 6 at each concentration. C. Rosmarinic acid concentration response curve. n=6 at each concentration. D. Piperine concentration response curve. n = 3 at each concentration. For all panels: * = $p < 0.05$ versus fMLP alone (0 concentration of plant compound). ** = $p < 0.01$ versus fMLP alone (0 concentration of plant compound).

vitro neutrophil movement, that is, on chemotaxis towards the potent chemoattractant of bacterial cell wall origin, f-met-leu-phe (fMLP). Recent studies have shown that curcumin exerts anti-cancer activities on multiple types of cancer (Deguchi, 2015). For this reason, curcumin is one of the most promising phytochemicals that targets cancers and inflammation-mediated diseases. In the present study, curcumin significantly inhibited neutrophil chemotaxis in a concentration-dependent manner with statistically significant inhibition at 50 and 100 µM (Figure 2A). Neutrophil chemotaxis to an IL-8 homologue in mice (MIP-2) proceeds through a signalling pathway that initiates at a G-protein-coupled receptor (CXCR2). Activation of this receptor renders an effect on F-actin polymerization in the lamellar region of the neutrophil through phosphoinositide 3-kinase (PI3K) and phosphatidylinositol(3,4,5)-trisphosphate ($PI(3,4,5)P_3$) pathway which includes protein kinase B (Akt/PKB) and guanosine triphosphatases Cdc42 and Rac 2. Larmonier et al. (2011), showed that curcumin inhibited actin formation at the leading edge of neutrophils during movement, an event that involved PI3K and PI ($3,4,5P_3$). The finding that ERK phosphorylation was not affected indicated that the curcumin effect was not targeted to initial stages of MIP-2/CXCR2 signal transduction in the neutrophil. The inhibitory effect herein reported may be due to regulation of F-actin polymerization through phosphoinositide 3-kinase (PI3K) and phosphatidylinositol(3,4,5)-trisphosphate ($PI(3,4,5)P_3$) in the lamellar region of a migrating neutrophil, all of which are vital components of leading edge formation (Larmonier et al, 2011).

Resveratrol, the polyphenol present in skins of red grapes and in red wines, has been linked with anti-inflammatory and anti-cancer activities (Inoue and Nakata, 2015; Wang et al., 2015). It is herein shown that resveratrol inhibited fMLP-induced chemotaxis in a concentration-dependent manner with statistically significant inhibition at 25, 50 and 100 µM (Figure 2B). This result confirms prior reports (Inoue and Nakata, 2015; Wang et al., 2015) that resveratrol has anti-inflammatory activities. Inoue and Nakata state that resveratrol is a phytoalexin indicating that it is an antimicrobic synthesized by plants in response to assault by pathogenic bacteria or environmental stresses with resultant resistance to infection and stresses. Other anti-inflammatory processes ascribed to resveratrol are cyclooxygenase inhibition (Inoue and Nakata, 2015) and prevention of cytokine-induced vascular leakage (Wang, Dabrosin et al. 2015).

Rosmarinic acid from *Rosmarinus officinalis* has been shown to be anti-inflammatory *in vivo* by reducing number of leukocytes that roll, adhere and migrate to an inflamed site after injection of inflammatory agents in a rat model (Nogueira de Melo et al., 2011). Following up on this report, the question was posed as to whether purified rosmarinic acid rendered a similar effect in vitro as rosemary essential oil did in vivo. As shown herein, rosmarinic aid displayed significant anti-chemotactic effect, albeit at a single concentration (100 uM: Figure 2C). To our knowledge, this is the first report of inhibition of chemotaxis of human neutrophils by rosmarinic acid.

While piperine from *Piper nigrum* has been reported to have anti-inflammatory (Mujumdar et al., 1990; Sunila and Kuttan, 2004) and pro-inflammatory properties (Mujumdar et al., 1990; Sunila and Kuttan, 2004), piperine exhibited no effect on fMLP-induced neutrophil chemotaxis at the doses tested (Figure 2D). Mujumdar and Dhuley assessed piperine action in *in vivo* acute and chronic models of inflammation and identified that an anti-inflammatory piperine action was significantly manifested during acute inflammation at early stages. However, Sunila and Kuttan assessed piperine effect on solid tumor development and found that piperine increased total leukocyte number at the tumor site thereby implicating phagocyte recruitment and pro-inflammatory processes at the site. In another study, chemotaxis of macrophages (cell line Raw 264.7 of murine origin) was inhibited by piperine in a dose-dependent manner at concentrations similar to those used in the current study (Woo et al., 2007). It was therefore of interest to define the effect of piperine on chemotaxis of human neutrophils.

The present study identified the use of a well-established and long-used method to assess anti-inflammatory effects of phytochemicals, specifically the anti-inflammatory effect of inhibition of neutrophil chemotaxis. Studies suggest that neutrophil and cancer cell movement share common features such as mechanisms of signal transduction, movement as receptor-mediated events and induction by chemokine chemoattractants (Soon, 2007; Wang, 2009). Therefore, prevention of chemotaxis by phytochemicals has the potential to alleviate disease conditions involving inflammation. As the inflammatory process becomes better elucidated, the list of diseases caused or affected by inflammation grows longer. Interestingly, links between cancer and inflammation have been identified, especially as related to cell movement (Lin and Karin, 2007). For this reason, effects of phytochemicals on cancer cell movement deserve assessment for anti-metastasis potential. Future studies focus on mechanistic actions of these phytochemicals relevant to neutrophil chemotaxis.

CONCLUSION

Plant-derived compounds, such as resveratrol, curcumin and rosmarinic acid, inhibit chemotaxis of human neutrophils. These results indicate that phytochemicals have the ability to inhibit neutrophil recruitment to sites of infection and injury, and therefore have potential as anti-inflammatory agents with mechanistic action targeted at initial step of the innate immune response.

ACKNOWLEDGEMENTS

This work was funded in part by the Saint Louis University President Research Fund to URE.

REFERENCES

Antonicelli F, Brown D, Parmentier M, Drost EM, Hirani N, Rahman I, Donaldson K, MacNee W (2004). Regulation of LPS-mediated inflammation in vivo and in vitro by the thiol antioxidant Nacystelyn. Am. J. Physiol. Lung Cell Mol. Physiol. 286:L1319-1327.

Bardoel BW, Kenny EF, Sollberger G, Zychlinsky A (2014). The balancing act of neutrophils. Cell Host Microb. 15:526-536.

Boyum A (1968). Isolation of mononuclear cells and granulocytes from human blood. Isolation of mononuclear cells by one centrifugation, and of granulocytes by combining centrifugation and sedimentation at 1 g. Scand. J. Clin. Lab. Invest. Suppl. 97:77-89.

Budhiraja A, Dhingra G (2014). Development and characterization of a novel antiacne niosomal gel of rosmarinic acid. Drug Deliv. [Epub ahead of print].

Costa RS, Carneiro TC, Cerqueira-Lima AT, Queiroz NV, Alcântara-Neves NM, Pontes-de-Carvalho LC, Velozo Eda S, Oliveira EJ, Figueiredo CA (2012). *Ocimum gratissimum* Linn. and rosmarinic acid, attenuate eosinophilic airway inflammation in an experimental model of respiratory allergy to Blomia tropicalis. Int. Immunopharmacol. 13:126-134.

Deguchi A (2015). Curcumin targets in inflammation and cancer. Endocr. Metab. Immune Disord. Drug Targets. 15:88-96.

den Broeder AA, Wanten GJ, Oyen WJ, Naber T, van Riel PL,

Barrera P (2003). Neutrophil migration and production of reactive oxygen species during treatment with a fully human anti-tumor necrosis factor-alpha monoclonal antibody in patients with rheumatoid arthritis. J. Rheumatol. 30:232-237.
Dong Y, Huihui Z, Li C (2015). Piperine inhibit inflammation, alveolar bone loss and collagen fibers breakdown in a rat periodontitis model. J Periodontal Res. [Epub ahead of print].
Fang L, Gao H, Zhang W, Zhang W, Wang Y (2015). Resveratrol alleviates nerve injury after cerebral ischemia and reperfusion in mice by inhibiting inflammation and apoptosis. Int. J. Clin. Exp. Med. 8:3219-3226.
Hassan-Khabbar S, Vamy M, Cottart CH, Wendum D, Vibert F, Savouret JF, Therond P, Clot JP, Waligora AJ, Nivet-Antoine V (2010). Protective effect of post-ischemic treatment with trans-resveratrol on cytokine production and neutrophil recruitment by rat liver. Biochimie 92:405-410.
Headland SE, Norling LV (2015). The resolution of inflammation: Principles and challenges. Semin. Immunol. 27(3):149-160
Heuertz RM, Tricomi SM, Ezekiel UR, Webster RO (1999). C-reactive protein inhibits chemotactic peptide-induced p38 mitogen-activated protein kinase activity and human neutrophil movement. J. Biol. Chem. 274:17968-17974.
Inoue H, Nakata R (2015). Resveratrol targets in inflammation. Endocr. Metab. Immune Disord. Drug Targets. J. Periodont. Res. [Epub ahead of print].
Kaur M, Singh D (2013). Neutrophil chemotaxis caused by chronic obstructive pulmonary disease alveolar macrophages: the role of CXCL8 and the receptors CXCR1/CXCR2. J. Pharmacol. Exp. Ther. 347:173-180.
Kinane DF, Cullen CF, Johnston FA, Evans CW (1989). Neutrophil chemotactic behaviour in patients with early-onset forms of periodontitis (I). Leading front analysis in Boyden chambers. J. Clin. Periodontol. 16:242-246.
Kolaczkowska E, Kubes P (2013). Neutrophil recruitment and function in health and inflammation. Nat. Rev. Immunol. 13:159-175.
Kruger P, Saffarzadeh M, Weber AN, Rieber N, Radsak M, von Bernuth H, Benarafa C, Roos D, Skokowa J, Hartl D (2015). Neutrophils: Between host defence, immune modulation, and tissue injury. PLoS Pathog. 11:e1004651.
Larmonier CB, Midura-Kiela MT, Ramalingam R, Laubitz D, Janikashvili N, Larmonier N, Ghishan FK, Kiela PR (2011). Modulation of neutrophil motility by curcumin: implications for inflammatory bowel disease. Inflamm. Bowel Dis. 17:503-515.
Lin WW, Karin M (2007). A cytokine-mediated link between innate immunity, inflammation, and cancer. J. Clin. Invest. 117:1175-1183.
McCrea CE, West SG, Kris-Etherton PM, Lambert JD, Gaugler TL, Teeter DL, Sauder KA, Gu Y, Glisan SL, Skulas-Ray AC (2015). Effects of culinary spices and psychological stress on postprandial lipemia and lipase activity: results of a randomized crossover study and *in vitro* experiments. J. Transl. Med. 13:7.
McNeely MC, Lawley TJ, Harvath L (1993). Monoclonal antibody modulates human neutrophil chemotaxis to N-formyl-methionyl-leucyl-phenylalanine (fMLP). J. Invest. Dermatol. 101:377-382.
Moghaddam SJ, Barta P, Mirabolfathinejad SG, Ammar-Aouchiche Z, Garza NT, Vo TT, Newman RA, Aggarwal BB, Evans CM, Tuvim MJ, Lotan R, Dickey BF (2009). Curcumin inhibits COPD-like airway inflammation and lung cancer progression in mice. Carcinogenesis 30:1949-1956.
Mujumdar AM, Dhuley JN, Deshmukh VK, Raman PH, Naik SR (1990). Anti-inflammatory activity of piperine. Jpn. J. Med. Sci. Biol. 43:95-100.
Narumoto O, Matsuo Y, Sakaguchi M, Shoji S, Yamashita N, Schubert D, Abe K, Horiguchi K, Nagase T, Yamashita N (2012). Suppressive effects of a pyrazole derivative of curcumin on airway inflammation and remodeling. Exp. Mol. Pathol. 93:18-25.
Nogueira de Melo GA, Grespan R, Fonseca JP, Farinha TO, Silva EL, Romero AL, Bersani-Amado CA, Cuman RK (2011). *Rosmarinus officinalis* L. essential oil inhibits *in vivo* and *in vitro* leukocyte migration. J. Med. Food 14:944-946.
Nonose N, Pereira JA, Machado PR, Rodrigues MR, Sato DT, Martinez CA (2014). Oral administration of curcumin (*Curcuma longa*) can attenuate the neutrophil inflammatory response in zymosan-induced arthritis in rats. Acta Cir Bras 29:727-734.
Pearson W, Fletcher RS, Kott LS (2012). Oral rosmarinic acid-enhanced Mentha spicata modulates synovial fluid biomarkers of inflammation in horses challenged with intra-articular LPS. J. Vet. Pharmacol. Ther. 35:495-502.
Rocha J, Eduardo-Figueira M, Barateiro A, Fernandes A, Brites D, Bronze R, Duarte CM, Serra AT, Pinto R, Freitas M, Fernandes E, Silva-Lima B, Mota-Filipe H, Sepodes B (2015). Anti-inflammatory effect of rosmarinic acid and an extract of Rosmarinus officinalis in rat models of local and systemic inflammation. Basic Clin. Pharmacol. Toxicol. 116:398-413.
Sabina EP, Nagar S, Rasool M (2011). A role of piperine on monosodium urate crystal-induced inflammation--an experimental model of gouty arthritis. Inflammation 34:184-192.
Soon LL (2007). A discourse on cancer cell chemotaxis: where to from here? IUBMB Life 59:60-67.
Sunila ES, Kuttan G (2004). Immunomodulatory and antitumor activity of Piper longum Linn. and piperine. J. Ethnopharmacol. 90:339-346.
Vaibhav K, Shrivastava P, Javed H, Khan A, Ahmed ME, Tabassum R, Khan MM, Khuwaja G, Islam F, Siddiqui MS, Safhi MM, Islam F (2012). Piperine suppresses cerebral ischemia- reperfusion-induced inflammation through the repression of COX- 2, NOS-2, and NF-κB in middle cerebral artery occlusion rat model. Mol. Cell Biochem. 367:73-84.
Wang F (2009). The signaling mechanisms underlying cell polarity and chemotaxis. Cold Spring Harb. Perspect. Biol. 1:4.
Wang Z, Dabrosin C, Yin X, Fuster MM, Arreola A, Rathmell WK, Generali D, Nagaraju GP, El-Rayes B, Ribatti D, Chen YC, Honoki K, Fujii H, Georgakilas AG, Nowsheen S, Amedei A, Niccolai E, Amin A, Ashraf SS, Helferich B, Yang X, Guha G, Bhakta D, Ciriolo MR, Aquilano K, Chen S, Halicka D, Mohammed SI, Azmi AS, Bilsland A, Keith WN, Jensen LD (2015). Broad targeting of angiogenesis for cancer prevention and therapy. Semin. Cancer Biol. pii:S1044-579X(15)00002-4.
Woo HM, Kang JH, Kawada T, Yoo H, Sung MK, Yu R (2007). Active spice-derived components can inhibit inflammatory responses of adipose tissue in obesity by suppressing inflammatory actions of macrophages and release of monocyte chemoattractant protein-1 from adipocytes. Life Sci. 80:926-931.
Zang N, Li S, Li W, Xie X, Ren L, Long X, Xie J, Deng Y, Fu Z, Xu F, Liu E (2015.) Resveratrol suppresses persistent airway inflammation and hyperresponsivess might partially via nerve growth factor in respiratory syncytial virus-infected mice. Int. Immunopharmacol. 28: 121-128.
Zigmond SH, Hirsch JG (1973.) Leukocyte locomotion and chemotaxis. New methods for evaluation, and demonstration of a cell-derived chemotactic factor. J. Exp. Med. 137:387-410.

17

Analysis of bioactive chemical compounds of *Euphorbia lathyrus* using gas chromatography-mass spectrometry and Fourier-transform infrared spectroscopy

Azhar Abduameer Sosa[1], Suhaila Husaein Bagi[1], and Imad Hadi Hameed[2]*

[1]College of Education for Women, Al-Qadisyia University, Iraq.
[2]College of Nursing, Babylon University, Iraq.

The aim of this study was determination the phytochemical composition of methanolic seeds extract of *Euphorbia lathyrus*. Gas chromatography-mass spectrometry (GC-MS) analysis of *E. lathyrus* revealed the existence of the Carbonic acid, (ethyl)(1,2,4-triazol-1-ylmethyl) diester, 1H-Pyrrole,2,5-dihydro-1-nitroso, Hexanal dimethyl acetal, Isosorbide dinitrate, DL-Arabinose, Cyclopropane,1-fluoro-1-(2-bromoethenyl)-2,2,3,3-tetramethyl, α-D-Glucopyranoside, O-α-D-glucopyranosyl-(1.fwdarw.3)-ß-d-fruc, Desulphosinigrin, D-Glucose, 6-O-α-D-galactopyranosyl, Octanoic acid, Benzofuran,2,3-dihydro, 6-Acetyl-ß-d-mannose, Estragole, Ascaridole epoxide, 3-Allyl-6-methoxyphenol, 4-Amino-1,5,pentandioic acid, l-Gala-l-ido-octonic lactone, y-Sitosterol, Tetradecanoic acid, l-(+)-Ascorbic acid 2,6-dihexadecanoate, Estra -1,3,5(10)-trien-17ß-ol, Propanoic acid,2-(3-acetoxy-4,4,14-trimethylandrost-8-en-17-yl), Cis-13-Eicosenoic acid, Eicosanoic acid, 3-Pyrinecarboxylic acid, 2,7,10-tris(acetyloxy)-1,1a,2,3,4,6,7,10, Oleic acid, eicosyl ester, Butanoic acid, 4-chloro-,1,1a,1b,4,4a,5,7a,7b,8,9-decahydro-4a, Ethyl iso–allocholate, Ethyl iso –allocholate, Olean-12-ene-3,15,16,21,22,28-hexol, (3ß,15α,16α,21ß,22α)- and 2,4,6-Decatrienoic acid,1a,2,5,5a,6,9,10,10a-octahydro-5,5a-dihy. The Fourier-transform infrared spectroscopy (FTIR) analysis of *E. lathyrus* seeds proved the presence of alkenes, aliphatic fluoro compounds, alcohols, ethers, carboxlic acids, esters, nitro compounds, alkanes, hydrogen bonded alcohols, and phenols.

Key words: Gas chromatography-mass spectrometry (GC/MS), bioactive compounds, Fourier-transform infrared spectroscopy (FT-IR), *Euphorbia lathyrus*.

INTRODUCTION

Medicinal plant parts (roots, leaves, branches/stems, barks, flowers, and fruits) are commonly rich in phenolic compounds, such as flavonoids, phenolic acids, stilbenes, tannins, coumarins, lignans and lignins (Cai et

*Corresponding author. E-mail: imad_dna@yahoo.com.

al., 2004; Altameme et al., 2015a; Al-Marzoqi et al., 2015). The seed of *Euphorbia lathyris* is a traditional Chinese medicine which has been used for the treatment of hydropsy, ascites, anuresis and constipation, amenorrhea, and scabies (Liu et al., 2011). Nowadays, traditional medicinal practices form an integral part of complementary or alternative medicine. Although their efficacy and mechanisms of action have not been tested scientifically in most cases, these simple medicinal preparations often mediate beneficial responses due to their active chemical constituents (Park and Pezzutto, 2002; Corro et al., 2014; Hameed et al., 2015a). In recent years, it was reported that the seeds of *Euphorbia* had a significant effect on leukemia, esophageal carcinoma, and skin cancer (Tapiero et al., 2002; Liu et al., 2011; Al-Marzoqi et al., 2016). The seed of *E. lathyris* is a kind of toxic traditional Chinese medicine, which is characterized by pungent, warm and poisonous in drug properties. It shows several side effects, such as irritation and inflammation intense on the skin, mouth and gastrointestinal tract irritation, carcinogenic, etc. (Buenz et al., 2004; Altameme et al., 2015b). The objective of this study was to analyse the chemical composition of seeds extract from methanol. The phytochemical compound was screened by gas chromatography-mass spectrometry (GC-MS) and Fourier-transform infrared spectroscopy (FT-IR) technique.

MATERIALS AND METHODS

Plant and preparation of extracts

E. lathyrus dried seeds were purchased from local market in hilla city, middle of Iraq. After thorough cleaning and removal of foreign materials, the fruits were stored in airtight container to avoid the effect of humidity and then stored at room temperature until further use. About 30 g of the plant sample powdered were soaked in 100 ml methanol for 16 h in a rotatory shaker (Hamza et al., 2015; Hussein et al., 2016a). Whatman No.1 filter paper was used to separate the extract of plant. The filtrates were used for further phytochemical analysis. It was again filtered through sodium sulphate in order to remove the traces of moisture (Altameme et al., 2015c; Hameed et al., 2015b).

Identification of component by GC-MS analysis

The physicochemical properties of *E. lathyrus* are shown in Table 1. Interpretation of mass spectroscopy (GC-MS) was conducted by using data base of National Institute Standard and Technology (NIST) having more than 62000 patterns. The spectrum of the unknown component was compared with the spectrum of the known component stored in the NIST library. The identity of the components in the extracts was assigned by the comparison of their retention indices and mass spectra fragmentation patterns with those stored on the computer library and also with published literatures (Hadi et al., 2016; Hameed et al., 2015c; Hussein et al., 2016b).The GC-MS analysis of the plant extract was made in an Agilent 7890 A instrument under computer control at 70 eV. About 1 µl of the methanol extract was injected into the GC-MS using a micro syringe and the scanning was done for 45 min. The fragments obtained were actually charged ions with a certain mass (Hameed et al., 2015d; Hussein et al., 2016c). Helium gas was used as a carrier as well as an eluent. The flow rate of helium was set to 1 ml/min. The electron gun of mass detector liberated electrons having energy of about 70 eV. The column employed here for the separation of components was Elite 1 (100% dimethyl poly siloxane).

Fourier transform infrared spectrophotometer (FTIR)

The powdered sample of *E. lathyrus* specimen was treated for FTIR spectroscopy (Shimadzu, IR Affinity 1, Japan). The sample was run at infrared region between 400 and 4000 nm (Hussein et al., 2016; Jasim et al., 2015).

RESULTS AND DISCUSSION

Gas chromatography and mass spectroscopy analysis of compounds was carried out in methanolic seed extract of *E. lathyrus* shown in Table 1. The GC-MS chromatogram of the 31 peaks of the compounds detected is as shown in Figure 1. Chromatogram GC-MS analysis of the methanol extract of *E. lathyrus* showed the presence of thirty one major peaks and the components corresponding to the peaks were determined as follows. The first set up peak was determined to be Carbonic acid, (ethyl)(1,2,4-triazol-1-ylmethyl) diester (Figure 2). The next peaks were considered to be 1H-Pyrrole,2,5-dihydro-1-nitroso, Hexanal dimethyl acetal, Isosorbide dinitrate, DL-Arabinose, Cyclopropane,1-fluoro-1-(2-bromoethenyl)-2,2,3,3-tetramethyl, α-D-Glucopyranoside, O-α-D-glucopyranosyl - (1.fwdarw.3) – ß - d-fruc, Desulphosinigrin, D-Glucose, 6-O-α-D-galactopyranosyl, Octanoic acid, Benzofuran,2,3-dihydro, 6-Acetyl-ß-d-mannose, Estragole, Ascaridole epoxide, 3-Allyl-6-methoxyphenol, 4-Amino-1,5,pentandioic acid, l-Gala-l-ido-octonic lactone, y-Sitosterol, Tetradecanoic acid, l-(+)-Ascorbic acid 2,6-dihexadecanoate, Estra-1,3,5(10)-trien-17ß-ol, Propanoic acid,2-(3-acetoxy-4,4,14-trimethylandrost-8-en-17-yl), Cis-13-Eicosenoic acid, Eicosanoic acid, 3-Pyrinecarboxylic acid , 2,7,10-tris(acetyloxy)-1,1a,2,3,4,6,7,10, Oleic acid, eicosyl ester, Butanoic acid, 4-chloro-,1,1a,1b,4,4a,5,7a,7b,8,9-decahydro-4a, Ethyl iso-allocholate, Ethyl iso – allocholate, Olean-12-ene-3,15,16,21,22,28-hexol, (3ß,15α,16α,21ß,22α)- and 2,4,6-Decatrienoic acid,1a,2,5,5a,6,9,10,10a-octahydro-5,5a-dihy (Figures 3 to 31). The FTIR analysis of *E. lathyrus* seeds proved the presence of alkenes, aliphatic fluoro compounds, alcohols, ethers, carboxlic acids, esters, nitro compounds, alkanes, hydrogen bonded alcohols and phenols which shows major peaks at 837.11, 918.12, 1037.70, 1145.72, 1232.51, 1261.45, 1317.38, 1409.96, 1519.91, 1625.99, 1741.72, 2682.98, 2854.65, 2924.09, 3082.25, and 3275.13 (Table 2 and Figure 32). *E. lathyris* L. active for disinfection is an herbaceous plant of Euphorbiaceae and has been extensively researched in the field of medicine. Phenolic compounds were isolated and identified from *E. lathyrus* using RP-HPLC under the

Table 1. Major phytochemical compounds identified in methanolic extract of *Euphorbia lathyrus*.

S/N	Phytochemical compound	RT (min)	Molecular Weight	Exact mass	Chemical structure	Pharmacological actions
1	Carbonic acid, (ethyl)(1,2,4-triazol-1-ylmethyl) diester	3.259	171	171.064391	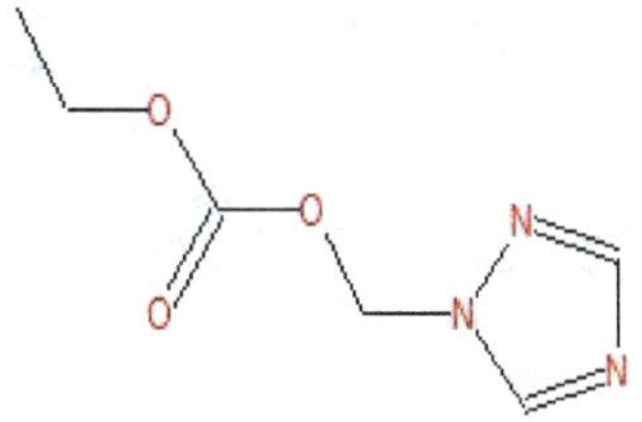	Pharmacological activities such as anti-microbial, anti-inflammatory
2	1H-Pyrrole,2,5-dihydro-1-nitroso-	3.367	98	98.0480127	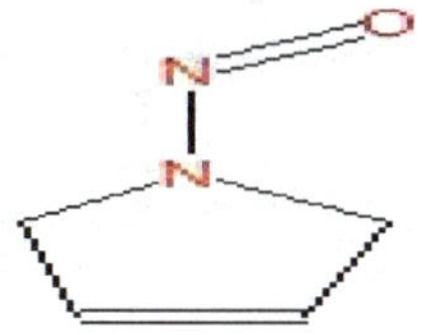	Antibacterial, antiviral, anticonvulsant and analgesic
3	Hexanal dimethyl acetal	3.533	146	146.13068	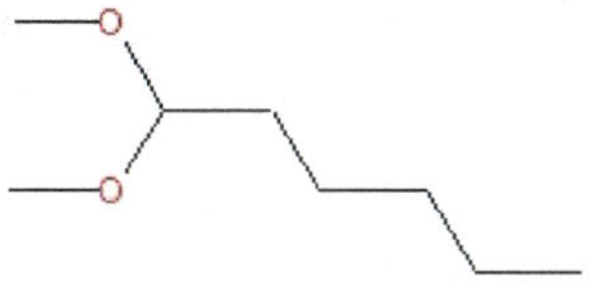	Antiviral and anti-inflammatory
4	Isosorbide dinitrate	4.546	236	236.028066	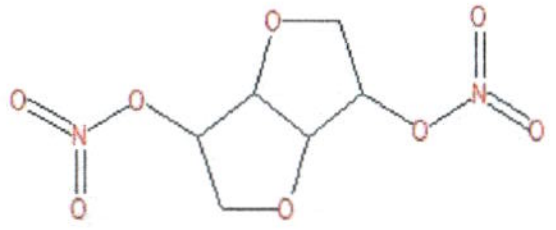	Relaxation
5	DL-Arabinose	4.878	150	150.052823	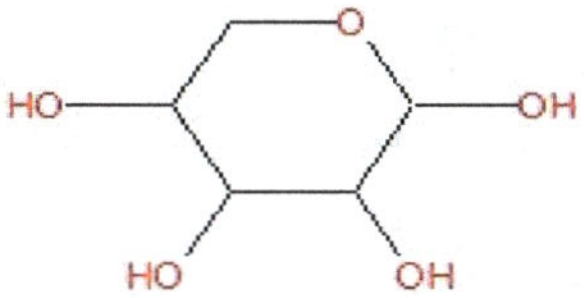	Anti-tumor activity
6	Cyclopropane,1-fluoro-1-(2-bromoethenyl)-2,2,3,3-tetramethyl-	5.010	220	220.026291	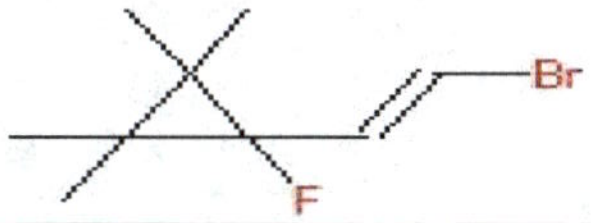	Many medicinal activities, which included anti-cancer and anti-cardiovascular

Table 1. cont'd

7	α-D-Glucopyranoside, O-α-D-glucopyranosyl-(1.fwdarw.3)-ß-d-fruc	5.261	504	504.169035	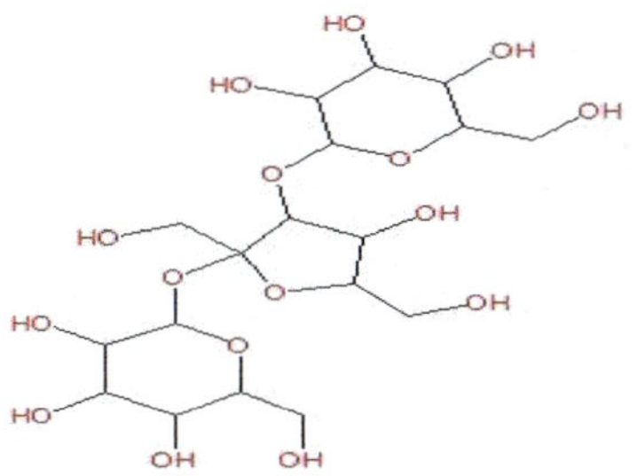	Anti-diabetic activity and anti-tumour
8	Desulphosinigrin	5.313	279	279.077658	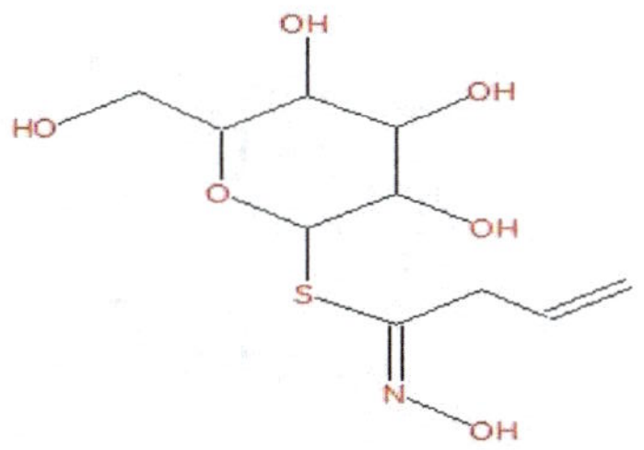	Antibacterial activity
9	D-Glucose, 6-O-α-D-galactopyranosyl	5.782	342	342.11621	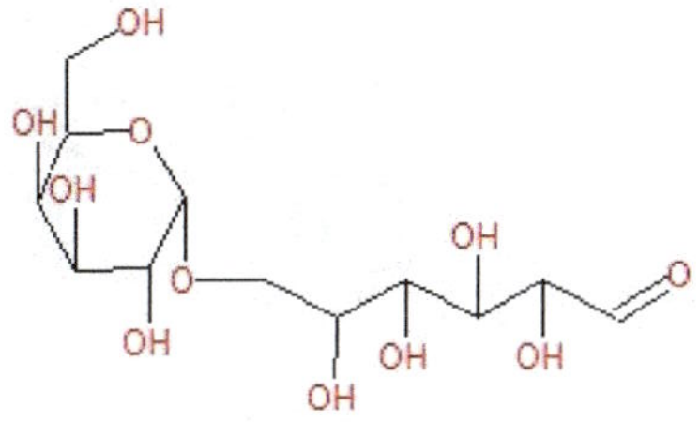	Anti-trypanosomal activity
10	Octanoic acid	6.137	144	144.115029	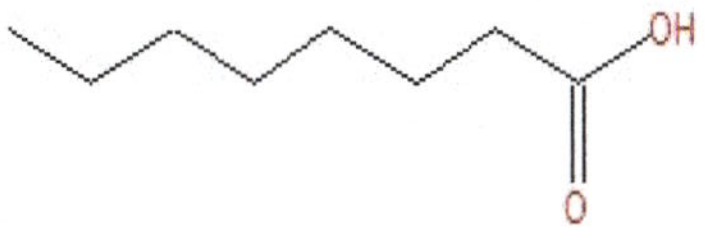	Anti-bacterial activity
11	Benzofuran,2,3-dihydro-	6.715	120	120.0575147	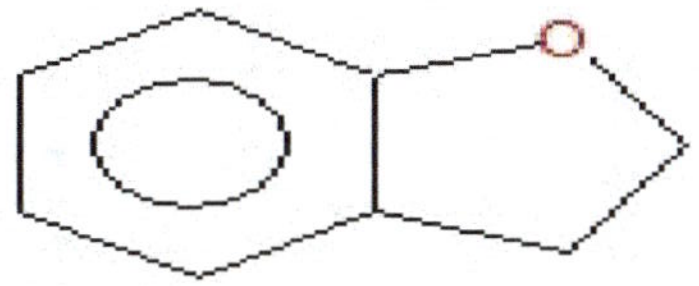	Anti-HIV, anticancer, antibacterial, and antifungal activities

Table 1. cont'd

12	6-Acetyl-ß-d-mannose	6.984	222	222.073953	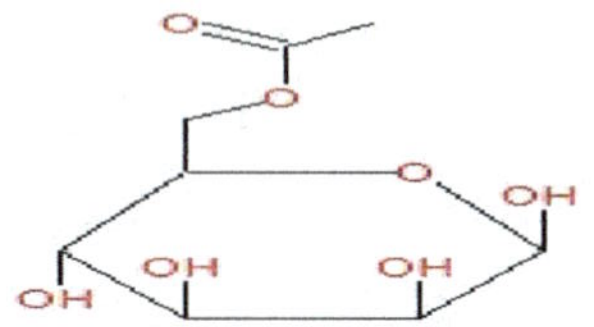	Anti-inflammatory and anti-oxidant
13	Estragole	7.481	148	148.088815	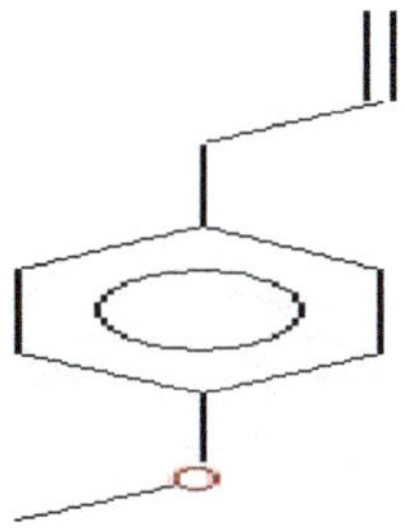	Estragole has been shown to have an anti-inflammatory activity
14	Ascaridole epoxide	7.727	184	184.109944	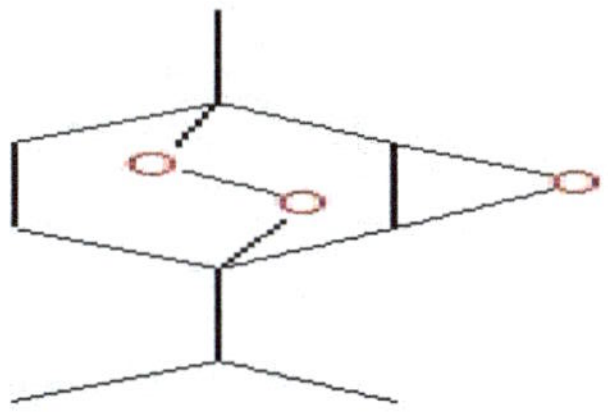	Anti-inflammatory
15	3-Allyl-6-methoxyphenol	8.443	164	164.08373	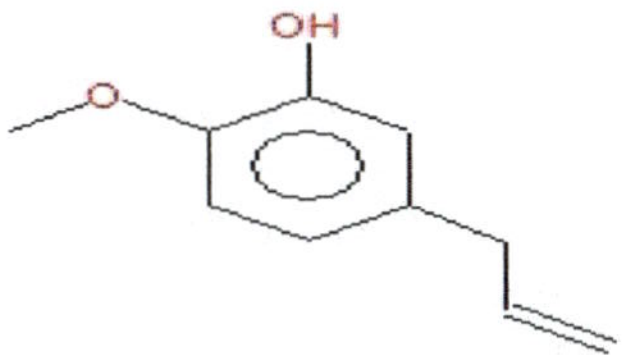	Anticancer activity
16	4-Amino-1,5,pentandioic acid	9.564	175	175.084458	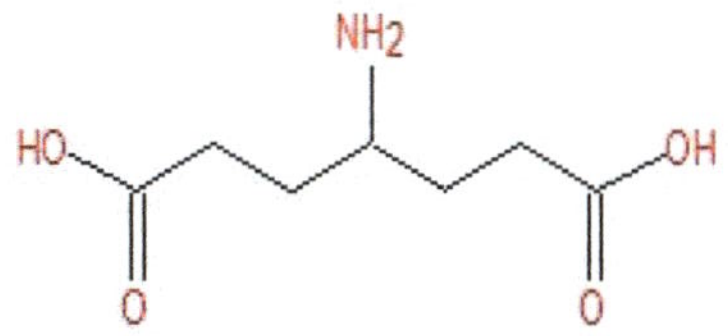	Anti-cancer agent

Table 1. cont'd

17	l-Gala-l-ido-octonic lactone	10.734	238	238.068868	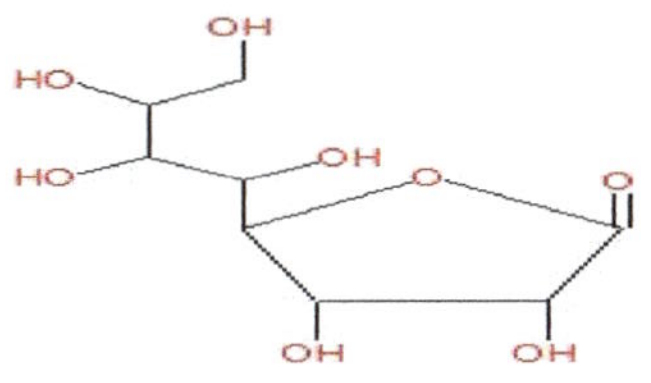	Antibacterial activity against Pseudomonas aerogenosa
18	y-Sitosterol	15.023	414	414.386166	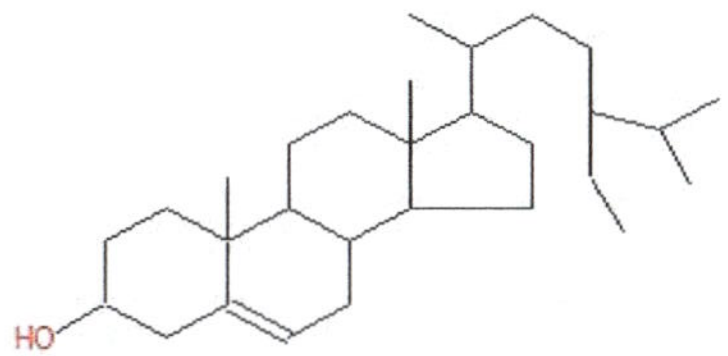	Anti-inflammatory activity
19	Tetradecanoic acid	13.455	228	228.20893	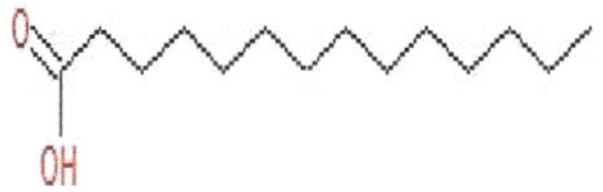	Antimicrobial, antispasmodic and *anti*-inflammatory effects
20	l-(+)-Ascorbic acid 2,6-dihexadecanoate	15.486	652	652.49142	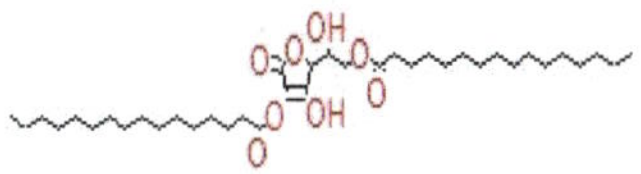	antioxidant
21	Estra -1,3,5(10)-trien-17ß-ol	16.007	256	256.182714	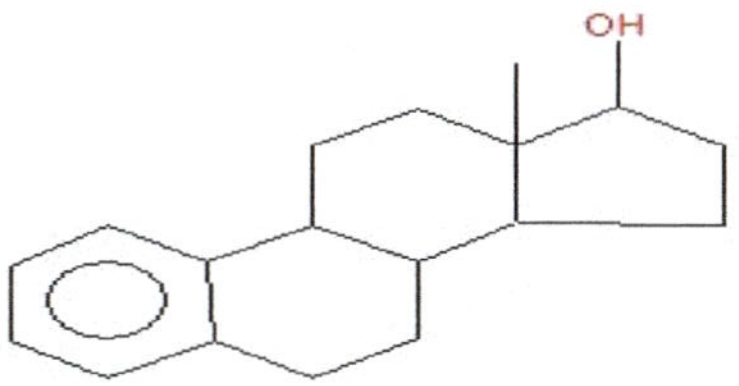	New chemical compound
22	Propanoic acid ,2-(3-acetoxy-4,4,14-trimethylandrost-8-en-17-yl)-	16.745	430	430.30831	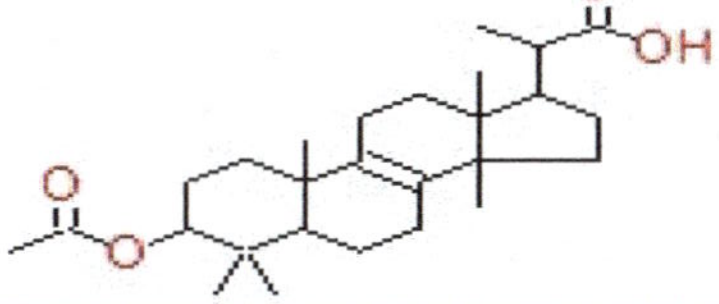	Anti-microbial and anti-tumor effects.

Table 1. cont'd

23	Cis-13-Eicosenoic acid	18.914	310	310.28718	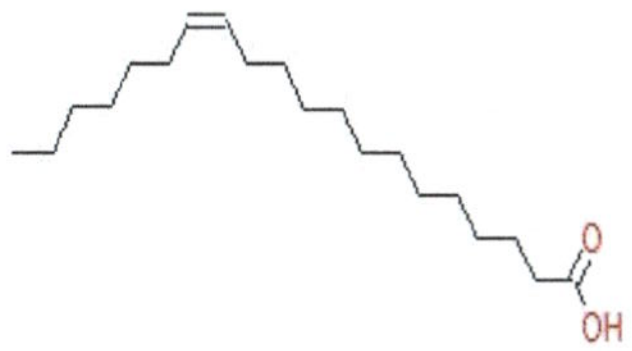	Anti-inflammatory activity
24	Eicosanoic acid	19.051	312	312.30283	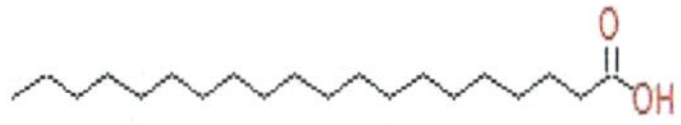	Anti-inflammatory effects
25	3-Pyrinecarboxylic acid , 2,7,10-tris(acetyloxy)-1,1a,2,3,4,6,7,10	19.246	597	597.257397	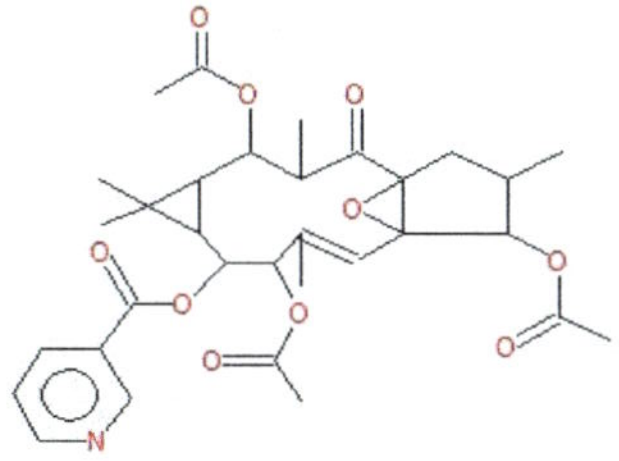	New chemical compound
26	Oleic acid, eicosyl ester	20.339	562	562.568882	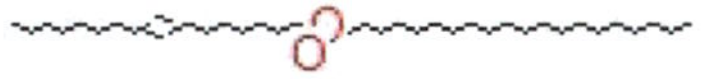	Anti-Candida activity
27	Butanoic acid, 4-chloro-,1,1a,1b,4,4a,5,7a,7b,8,9-decahydro-4a	21.083	572	572.194374	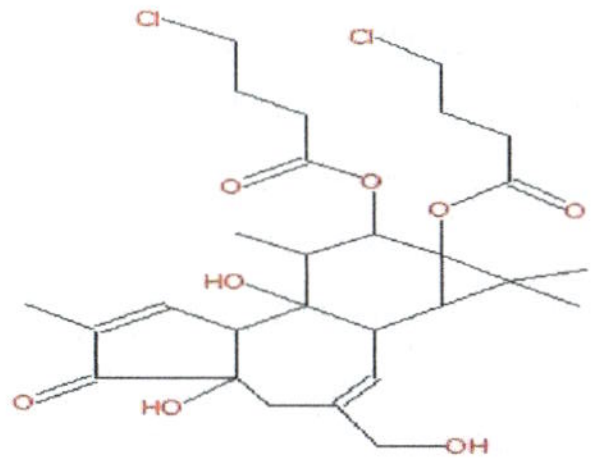	Antiviral, antitumor, anti-HIV and antinociceptive activities
28	Ethyl iso –allocholate	21.134	436	436.318874	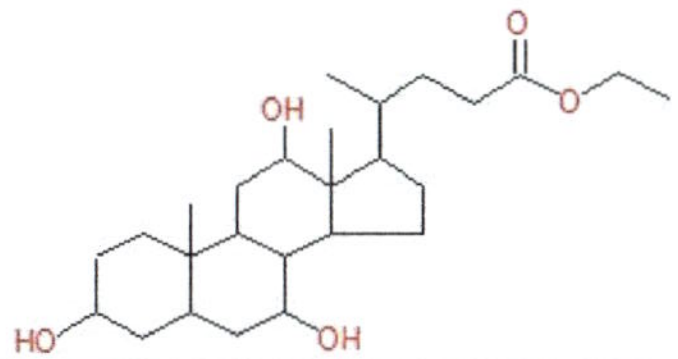	Anti-inflammatory activity

Table 1. cont'd

29	Olean-12-ene-3,15,16,21,22,28-hexol, (3ß,15α,16α,21ß,22α)-	21.603	506	506.360739	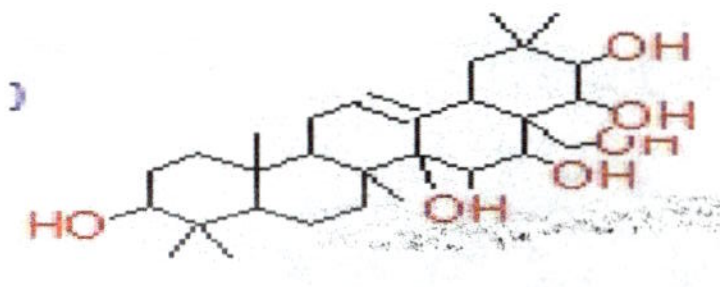	Anti-inflammatory
30	2,4,6-Decatrienoic acid ,1a,2,5,5a,6,9,10,10a-octahydro-5,5a-dihy	21.878	594	594.319267	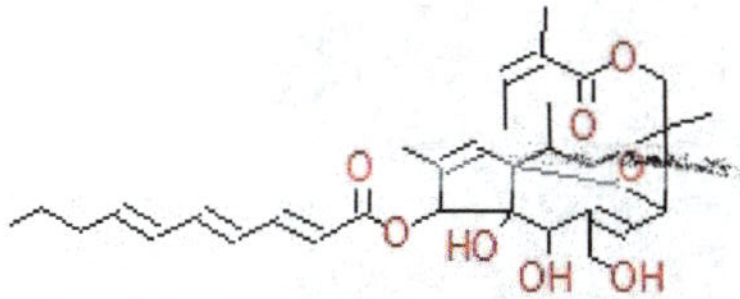	Anticancer

Table 2. FT-IR peak values of *Euphorbia lathyrus.*

No.	Peak (Wave number cm^{-1})	Intensity	Bond	Functional group assignment	Group frequency
1	659.66	59.626	-	Unknown	-
2	837.11	74.522	C-H	Alkenes	675-995
3	898.83	73.438	C-H	Alkenes	675-995
4	918.12	73.336	C-H	Alkenes	675-995
5	1037.7	54.275	C-F stretch	Aliphatic fluoro compounds	1000-1050
6	1145.7	65.485	C-O	Alcohols, Ethers, Carboxlic acids, Esters	1050-1300
7	1232.5	69.798	C-O	Alcohols, Ethers, Carboxlic acids, Esters	1050-1300
8	1261.5	72.924	C-O	Alcohols, Ethers, Carboxlic acids, Esters	1050-1300
9	1317.4	73.54	NO2	Nitro Compounds	1300-1370
10	1377.2	73.54	C-H	Alkanes	1340-1470
11	1410	74.741	C-H	Alkanes	1340-1470
12	1456.3	74.929	C-H	Alkanes	1340-1470
13	1519.9	70.721	-	Unknown	-
14	1626	62.255	-	Unknown	-
15	1741.7	79.565	-	Unknown	-
16	2683	92.491	-	Unknown	-
17	2854.7	80.11	C-H	Alkanes	2850-2970
18	2924.1	73.299	C-H	Alkanes	2850-2970
19	3082.3	86.714	H-O	H-bonded H-X group	2500-3500
20	3275.1	79.255	O-H	Hydrogen bonded Alcohols, Phenols	3200-3600

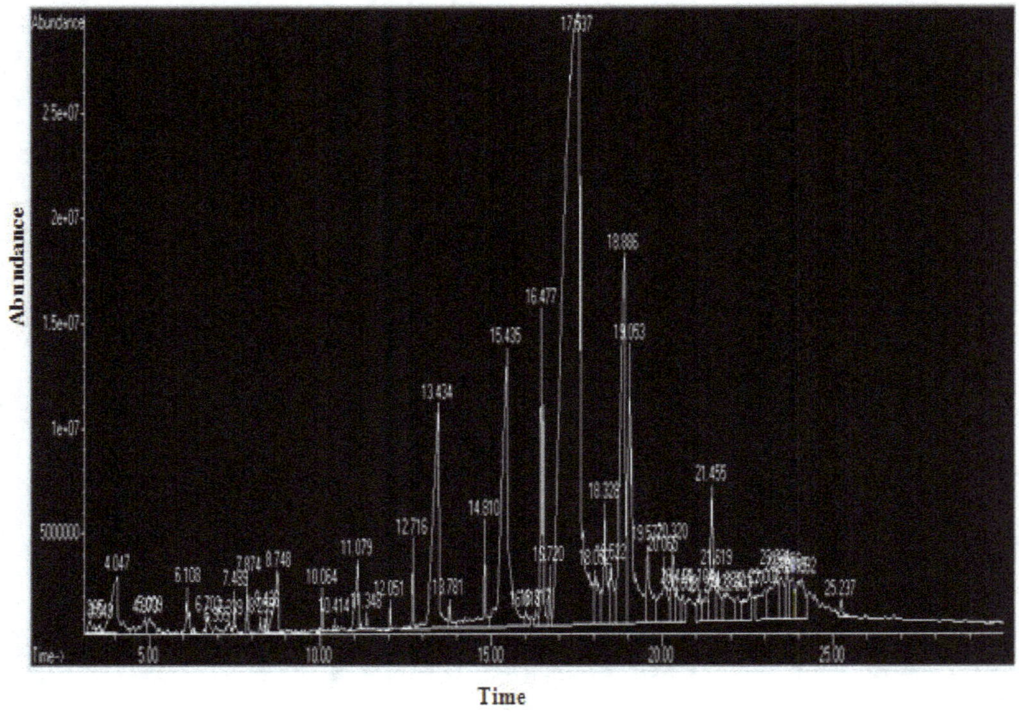

Figure 1. GC-MS chromatogram of methanolic extract of *Euphorbia lathyrus*.

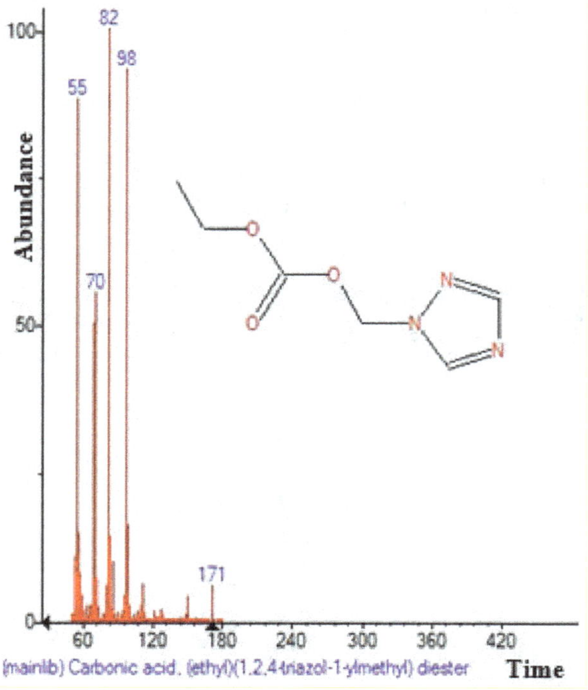

Figure 2. Structure of Carbonic acid , (ethyl)(1,2,4-triazol-1-ylmethyl) diester with 3.259 (RT) present in *Euphorbia lathyrus*.

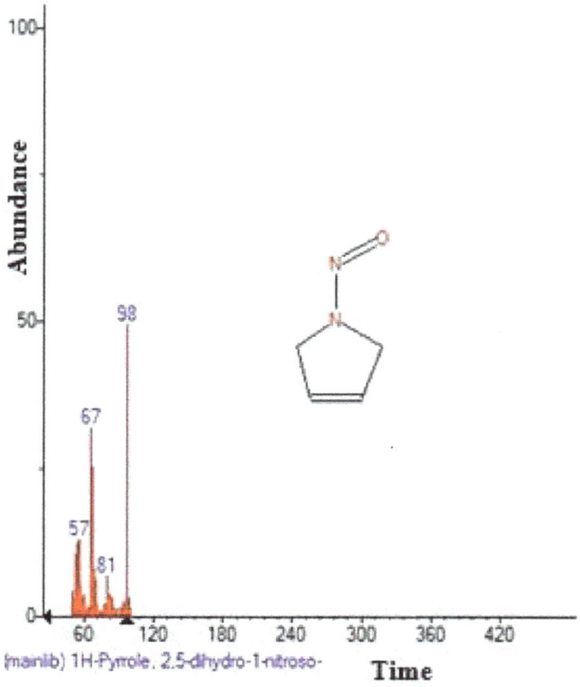

Figure 3. Structure of 1H-Pyrrole ,2,5-dihydro-1-nitroso with 3.367 (RT) present in *Euphorbia lathyrus*.

chromatographic conditions (Shahat et al., 2003; Reddy et al., 2003). *E. lathyris* L. oil (ELO) contains large amounts of FFAs and needs to determine acid value (Wei et al., 2007; Liu et al., 2011).

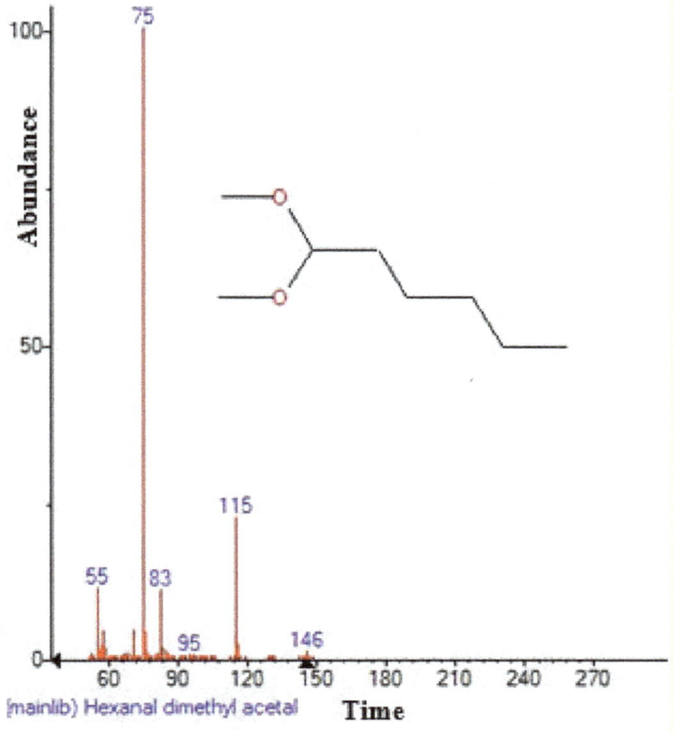

Figure 4. Structure of Hexanal dimethyl acetal with 3.533 (RT) present in *Euphorbia lathyrus*.

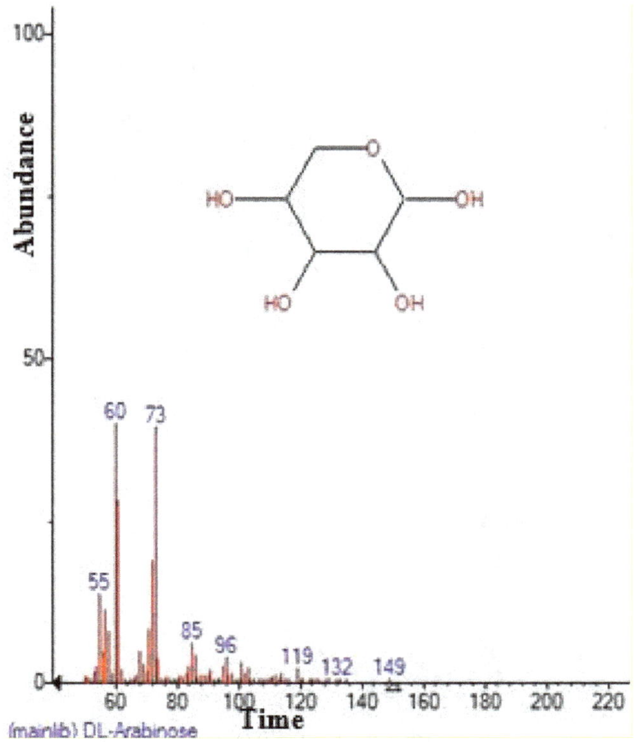

Figure 6. Structure of DL-Arabinose with 4.878 (RT) present in *Euphorbia lathyrus*

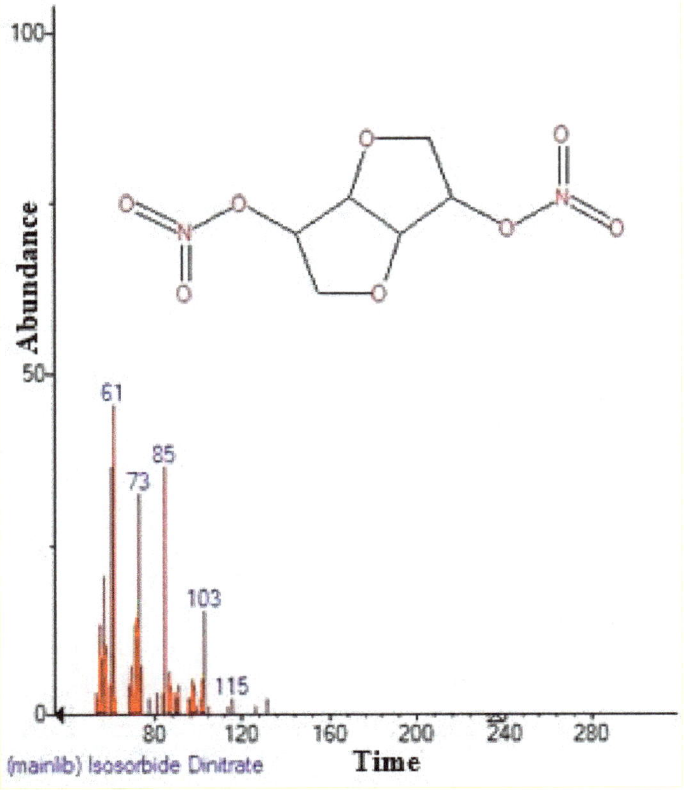

Figure 5. Structure of Isosorbide dinitrate with 4.546 (RT) present in *Euphorbia lathyrus*.

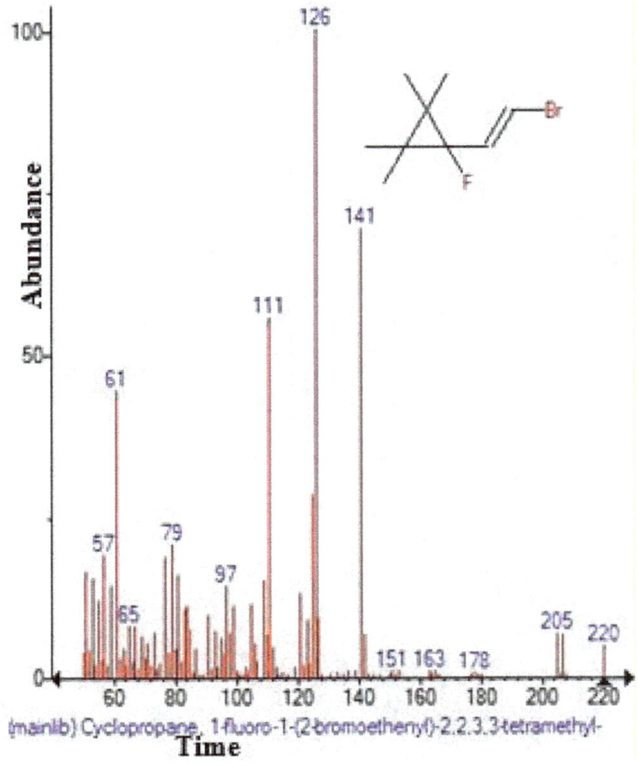

Figure 7. Structure of Cyclopropane ,1-fluoro-1-(2-bromoethenyl)-2,2,3,3-tetramethyl with 5.010 (RT) present in *Euphorbia lathyrus*.

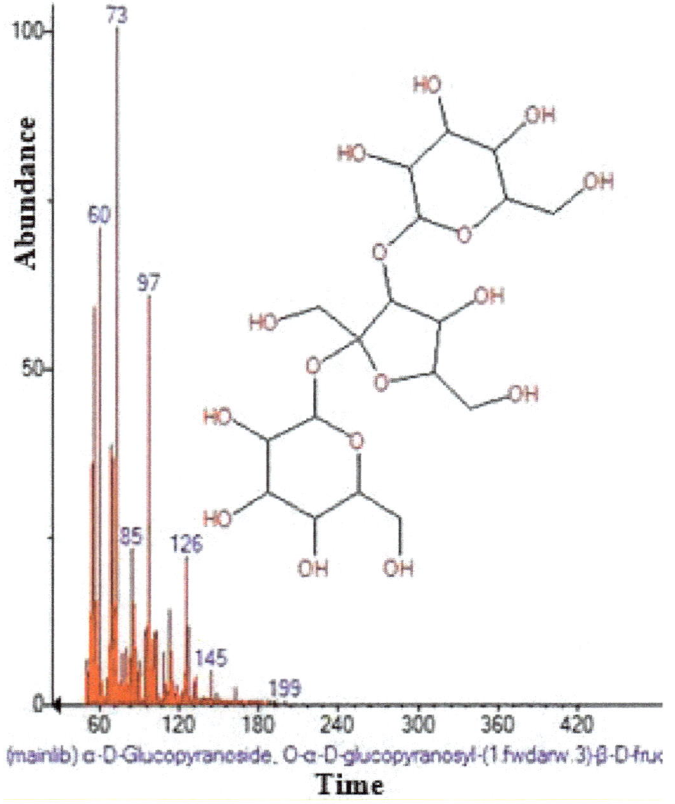

Figure 8. Structure of α-D-Glucopyranoside , O-α-D-glucopyranosyl-(1.fwdarw.3)-ß-d-fruc with 5.261 (RT) present in *Euphorbia lathyrus*.

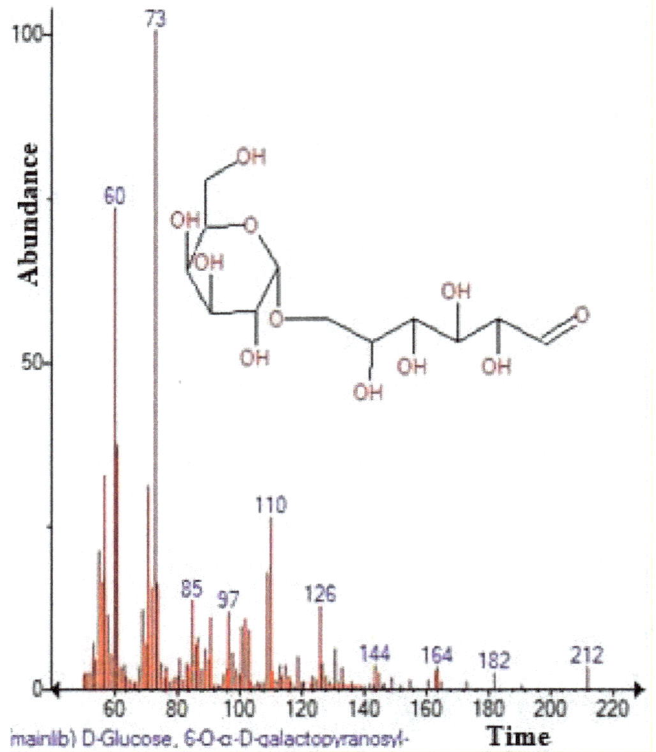

Figure 10. Structure of D-Glucose , 6-O-α-D-galactopyranosyl with 5.782 (RT) present in *Euphorbia lathyrus*.

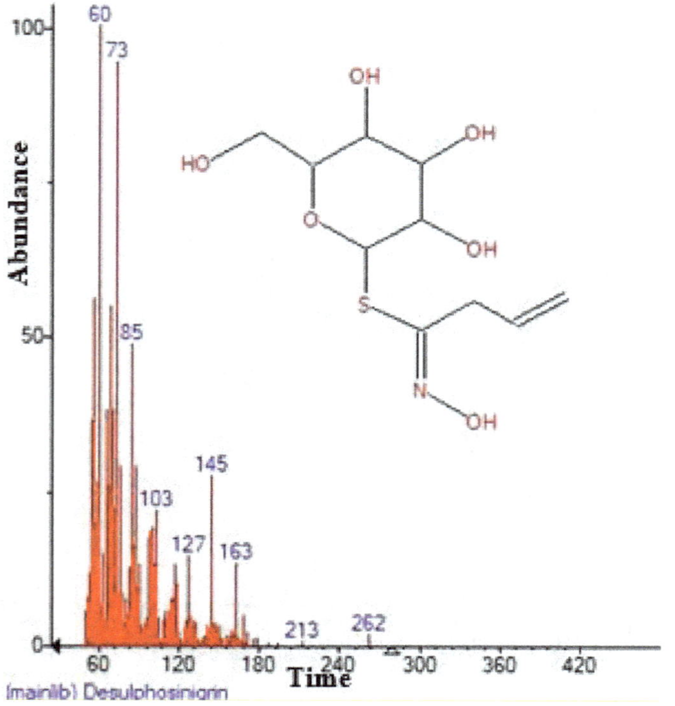

Figure 9. Structure of Desulphosinigrin with 5.313 (RT) present in *Euphorbia lathyrus*.

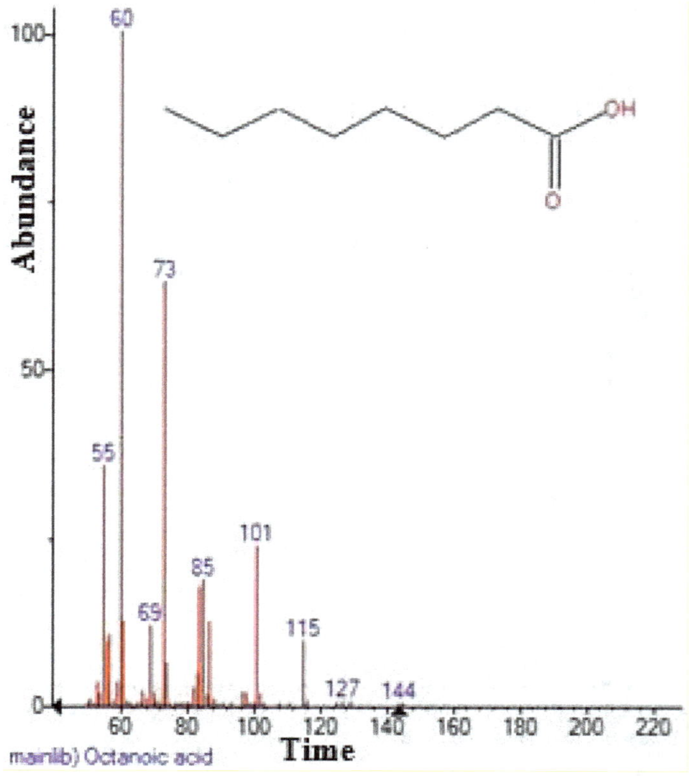

Figure 11. Structure of Octanoic acid with 6.137 (RT) present in *Euphorbia lathyrus*.

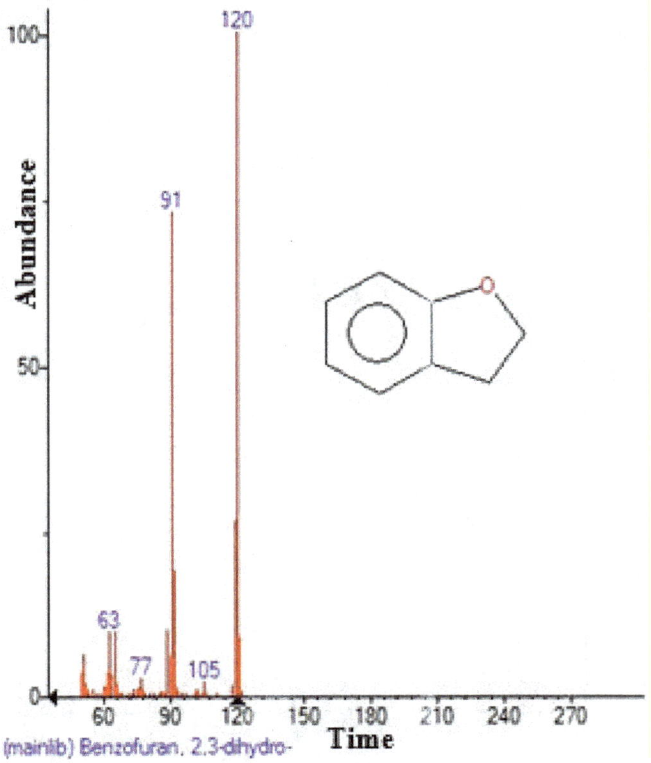

Figure 12. Structure of Benzofuran ,2,3-dihydro with 6.715 (RT) present in *Euphorbia lathyrus*.

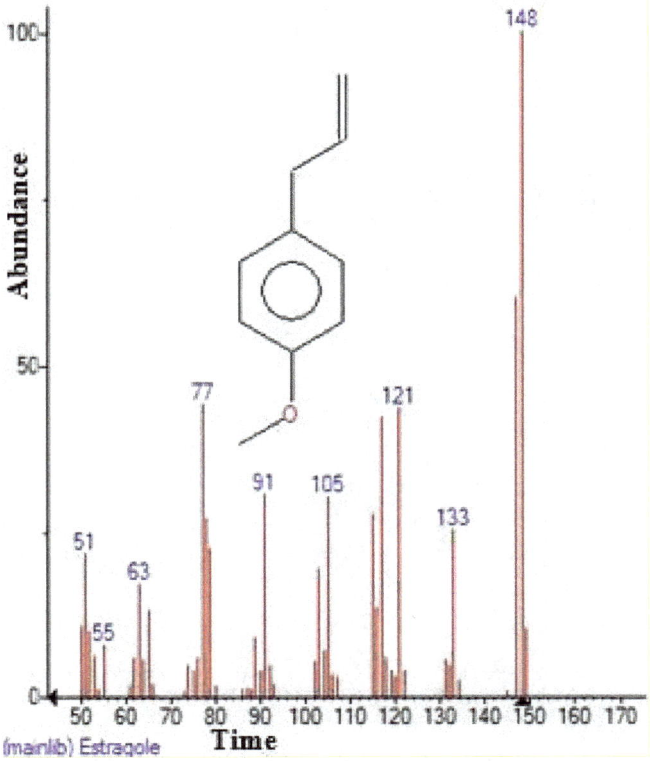

Figure 14. Structure of Estragole with 7.481 (RT) present in *Euphorbia lathyrus*.

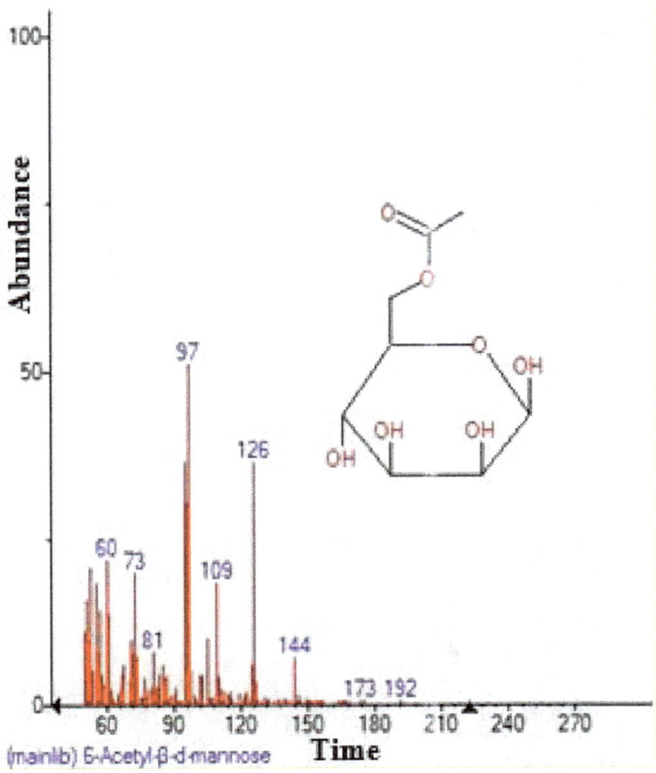

Figure 13. Structure of 6-Acetyl-ß-d-mannose with 6.984 (RT) present in *Euphorbia lathyrus*.

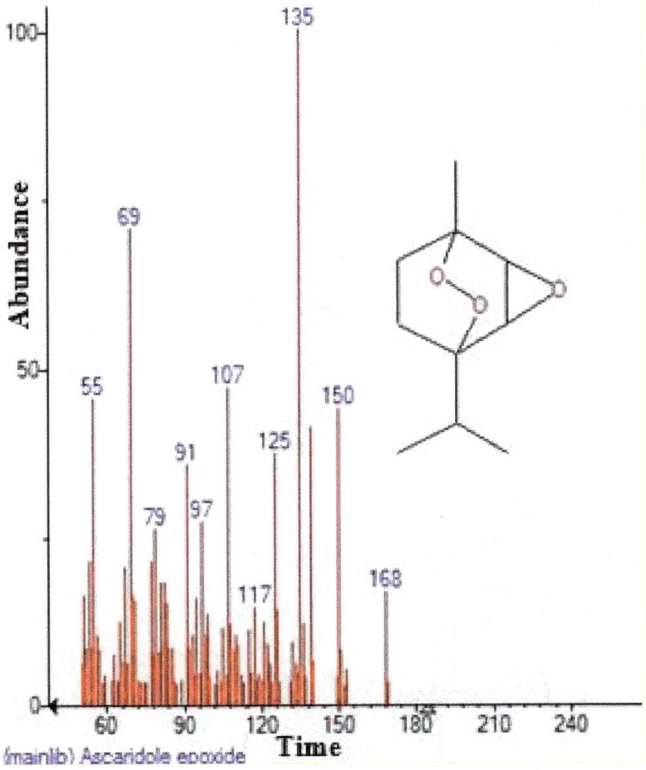

Figure 15. Structure of Ascaridole epoxide with 7.727 (RT) present in *Euphorbia lathyrus*.

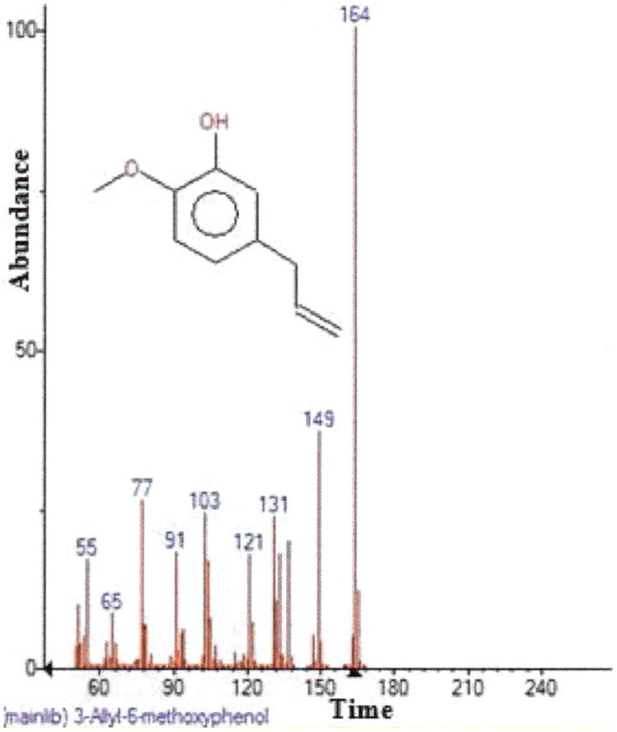

Figure 16. Structure of 3-Allyl-6-methoxyphenol with 8.443 (RT) present in *Euphorbia lathyrus*.

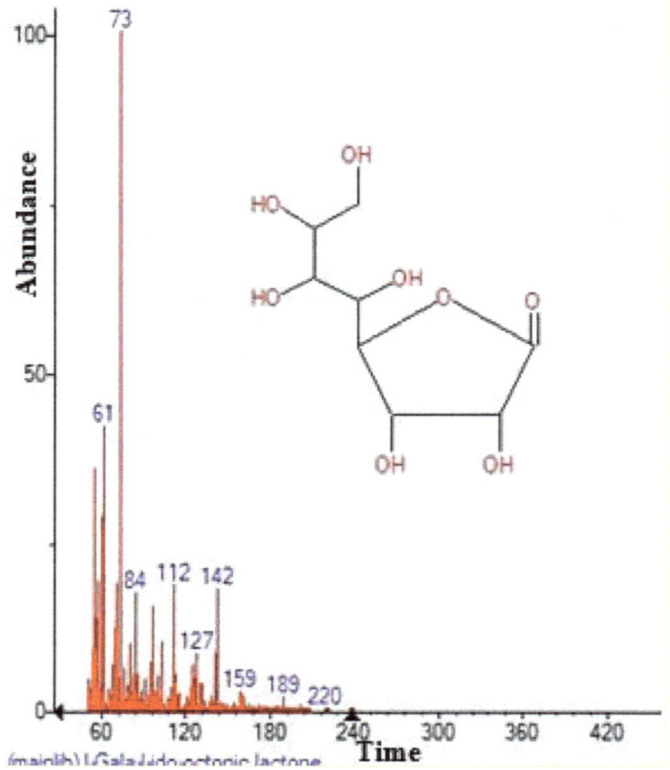

Figure 18. Structure of l-Gala-l-ido-octonic lactone with 10.743 (RT) present in *Euphorbia lathyrus*.

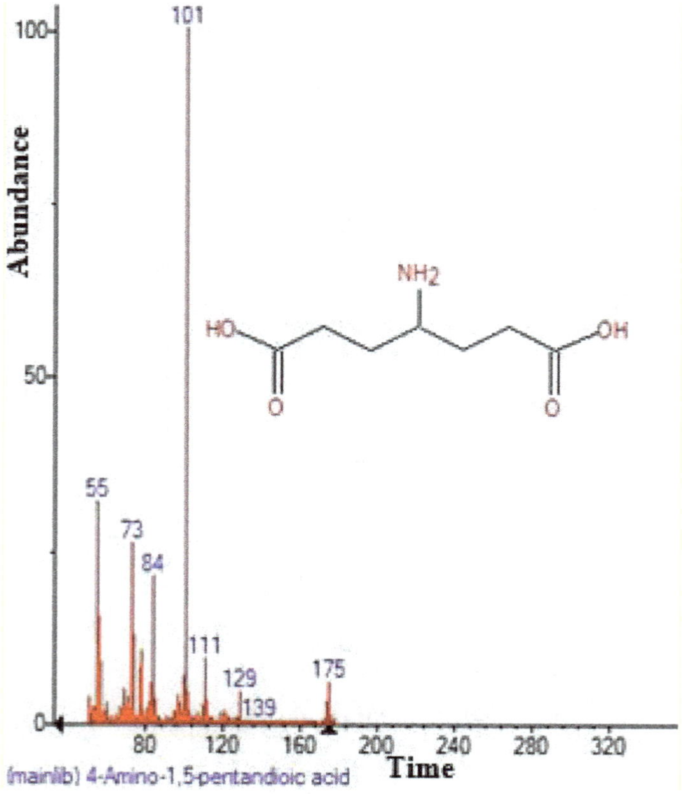

Figure 17. Structure of 4-Amino-1,5,pentandioic acid with 9.564 (RT) present in *Euphorbia lathyrus*.

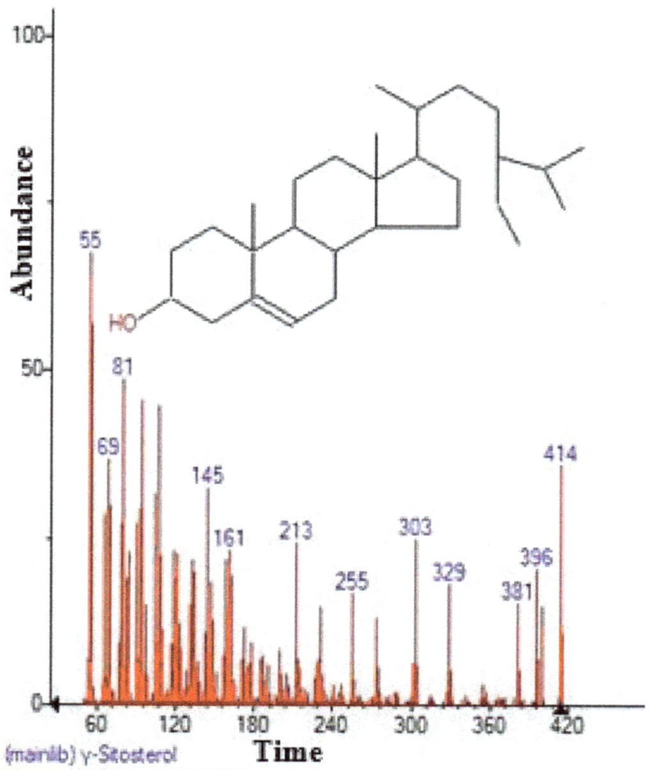

Figure 19. Structure of γ-Sitosterol with 15.023 (RT) present in *Euphorbia lathyrus*.

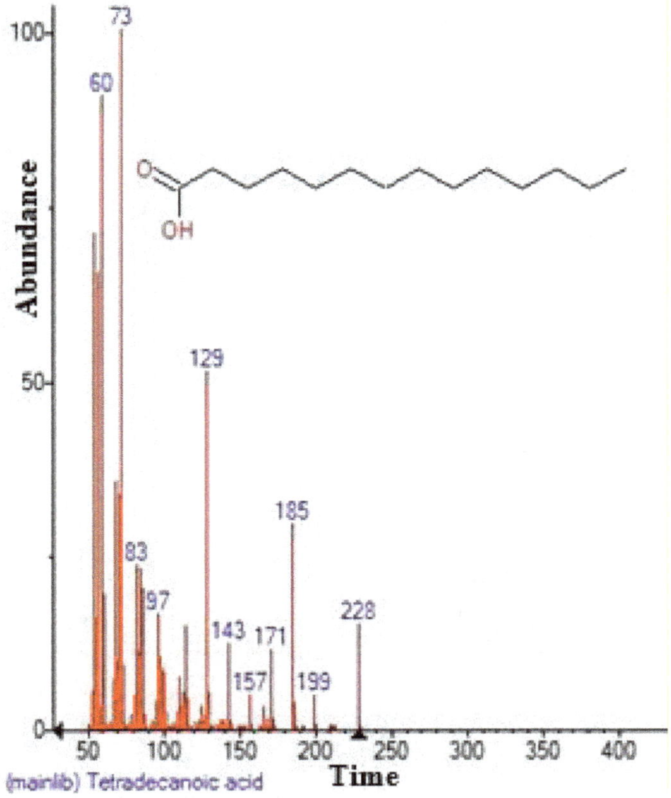

Figure 20. Structure of Tetradecanoic acid with 13.455 (RT) present in *Euphorbia lathyrus*.

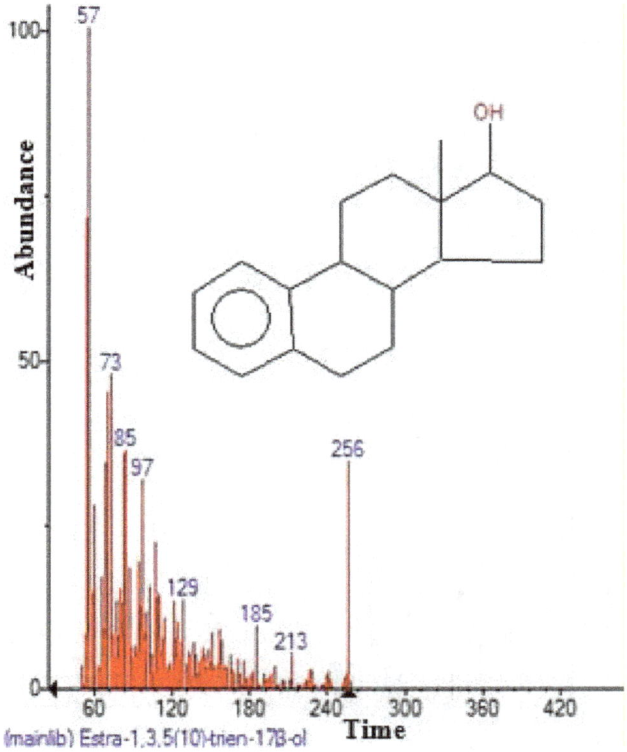

Figure 22. Structure of Estra -1,3,5(10)-trien-17ß-ol with 16.007 (RT) present in *Euphorbia lathyrus*.

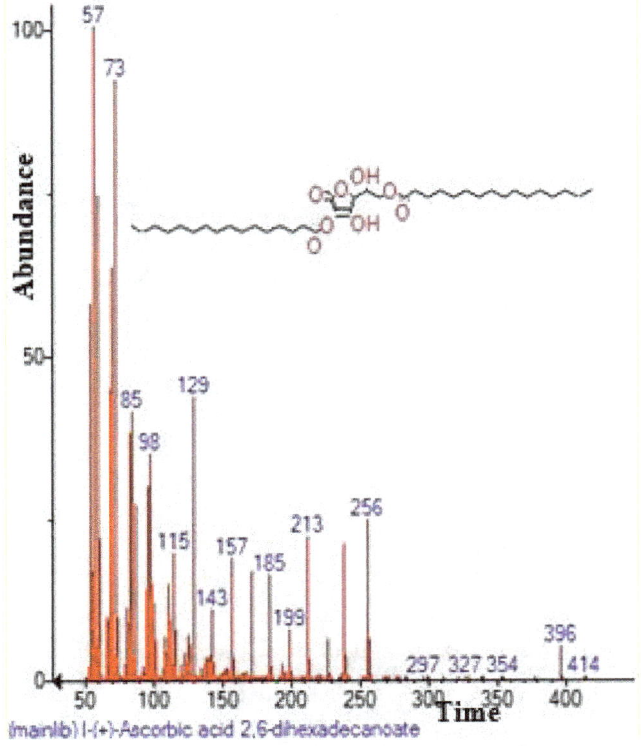

Figure 21. Structure of l-(+)-Ascorbic acid 2,6-dihexadecanoate with 15.486 (RT) present in *Euphorbia lathyrus*.

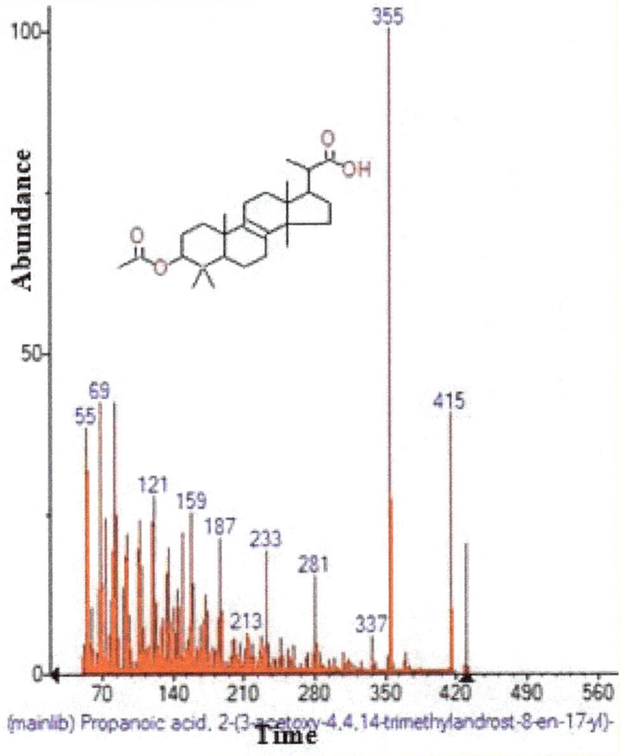

Figure 23. Structure of Propanoic acid ,2-(3-acetoxy-4,4,14-trimethylandrost-8-en-17-yl) with 16.745 (RT) present in *Euphorbia lathyrus*.

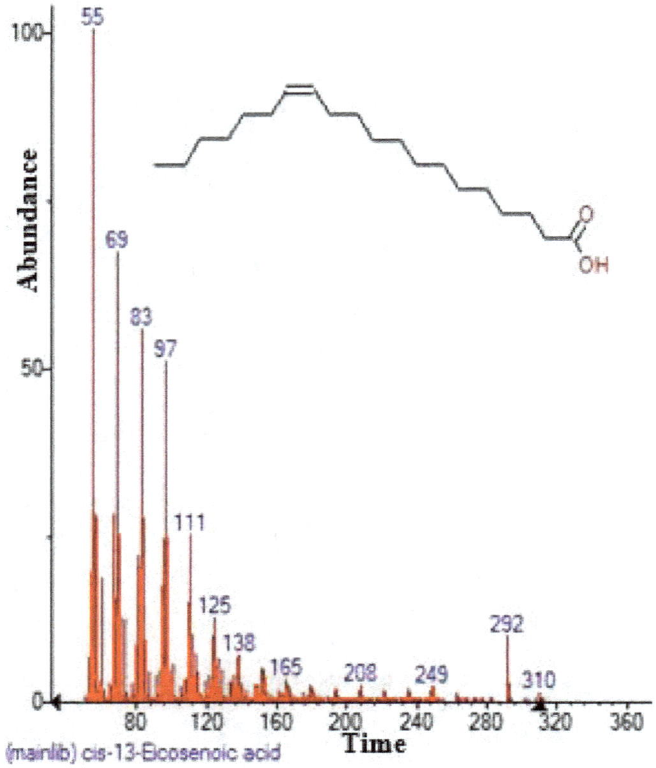

Figure 24. Structure of Cis-13-Eicosenoic acid with 18.914 (RT) present in *Euphorbia lathyrus*.

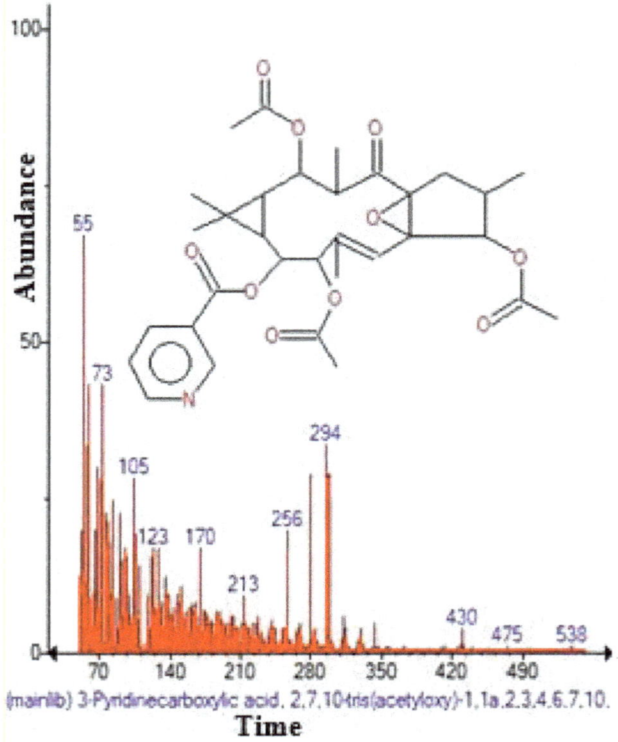

Figure 26. Structure of 3-Pyrinecarboxylic acid , 2,7,10-tris(acetyloxy)-1,1a,2,3,4,6,7,10 with 19.246 (RT) present in *Euphorbia lathyrus*.

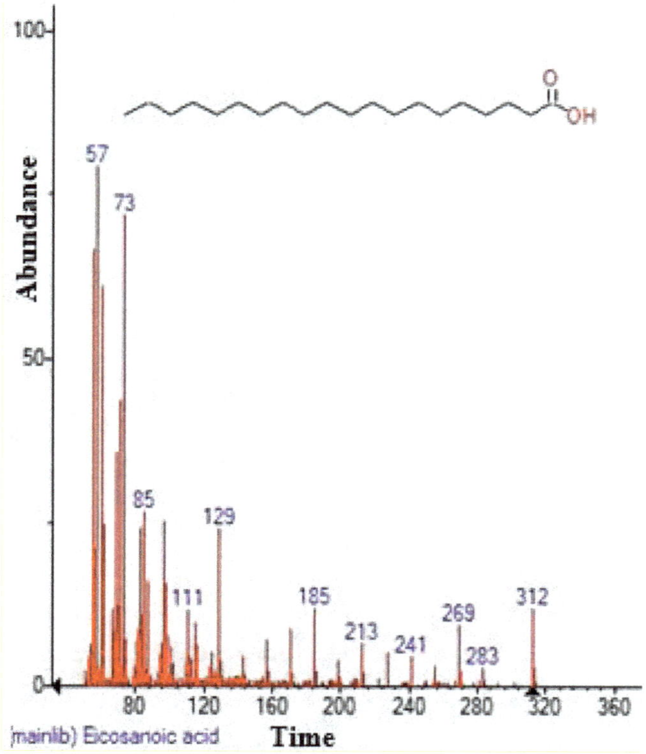

Figure 25. Structure of Eicosanoic acid with 19.051 (RT) present in *Euphorbia lathyrus*.

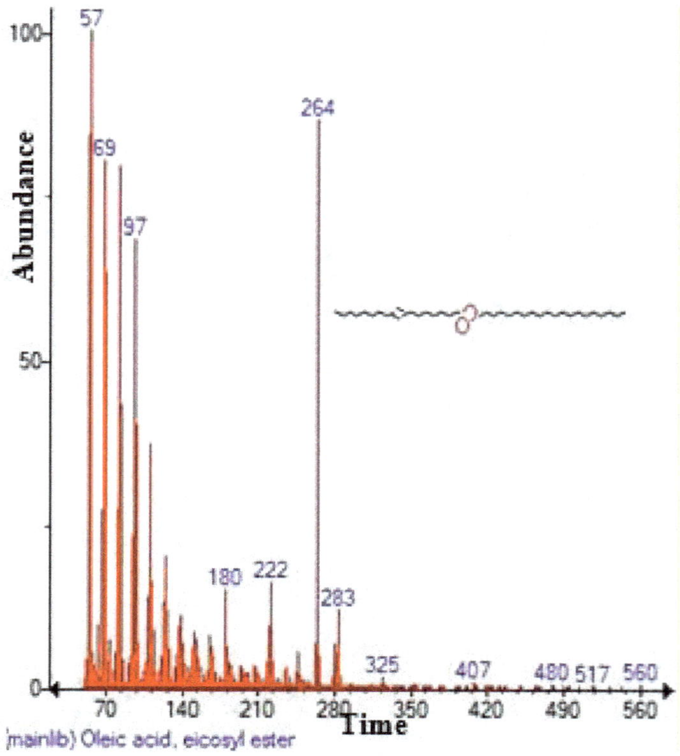

Figure 27. Structure of Oleic acid , eicosyl ester with 20.339 (RT) present in *Euphorbia lathyrus*.

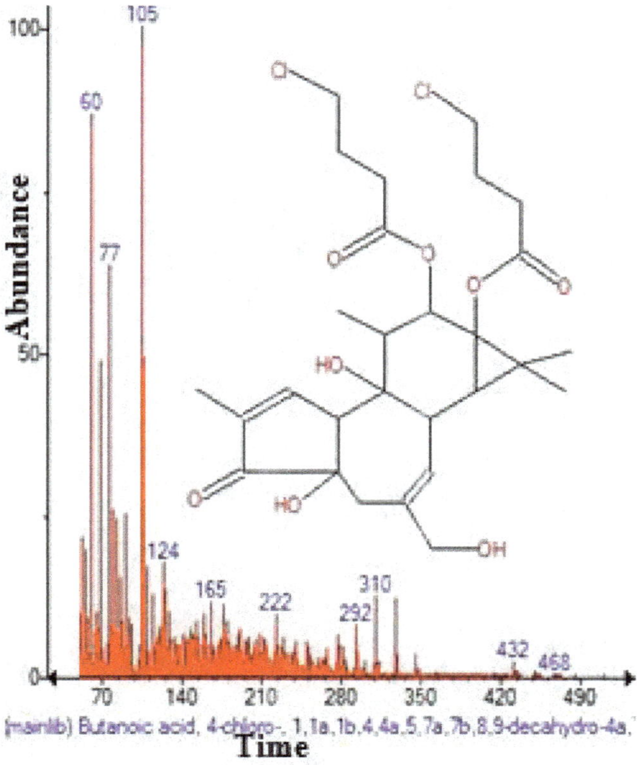

Figure 28. Structure of Butanoic acid , 4-chloro- ,1,1a,1b,4,4a,5,7a,7b,8,9-decahydro-4a with 21.083 (RT) present in *Euphorbia lathyrus*.

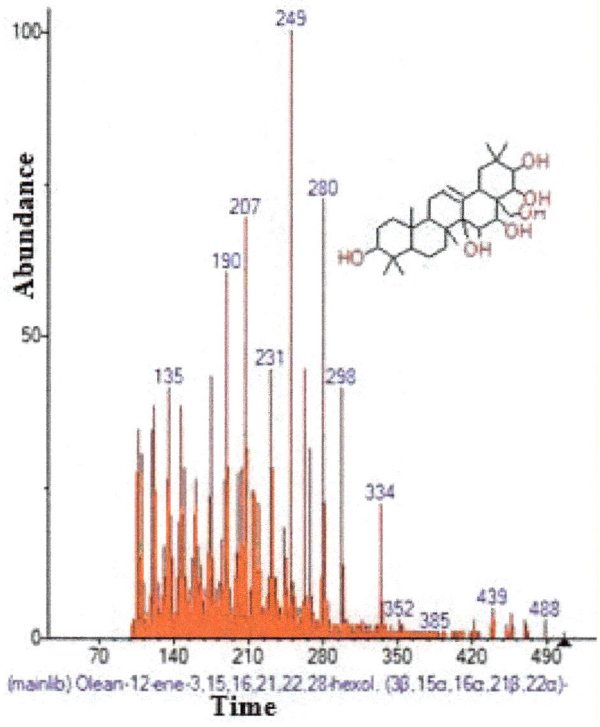

Figure 30. Structure of Olean -12-ene-3,15,16,21,22,28-hexol, (3ß,15α,16α,21ß,22α) with 21.603 (RT) present in *Euphorbia lathyrus*.

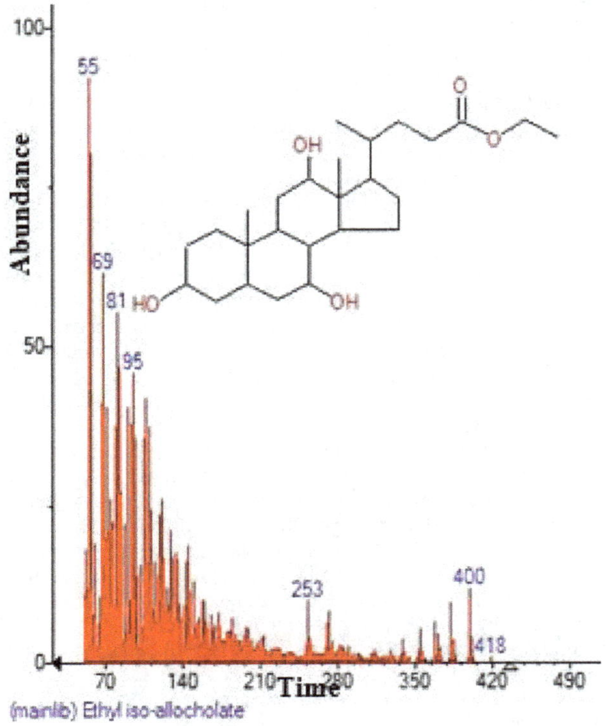

Figure 29. Structure of Ethyl iso –allocholate with 21.134 (RT) present in *Euphorbia lathyrus*.

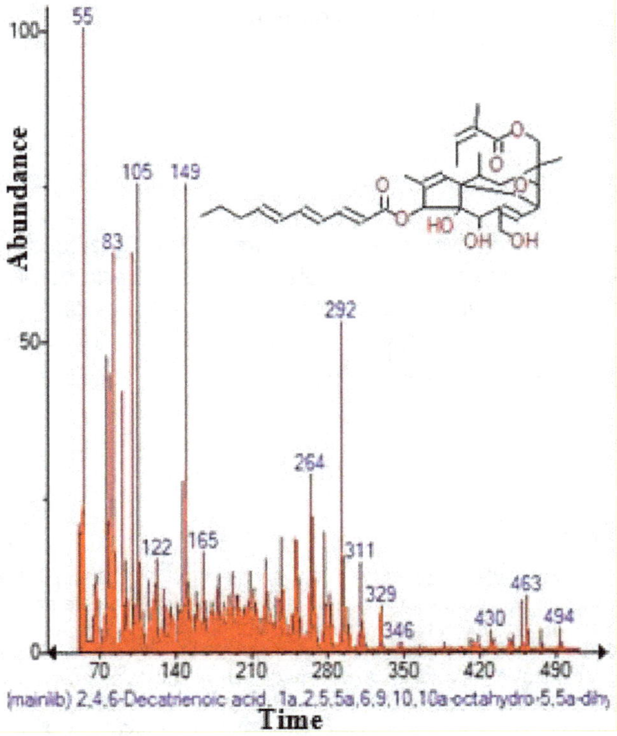

Figure 31. Structure of 2,4,6-Decatrienoic acid ,1a,2,5,5a,6,9,10,10a-octahydro-5,5a-dihy with 21.878 (RT) present in *Euphorbia lathyrus*.

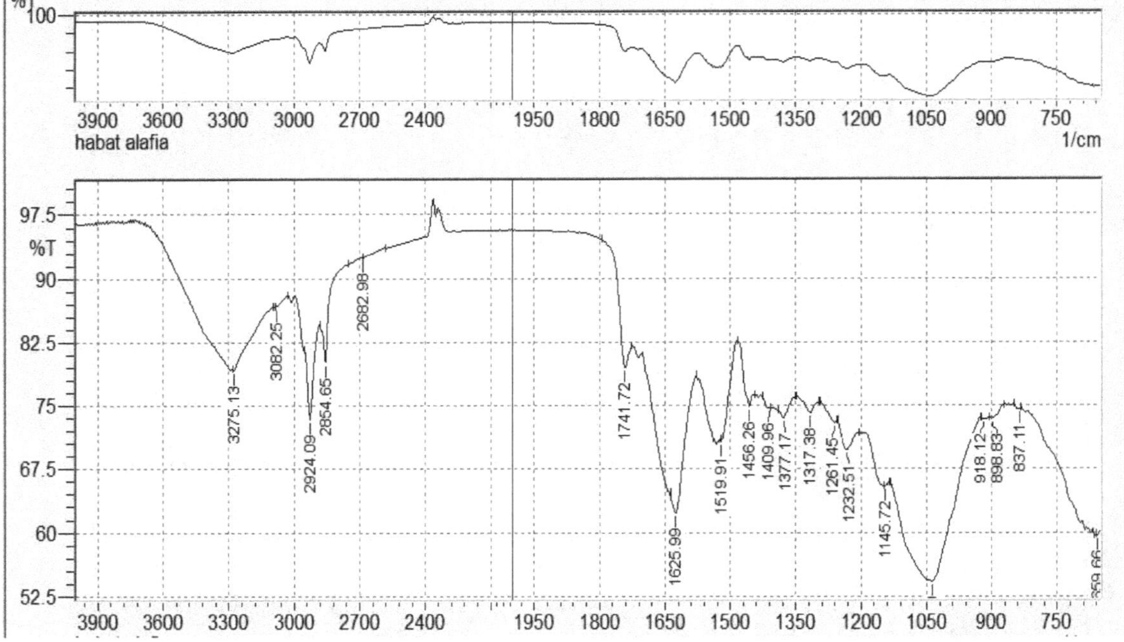

Figure 32. FT-IR profile of *Euphorbia lathyrus.*

Conclusion

E. lathyrus is native plant of Iraq. It contains chemical constitutions which may be useful for various herbal formulation as anti-inflammatory, analgesic, antipyretic, cardiac tonic, and antiasthamatic.

ACKNOWLEDGEMENTS

The authors would like to express their gratitude to Dr. Abdul-ghafar for his valuable suggestions and comments. They also which to express their deepest gratitude to Prof. Dr. Adul-Kareem for his valuable contributions and support throughout the study.

REFERENCES

Al-Marzoqi AH, Hadi MY, Hameed IH (2016). Determination of metabolites products by *Cassia angustifolia* and evaluate antimicobial activity. J. Pharmacogn. Phytother. 8(2):25-48.

Al-Marzoqi AH, Hameed IH, Idan SA (2015). Analysis of bioactive chemical components of two medicinal plants (*Coriandrum sativum* and *Melia azedarach*) leaves using gas chromatography-mass spectrometry (GC-MS). Afr. J. Biotechnol. 14(40):2812-2830.

Altameme H J, Hadi MY, Hameed IH (2015a). Phytochemical analysis of *Urtica dioica* leaves by fourier-transform infrared spectroscopy and gas chromatography-mass spectrometry. J. Pharmacogn. Phytother. 7(10):238-252.

Altameme HJ, Hameed IH, Abu-Serag NA (2015b). analysis of bioactive phytochemical compounds of two medicinal plants, *Equisetum arvense* and *Alchemila valgaris* seed using gas chromatography-mass spectrometry and fourier-transform infrared spectroscopy. Malays. Appl. Biol. 44(4):47–58.

Altameme HJ, Hameed IH, Idan SA, Hadi MY (2015c). Biochemical analysis of *Origanum vulgare* seeds by fourier-transform infrared (FT-IR) spectroscopy and gas chromatography-mass spectrometry (GC-MS). J. Pharmacogn. Phytother. 7(9):221-237.

Buenz EJ, Schnepple DJ, Bauer BA, Elkin PL, Riddle JM, Motley TJ (2004). Techniques: bioprospecting historical herbal texts by hunting for new leads in old tomes. Trends Pharmacol. Sci. 25:494-498.

Cai YZ, Luo Q, Sun M, Corke H (2004). Antioxidant activity and phenolic compounds of 112 Chinese medicinal plants associated with anticancer. Life Sci. 74:2157-2184.

Corro G, Bañuelos F, Vidal E, Cebada S (2014). Measurements of Surface Acidity of Solid Catalysts for Free Fatty Acids Esterification in *Jatropha curcas* crude oil for biodiesel production. Fuel. 115:625-628.

Hadi MY, Mohammed GJ, Hameed IH (2016). Analysis of bioactive chemical compounds of *Nigella sativa* using gas chromatography-mass spectrometry. J. Pharmacogn. Phytother. 8(2):8-24.

Hameed IH, Abdulzahra AI, Jebor MA, Kqueen CY, Ommer AJ (2015a). Haplotypes and variable position detection in the mitochondrial DNA coding region encompassing nucleotide positions. Mitochondrial DNA. 26(4):544-9.

Hameed IH, Hamza LF, Kamal SA (2015b). Analysis of bioactive chemical compounds of *Aspergillus niger* by using gas chromatography-mass spectrometry and fourier-transform infrared spectroscopy. J. Pharmacogn. Phytother. 7(8):132-163.

Hameed IH, Hussein HJ, Kareem MA, Hamad NS (2015c). Identification of five newly described bioactive chemical compounds in methanolic extract of *Mentha viridis* by using gas chromatography-mass spectrometry (GC-MS). J. Pharmacogn. Phytother. 7(7):107-125.

Hameed IH, Ibraheam IA, Kadhim HJ (2015d). Gas chromatography mass spectrum and fourier-transform infrared spectroscopy analysis of methanolic extract of *Rosmarinus oficinalis* leaves. J. Pharmacogn. Phytother. 7(6):90-106.

Hamza LF, Kamal SA, Hameed IH (2015). Determination of metabolites products by *Penicillium expansum* and evaluating antimicrobial activity. J. Pharmacogn. Phytother. 7(9):194-220.

Hussein AO, Mohammed GJ, Hadi MY, Hameed IH (2016a). Phytochemical screening of methanolic dried galls extract of *Quercus infectoria* using gas chromatography-mass spectrometry (GC-MS) and Fourier transform-infrared (FT-IR). J. Pharmacogn. Phytother. 8(3):49-59.

Hussein HJ, Hadi MY, Hameed IH (2016b). Study of chemical composition of *Foeniculum vulgare* using Fourier transform infrared spectrophotometer and gas chromatography - mass spectrometry. J. Pharmacogn. Phytother. 8(3):60-89.

Hussein HM, Hameed IH, Ibraheem OA (2016c). Antimicrobial activity and spectral chemical analysis of methanolic leaves extract of *Adiantum capillus-veneris* using GC-MS and FT-IR spectroscopy. Int. J. Pharmacogn. Phytochem. Res. 8(3).

Jasim H, Hussein AO, Hameed IH, Kareem MA (2015). Characterization of alkaloid constitution and evaluation of antimicrobial activity of *Solanum nigrum* using gas chromatography mass spectrometry (GC-MS). J. Pharmacogn. Phytother. 7(4):56-72.

Liu H, Hong LZ, Wang MW (2011). Progress of Study on Energy Plant *Euphorbia lathyris* L. Anhui Agric. Sci. Bull. 17:119-120.

Park EJ, Pezzutto JM (2002). Botanicals in cancer chemoprevention. Cancer Metastasis Rev. 21:231-255.

Reddy VBM, Reddy K, Gunasekar D, Murthy M, Caux C, Bodo B (2003). A new sesquiterpene lactone from *Bombax malabaricum*. Chem. Pharm. Bull. 51:458-459.

Shahat AA, Hassan RA, Nazif NM, Van MS, Pieters L, Hammuda FM (2003). Isolation of mangiferin from *Bombax malabaricum* and structure revision of shamimin. Planta Med. 69:1068-1070.

Tapiero H, Tew KD, Ba N, Mathe G (2002). Polyphenols: do they play a role in the prevention of human pathologies? Biomed. Pharmacother. 56:200-207.

Wei WL, Jin MY, Ma C (2007) Fatty Acid Composition Analysis of *Euphorbia lathyris* L. Seed Oil. China Oils Fats 32:70-71.

18

Determination of metabolites products by *Penicillium expansum* and evaluating antimicobial activity

Lena Fadhil Hamza, Sabreen A. Kamal and Imad Hadi Hameed*

Department of Biology, Babylon University, Hilla City, Iraq.

The objectives of this study were to analyze the secondary metabolites of *Penicillium expansum* and evaluate antibacterial activity. Twenty eight bioactive compounds were identified in the methanolic extract of *P. expansum*. The identification of bioactive chemical compounds is based on the peak area, retention time molecular weight and molecular formula. Gas chromatography mass spectrometry (GC/MS) analysis of *P. expansum* revealed the existence of the Levoglucosenone, Edulan II, 4-[Dichloromethyl]-2-[[2-[1-methyl-2-pyrrolidinyl]ethyl]amino-6-trichloro, 1,2-Cyclopentanedione, Ethanethiol, 2-(5-(4-methyl-2-pyridyloxy)pentyl)amino-hydrogen su, Imidazole,2-amino-5-[(2-carboxy)vinyl], D-Glucose,6-O-α-D-galactopyranosyl, Eicosanoic acid , phenylmethyl ester, Dodecanoic acid, 3- hydroxyl, DL-Leucine,N-glycyl, Cyclohexene,1,5,5-trimethyl-6-acetylmethyl, 1,2-Nonadecanediol, Bicyclo[2.2.1]heptane-2-carboxylic acid isobutyl-amide, 6-Acetyl-ß-d-mannose, α-D-Glucopyranoside,O-α-D-glucopyranosyl-(1.fwdarw.3)-ß-D-fruc, propanedioic acid, amino-diethyl ester, 4H-Pyran-4-one,2,3-dihydro-3,5-dihydroxy-6-methyl, valeric acid, dodecyl ester, deoxyspergualin, l-Gala-l-ido-octonic lactone, 5-Hydroxymethylfurfural, paromomycin, 16-Nitrobicyclo[10.4.0]hexadecane-1-ol-13-one, cis-Vaccenic acid, 2-Bromotetradecanoic acid, phthalic acid, butyl undecyl ester, picrotoxin, D-Fructose and diethyl mercaptal. The FTIR analysis of *P. expansum* proved the presence of aliphatic fluoro compounds, tetiary amine, C-N stretch and methylene-CH. asym which shows major peaks at 1028.06, 1151.50 and 2852.72, respectively. Methanolic extract of bioactive compounds of *P. expansum* were assayed for *in vitro* antibacterial activity against *Proteus mirabilis, Pseudomonas aerogenosa, Escherichia coli*, *Staphylococcus aureus* and *Klebsiella pneumonia* by using the diffusion method in agar. The zones of inhibition were compared with different standard antibiotics. *S. aureus* has maximum zone formation (7.01±0.141) mm.

Key words: Antimicrobial activity, metabolites, bioactive compounds, GC-MS, FT-IR, *P. expansum*.

INTRODUCTION

The genus *Penicillium* is known worldwide for the production of secondary metabolites (Pitt and Hocking, 1997). *Penicillium expansum* has been demonstrated to produce extracellular enzymes of commercial value, including the pectinases, utilized in fruit juice industry during the stage of pulp maceration, juice liquefaction or depectinization (Rosenberger et al., 1991; Baracat-Pereira et al., 1989), Patulin, a mutagenic, immunoitoxic

*Corresponding author. E-mail: imad_dna@yahoo.com.

and neurotoxic mycotoxin, particularly unacceptable to apple juice industry (Bracket and Marth, 1979). Most *Penicillium* species are considered ubiquitous, opportunistic saprophytes. Blue mold decay caused by *P. expansum* link is the most important postharvest disease of apple worldwide (Pierson et al., 1971). The genus *Penicillium* is subdivided into four subgenera (*Aspergilloides, Penicillium, Biverticillium* and *Furcatum*), determined by the number of branch points between phialide and stipe, down the main axis of the penicillus and others characters, like ratio of metula length to phialide, length and colony diameter on G25N and when the number of branch points is the same (Grassin and Fauquembergue, 1996).

Nutritionally, they are supremely undemanding being able to grow in almost any environment with a sprinkling of mineral salts, any but with the most complex forms of organic carbon, and a wide range of physical-chemical environments, temperature, pH and redox potential. The taxonomy of this genus is hard as its classification is based mainly on conidiophore and conidia structure, although the colony diameter after incubation under standardized conditions has greater importance for classification (Amiri and Bompeix, 2005; Morales et al., 2008; Hameed et al., 2015a). *P. expansum* is one of most important fungal pathogen of stored pome fruits and responsible for 50% of losses in all pome fruit and pear (Mattheis and Roberts, 1992; Andersen et al., 2004; Murphy et al., 2006; Hameed et al., 2015b).

It is reported to produce different secondary metabolites such as expansolides A and B (Massias et al., 1990), citrinin, ochratoxin A, chaetoglobosins A and C (Frisvad, 1992), rubratoxin B (Paterson et al., 1987; Hameed et al., 2015), roquefortine C, penitrem A (Bridge et al., 1989), patulin (Andersen et al., 2004; Altameme et al., 2015) and others like cyclopiazonic acid, brevianamide A, gentisyl alcohol, griseofulvin, mycophenolic acid and raistrick phenols (Frisvad and Filtenborg., 1989). The aims of this study were to analyze the secondary metabolites and evaluation of antibacterial activity.

MATERIALS AND METHODS

Collection, extraction and determination of metabolites

P. expansum was isolated from dried fruit. After the species were identified by the identification key, spores were grown in a liquid culture of potato dextrose broth (PDB) and incubated at 25°C in a shaker for 16 days at 130 rpm (Usha and Masilamani, 2013). The metabolites were determined and extracted for GC analysis using the method of Jasim et al. (2015). The extraction was performed by adding 25 ml methanol to 100 ml liquid culture in an Erlenmeyer flask after the infiltration of the culture. The mixture was incubated at 4°C for 10 min and then shook for 10 min at 130 rpm. Metabolites was separated from the liquid culture and evaporated to dryness with a rotary evaporator at 45°C. The residue was dissolved in 1 ml methanol, filtered through a 0.2 µm syringe filter, and stored at 4°C for 24 h before being used for GC-MS.

Gas chromatography-mass spectrometry (GC-MS)

Bioactive compound were examined for the chemical composition using GC-MS (Agilent 789N) equipped with a DB-5MS column (30 m×0.25 mm i.d., 0.25 um film thickness, J&W Scientific, Folsom, CA). The oven temperature was programmed (Imad et al., 2014a; Hussein et al., 2015). Helium was used as the carrier gas at the rate of 1.0 ml/min. Effluent of the GC column was introduced directly into the source of the MS via a transfer line (250°C). Ionization voltage was 70 eV and ion source temperature was 230°C. Scan range was 41 to 450 amu. The constituents were identified after being compared with available data in the GC-MS library in the literatures of Kareem et al. (2015) and Imad et al. (2014b).

Fourier transform infrared spectrophotometer (FTIR)

The sample was run at infrared region between 400 and 4000 nm. The powdered sample of the *P. expansum* specimen was treated for fourier transform infrared spectroscopy (Shimadzu, IR Affinity 1, Japan) (Imad et al., 2014c).

Determination of antibacterial activity of crude fraction of *P. expansum* compounds.

The test pathogens (*E. coli, Pseudomonas aeruginosa, Klebsiella pneumoniae* and *Staphylococcus aureus)* were swabbed in Muller Hinton agar plates. 50µl of fungal extracts was loaded on the bored wells. The wells were bored in 0.5 cm in diameter. The plates were incubated at 37°C for 24 h and examined. After the incubation the diameter of inhibition zones around the discs was measured.

Statistical analysis

Data were analyzed using analysis of variance (ANOVA), and differences among the means were determined for significance at $P < 0.05$ using Duncan's multiple range test (by SPSS software)Version 9.1 (Mohammed and Imad, 2013)

RESULTS AND DISCUSSION

Fungus identification and secondary metabolites production

The fungi were isolated by serial dilution method. Morphological, microscopical and microscopical characteristics of fungal strains were determined using specific media light and compound microscope (Figures 1 and 2). After fermentation, the secondary metabolites were produced by isolated microorganisms.

Identify the secondary metabolites from the methanolic crude extract of *P. expansum* by (GC-MS)

Gas chromatography and mass spectroscopy analysis of compounds was carried out in methanolic extract of *P. expansum*, shown in Table 1. The GC-MS chromatogram of the twenty eight peaks of the compounds detected was shown in Figure 2. Chromatogram GC-MS analysis of the

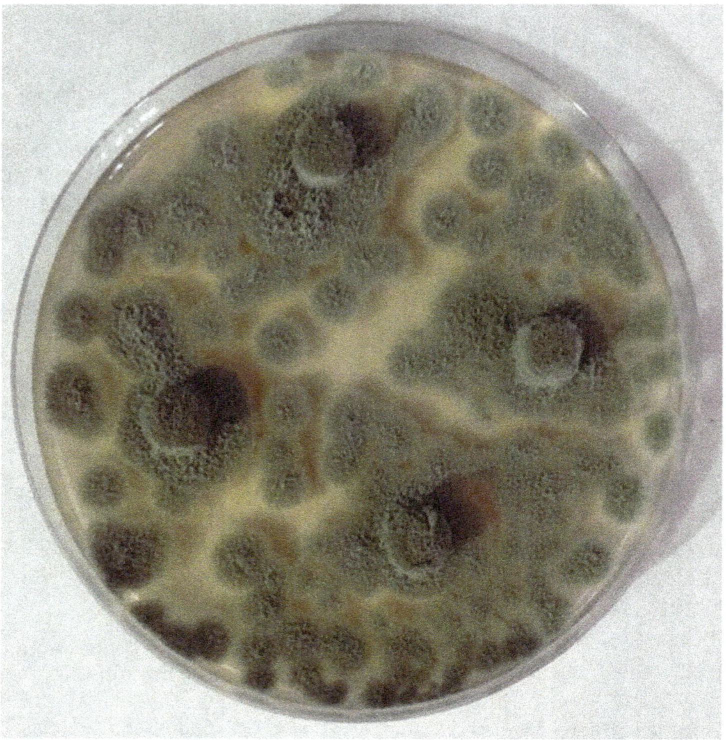

Figure 1. Morphological characterization of *P. expansum*.

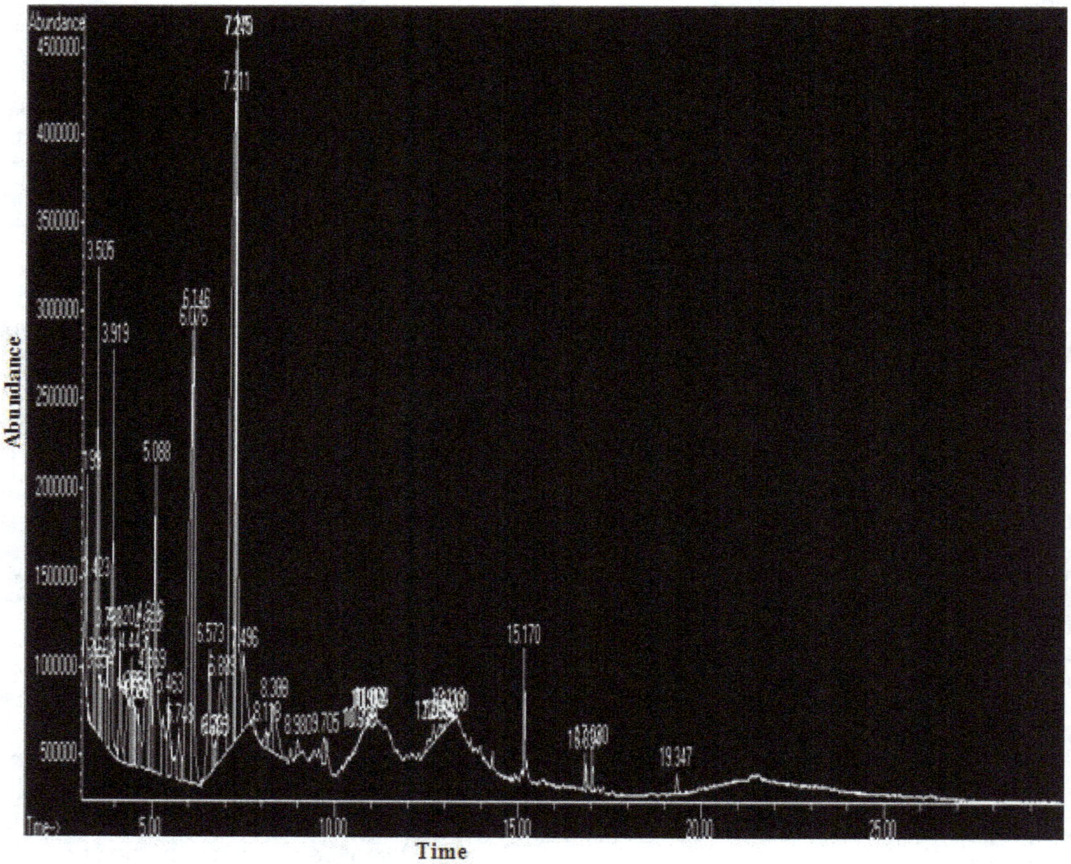

Figure 2. GC-MS chromatogram of methanolic extract of *P. expansum*.

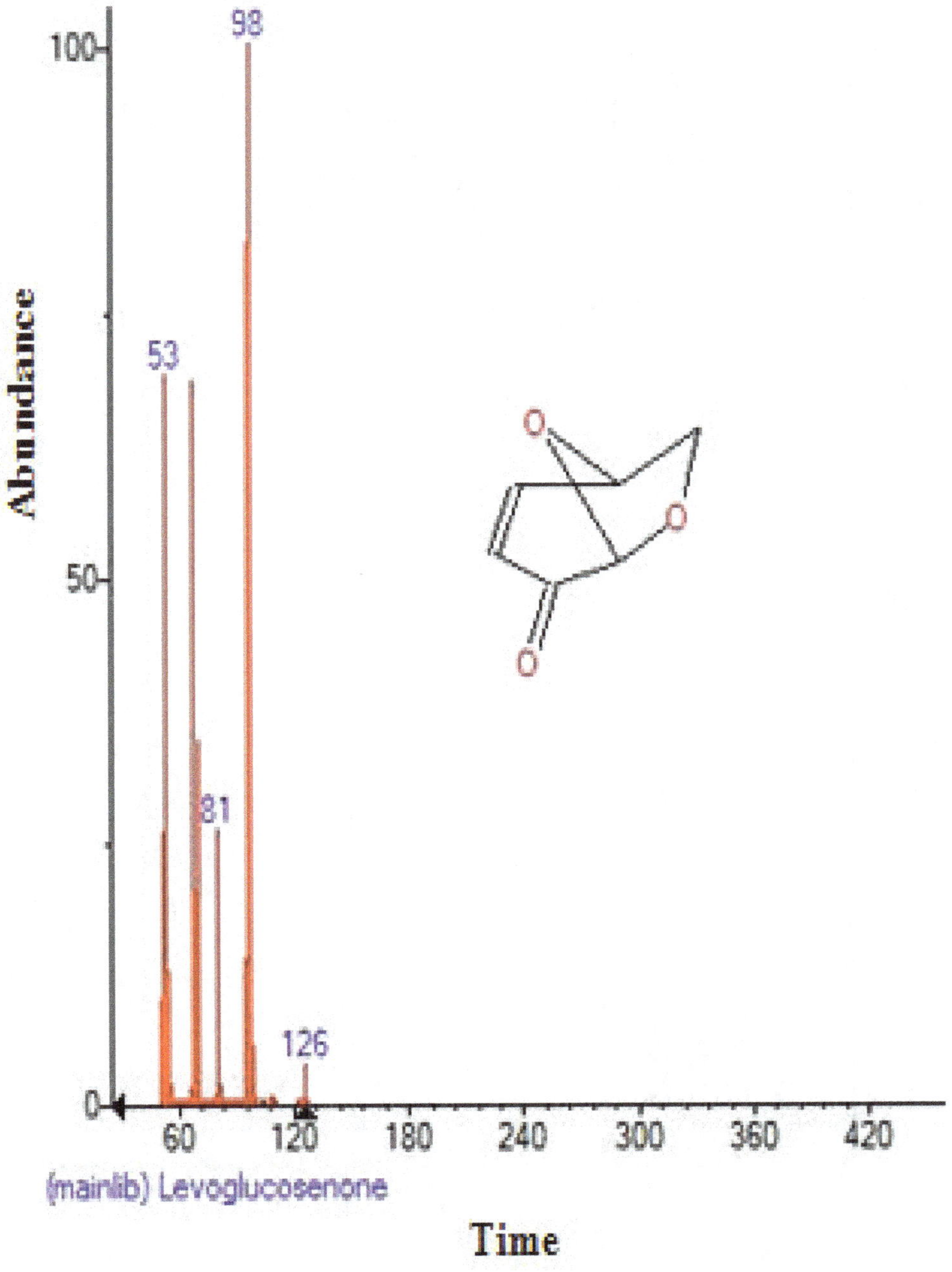

Figure 3. Mass spectrum of Levoglucosenone with Retention Time (RT)= 3.230.

methanol extract of *P. expansum* showed the presence of twenty eight major peaks, and the components corresponding to the peaks were determined as follows. The first set up peak was determined to be levoglucosenone, Edulan II, (Figure 3). The second peak indicated to be 4-[Dichloromethyl]-2-[[2-[1-methyl-2-pyrrolidinyl]ethyl]amino-6-trichloro (Figure 4). The next peaks were considered to be 1,2-Cyclopentanedione, ethanethiol, 2-(5-(4-methyl-2-pyridyloxy)pentyl) amino,hydrogen su, imidazole, 2-amino-5-[(2-carboxy)vinyl], D-Glucose,6-O-α-D-galactopyranosyl, eicosanoic acid, phenylmethyl ester, dodecanoic acid, 3-hydroxyl, DL-Leucine, N-glycyl, Cyclohexene,1,5,5-trimethyl-6-acetylmethyl, 1,2-Nonadecanediol, Bicyclo[2.2.1]heptane-2-carboxylic acid isobutyl-amide, 6-Acetyl-ß-d-mannose, α-D-Glucopyranoside,O-α-D-glucopyranosyl-(1.fwdarw.3)-ß-D-fruc, Propanedioic acid, amino-, diethyl ester, 4H-Pyran-4-one,2,3-dihydro-3,5-dihydroxy-6-methyl, valeric acid, dodecyl ester, deoxyspergualin, l-Gala-l-ido-octonic lactone, 5-Hydroxymethylfurfural, Paromomycin, 16-Nitrobicyclo [10.4.0]hexadecane-1-ol-13-one, cis-Vaccenic acid, 2-

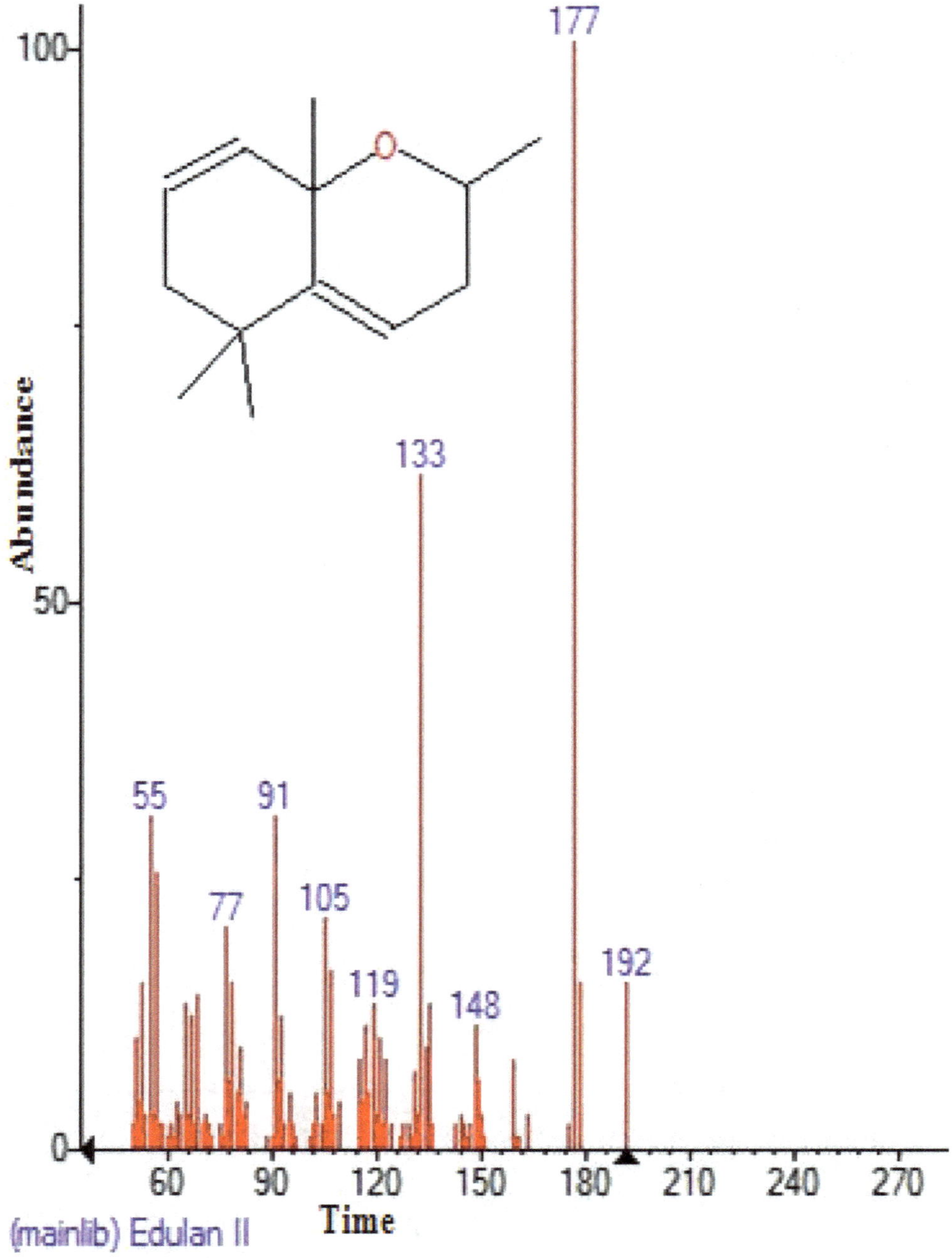

Figure 4. Mass spectrum of Edulan II with retention time (RT)= 3.613.

Bromotetradecanoic acid, Phthalic acid, butyl undecyl ester, Picrotoxin, D-Fructose and diethyl mercaptal (Figure 5 to 30).

Identify the secondary metabolites from the methanolic crude extract of *P. expansum* by (FTIR)

Fourier-transform infrared analysis of dry methanolic extract of *P. expansum* proved the presence of aliphatic fluoro compounds, tetiary amine, C-N stretch and methylene-CH. asym which shows major peaks at 1028.06, 1151.50 and 2852.72, respectively (Table 2 and Figure 31).

Antibacterial activity

K. pneumoniae, Pseudomonas aeroginosa, E. coli and *S.aeureus* are four clinical pathogens selected forantibacterial activity, and maximum zone formation against *S. aureus* (Table 3 and Figure 32).

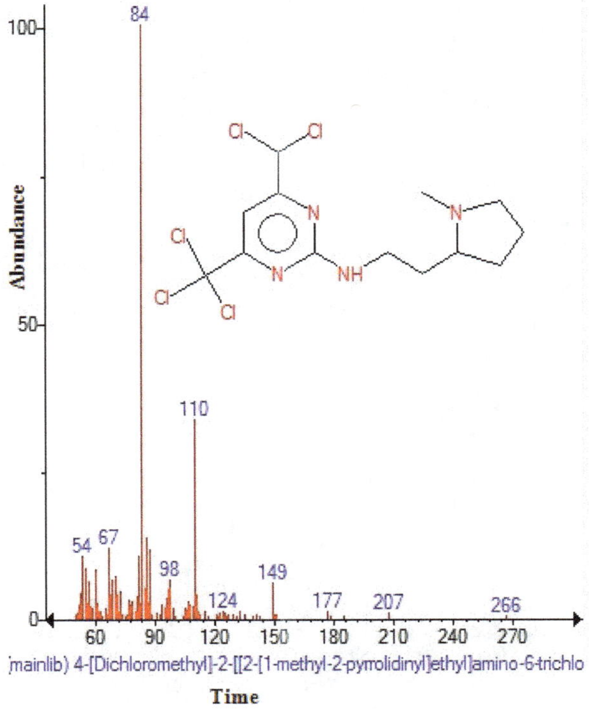

Figure 5. Mass spectrum of 4-[Dichloromethyl]-2-[[2-[1-methyl-2-pyrrolidinyl]ethyl]amino-6-trichloro with retention time (RT)= 3.693.

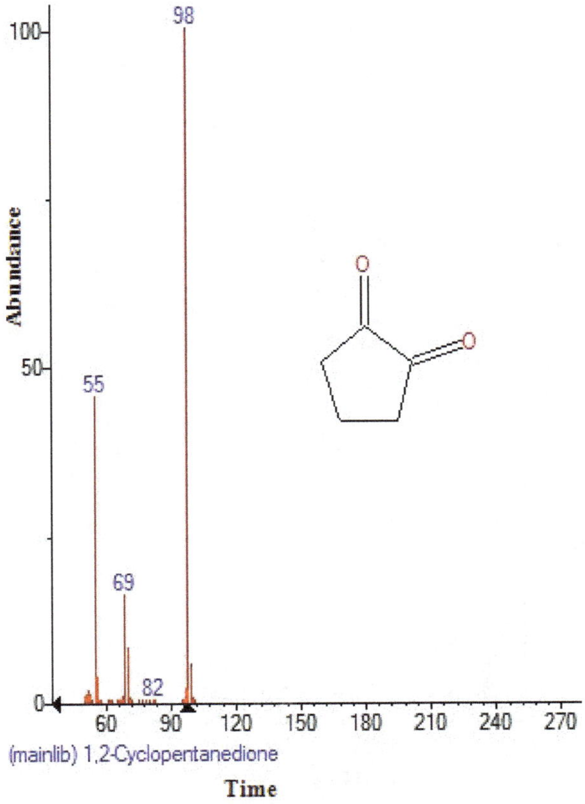

Figure 6. Mass spectrum of 1,2-Cyclopentanedione with retention time (RT)= 3.750.

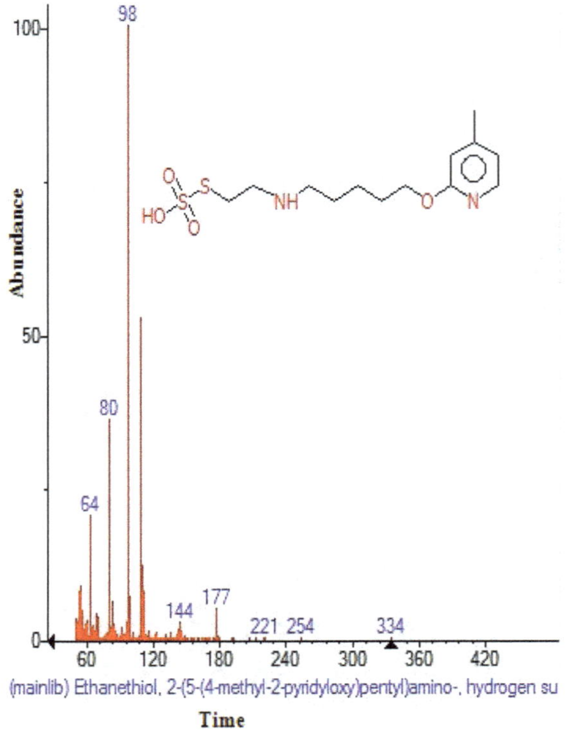

Figure 7. Mass spectrum of Ethanethiol , 2-(5-(4-methyl-2-pyridyloxy)pentyl)amino-,hydrogen su with retention time (RT)= 3.779.

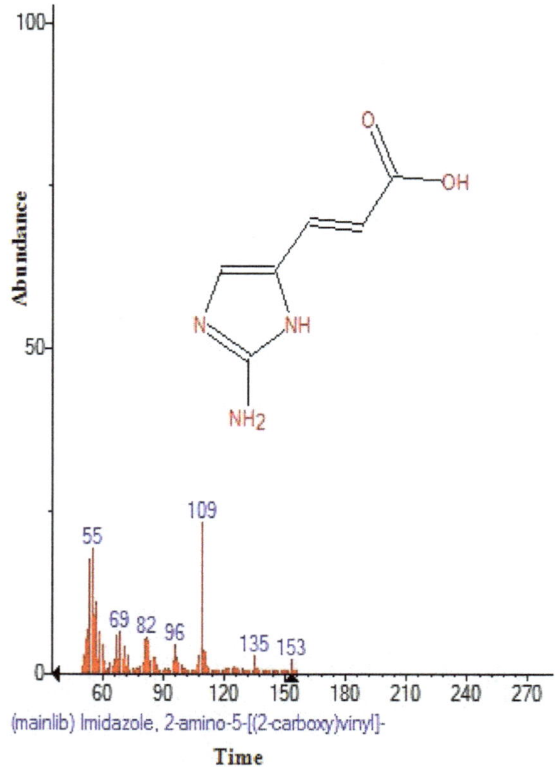

Figure 8. Mass spectrum of Imidazole,2-amino-5-[(2-carboxy)vinyl] with retention time (RT)= 3.859.

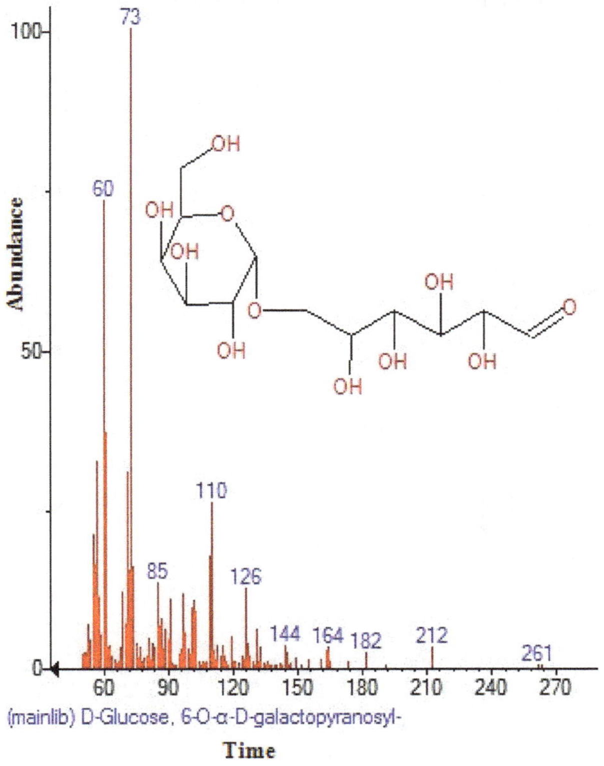

Figure 9. Mass spectrum of D-Glucose,6-O-α-D-galactopyranosyl with retention time (RT)= 3.997.

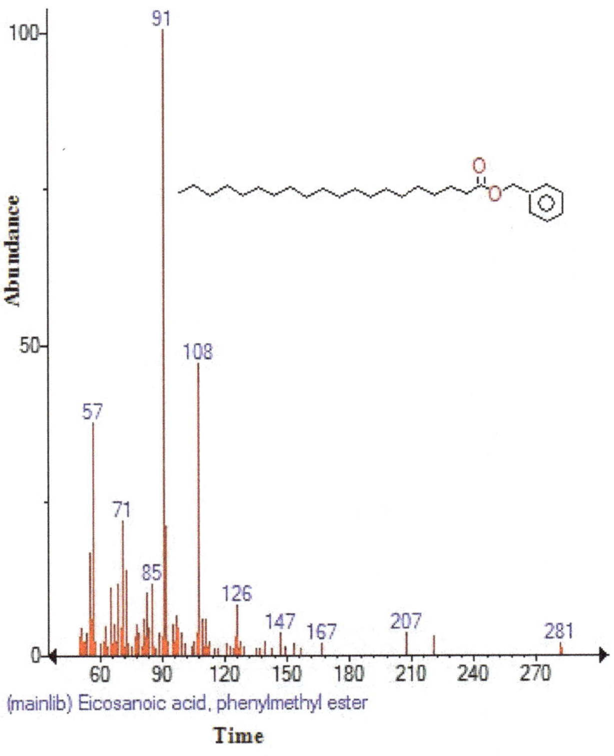

Figure 10. Mass spectrum of eicosanoic acid, phenylmethyl ester with retention time (RT)= 4.546.

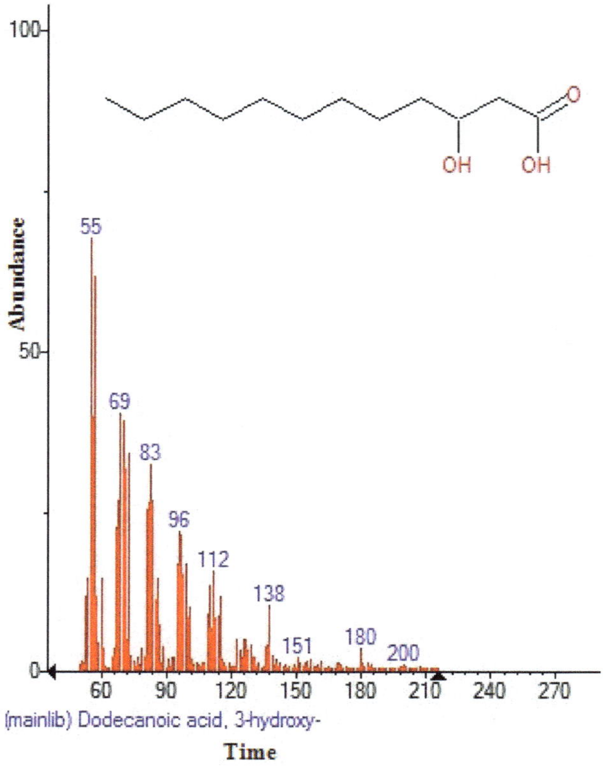

Figure 11. Mass spectrum of dodecanoic acid , 3-hydroxyl with retention time (RT)= 4.626.

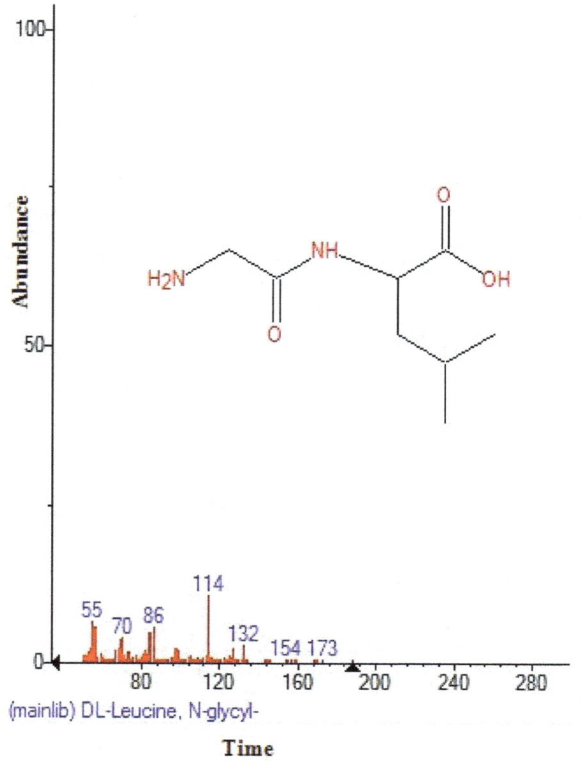

Figure 12. Mass spectrum of DL-Leucine,N-glycyl with retention time (RT)= 4.763.

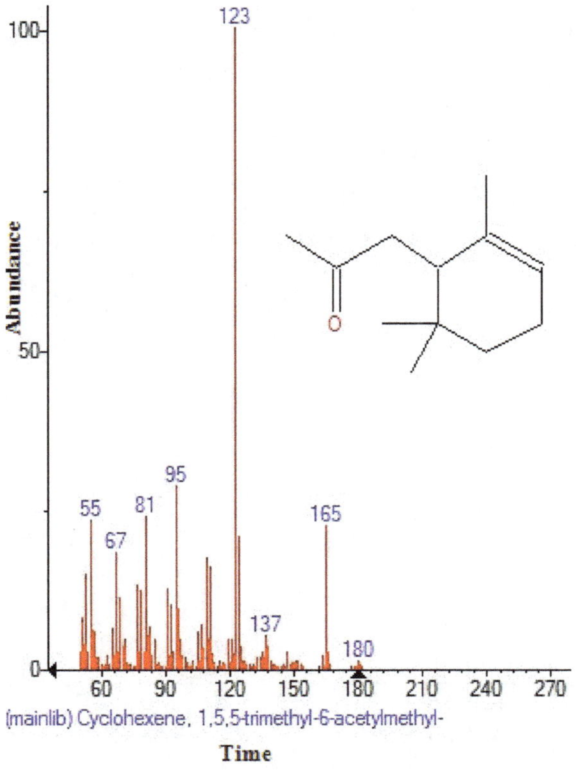

Figure 13. Mass spectrum of cyclohexene,1,5,5-trimethyl-6-acetylmethyl with retention time (RT)= 5.124.

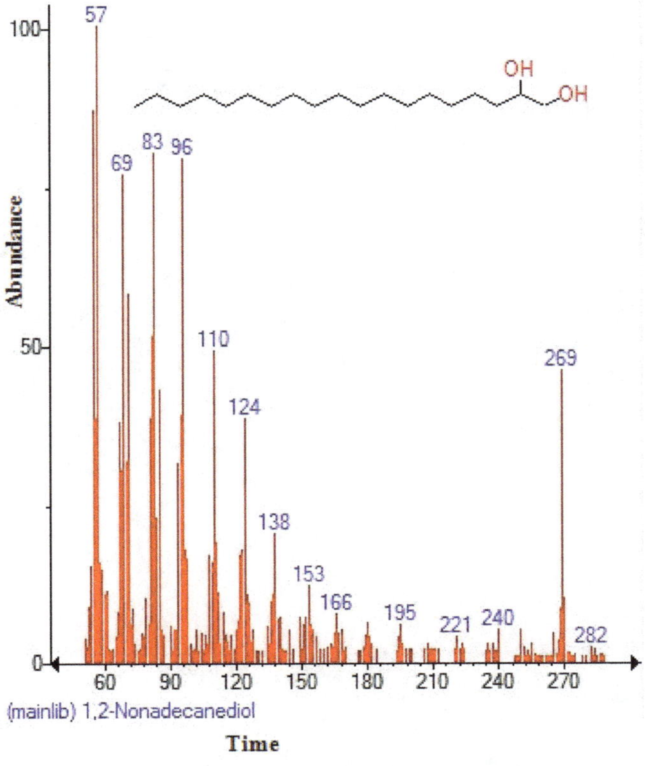

Figure 14. Mass spectrum of 1,2-Nonadecanediol with retention time (RT)= 5.095.

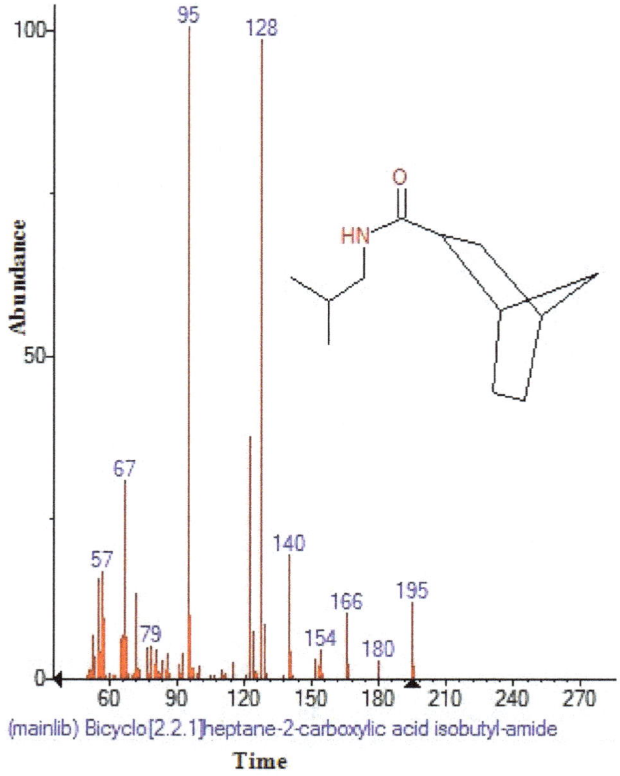

Figure 15. Mass spectrum of bicyclo[2.2.1]heptane-2-carboxylic acid isobutyl-amide with retention time (RT)= 5.232.

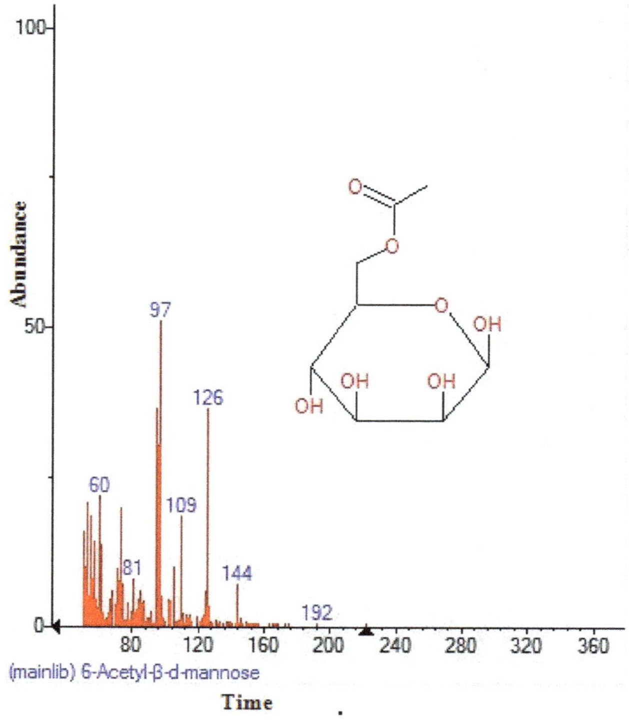

Figure 16. Mass spectrum of 6-Acetyl-ß-d-mannose with retention time (RT)= 5.536.

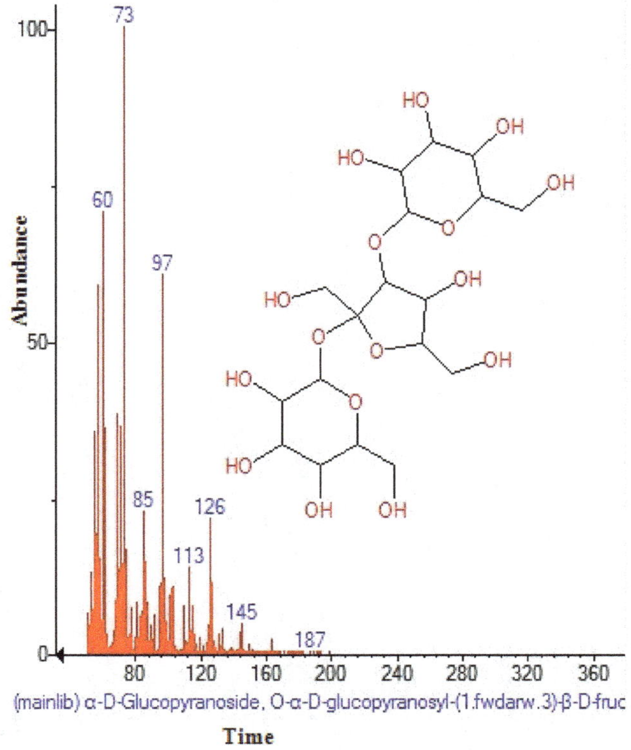

Figure 17. Mass spectrum of α-D-Glucopyranoside,O-α-D-glucopyranosyl-(1.fwdarw.3)-ß-D-fruc with retention time (RT)= 5.805.

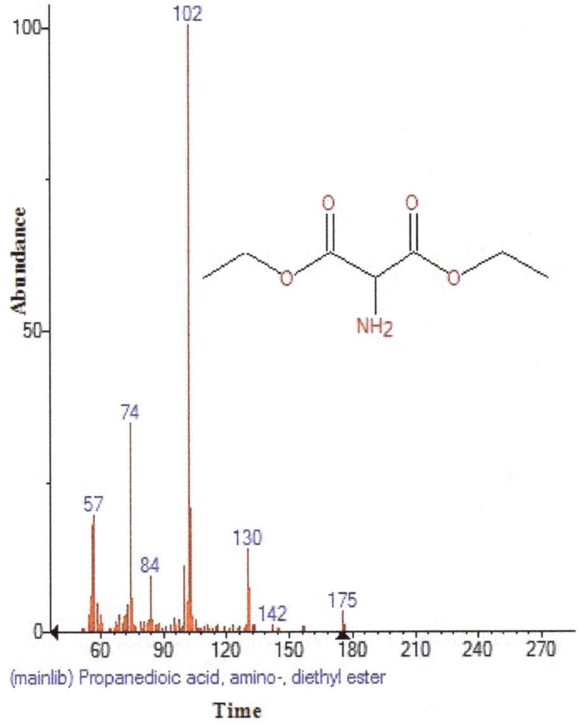

Figure 18. Mass spectrum of Propanedioic acid , amino -, diethyl ester with retention time (RT)= 5.862.

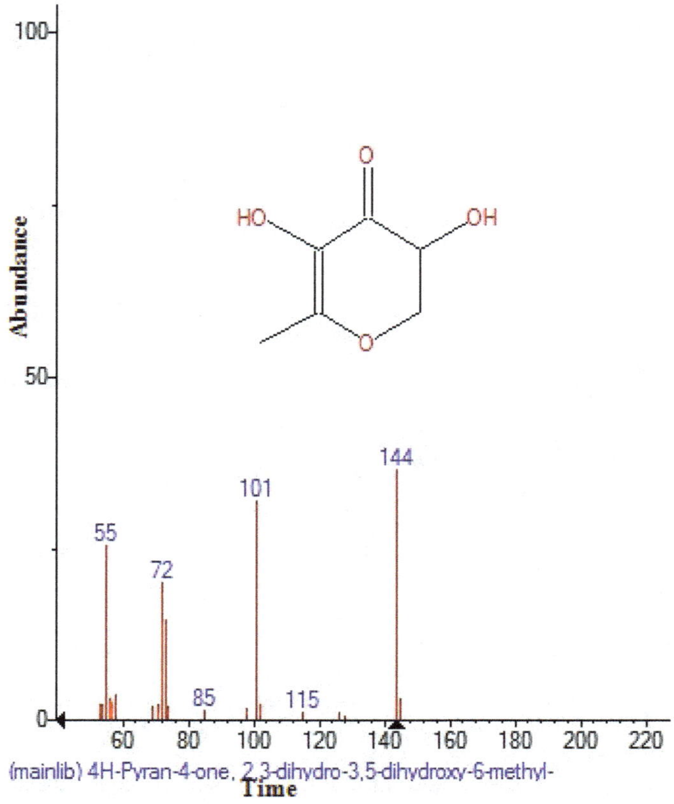

Figure 19. Mass spectrum of 4H-Pyran-4-one,2,3-dihydro-3,5-dihydroxy-6-methyl with retention time (RT)= 5.942.

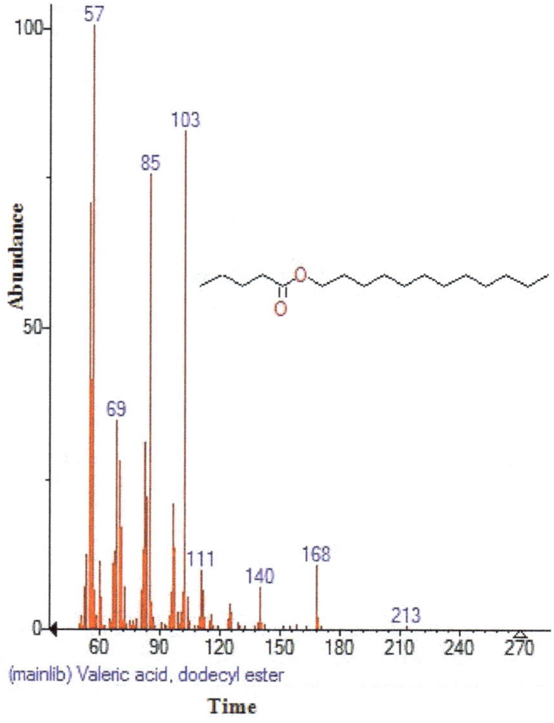

Figure 20. Mass spectrum of valeric acid, dodecyl ester with retention time (RT)= 6.600.

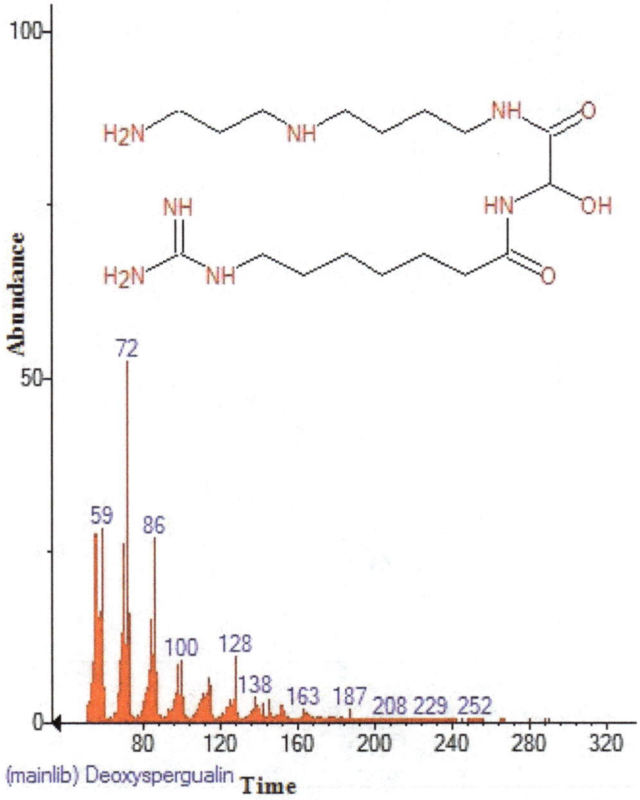

Figure 21. Mass spectrum of Deoxyspergualin with retention time (RT)= 6.852.

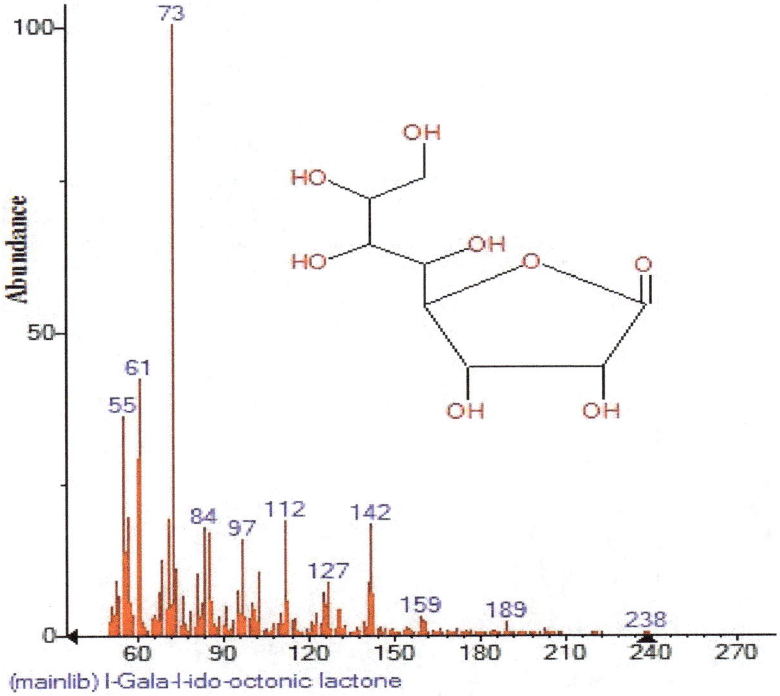

Figure 22. Mass spectrum of l-Gala-l-ido-octonic lactone with retention time (RT)= 6.766.

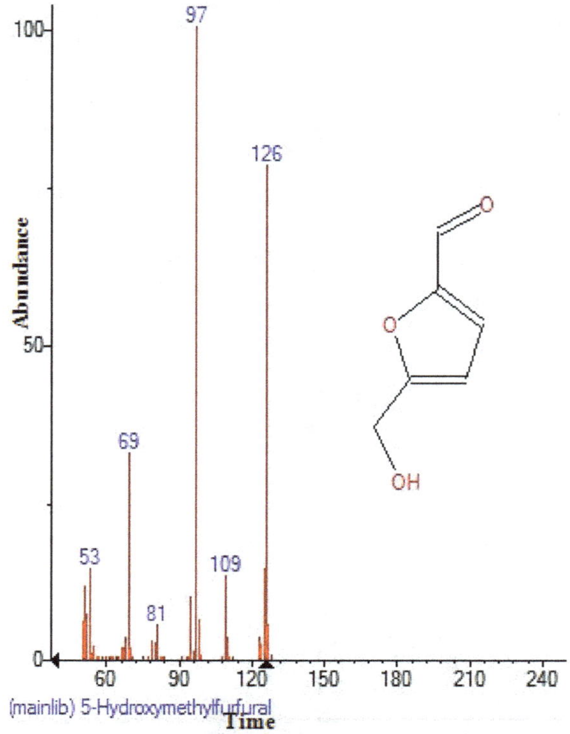

Figure 23. Mass spectrum of 5-Hydroxymethylfurfural with retention time (RT)= 6.983.

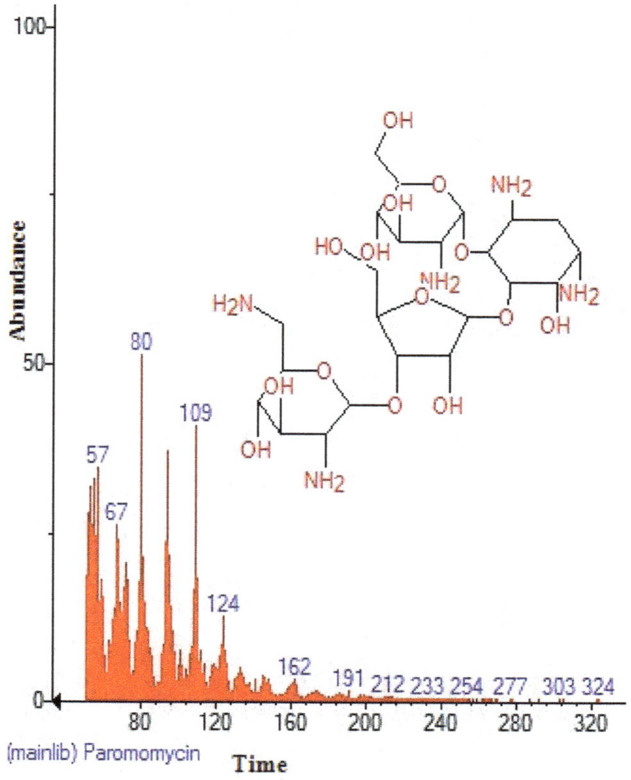

Figure 24. Mass spectrum of paromomycin with retention time (RT)= 7.807.

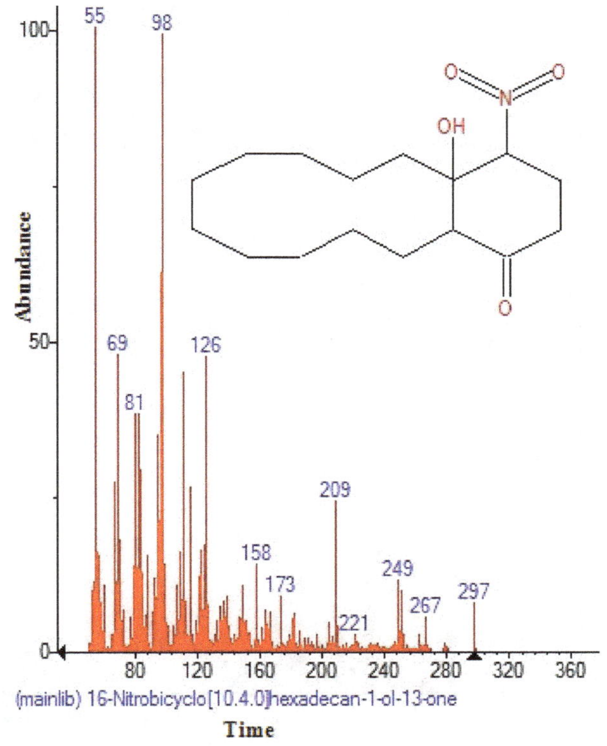

Figure 25. Mass spectrum of 16-Nitrobicyclo[10.4.0]hexadecane-1-ol-13-one with retention time (RT)= 8.797.

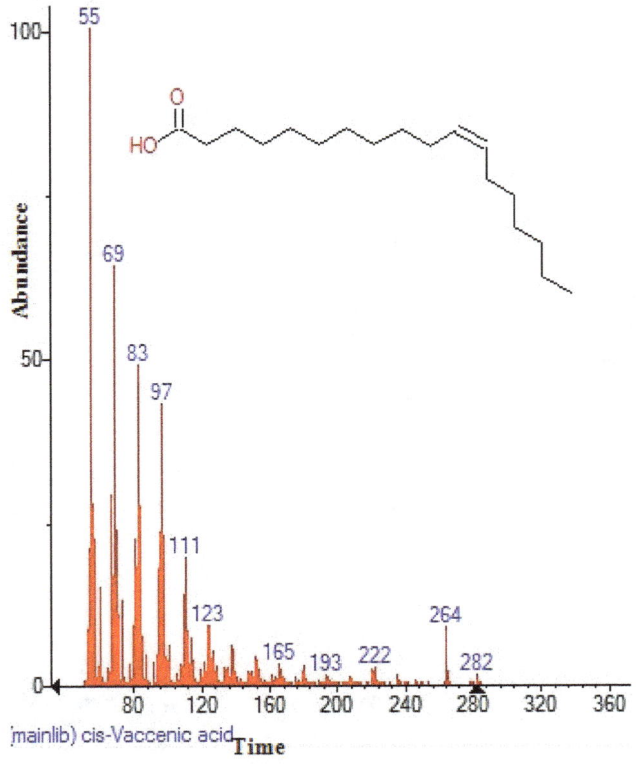

Figure 26. Mass spectrum of Cis-Vaccenic acid with retention time (RT)= 10.085.

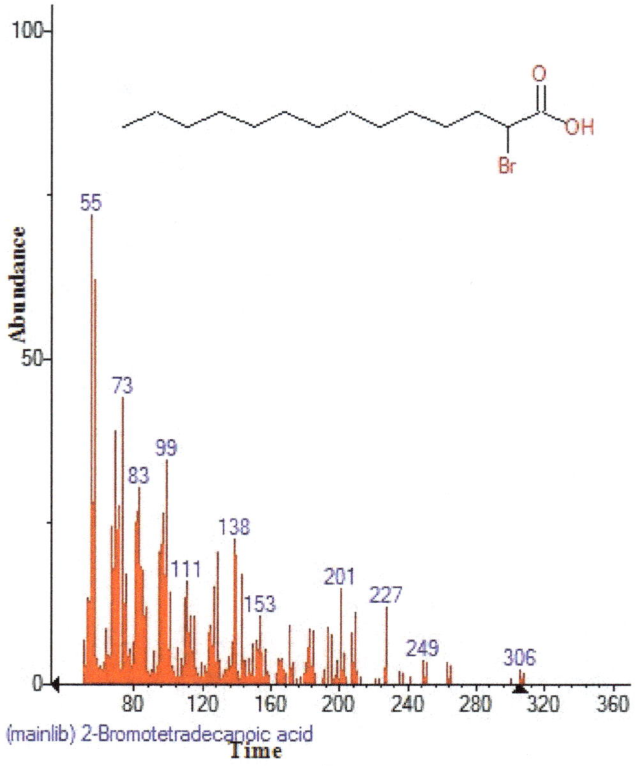

Figure 27. Mass spectrum of 2-Bromotetradecanoic acid with retention time (RT)= 11.567.

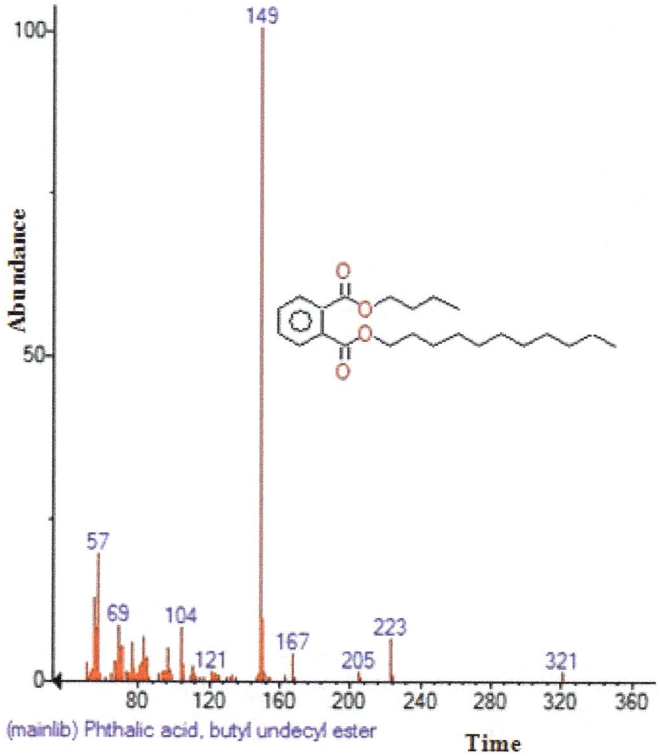

Figure 28. Mass spectrum of Phthalic acid , butyl undecyl ester with retention time (RT)= 14.279.

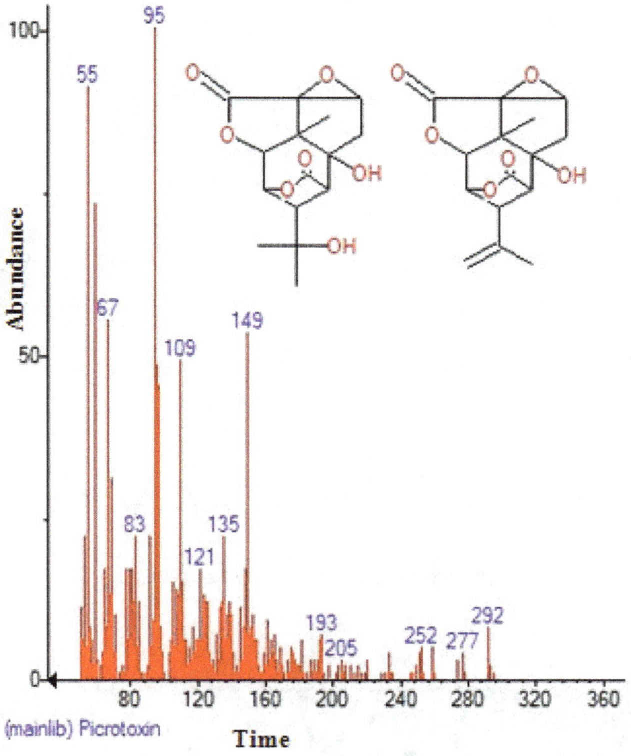

Figure 29. Mass spectrum of picrotoxin with retention time (RT)= 14.582.

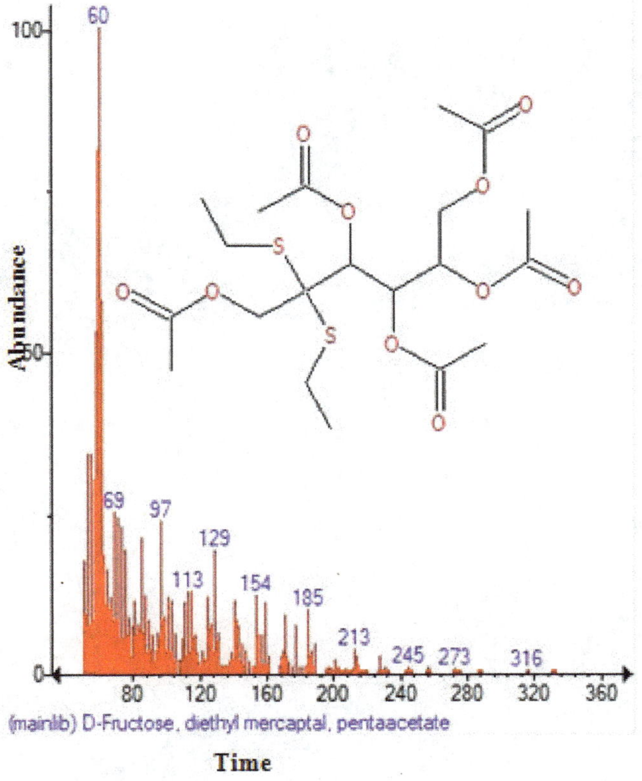

Figure 30. Mass spectrum of D-Fructose, diethyl mercaptal and pentaacetate with retention time (RT)= 15.046.

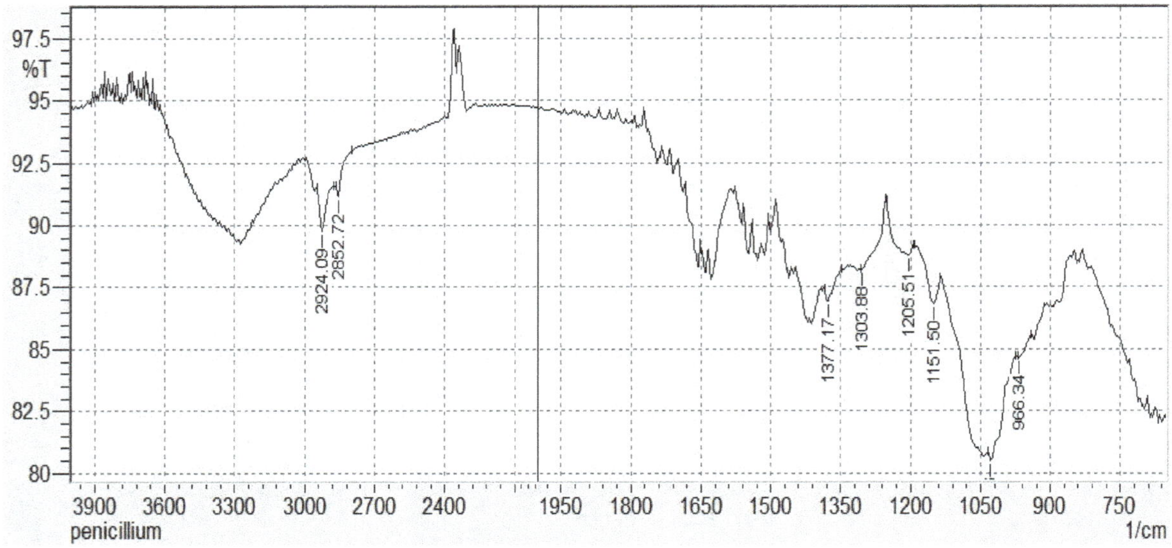

Figure 31. Fourier-transform infrared spectroscopy peak values of *P. expansum.*

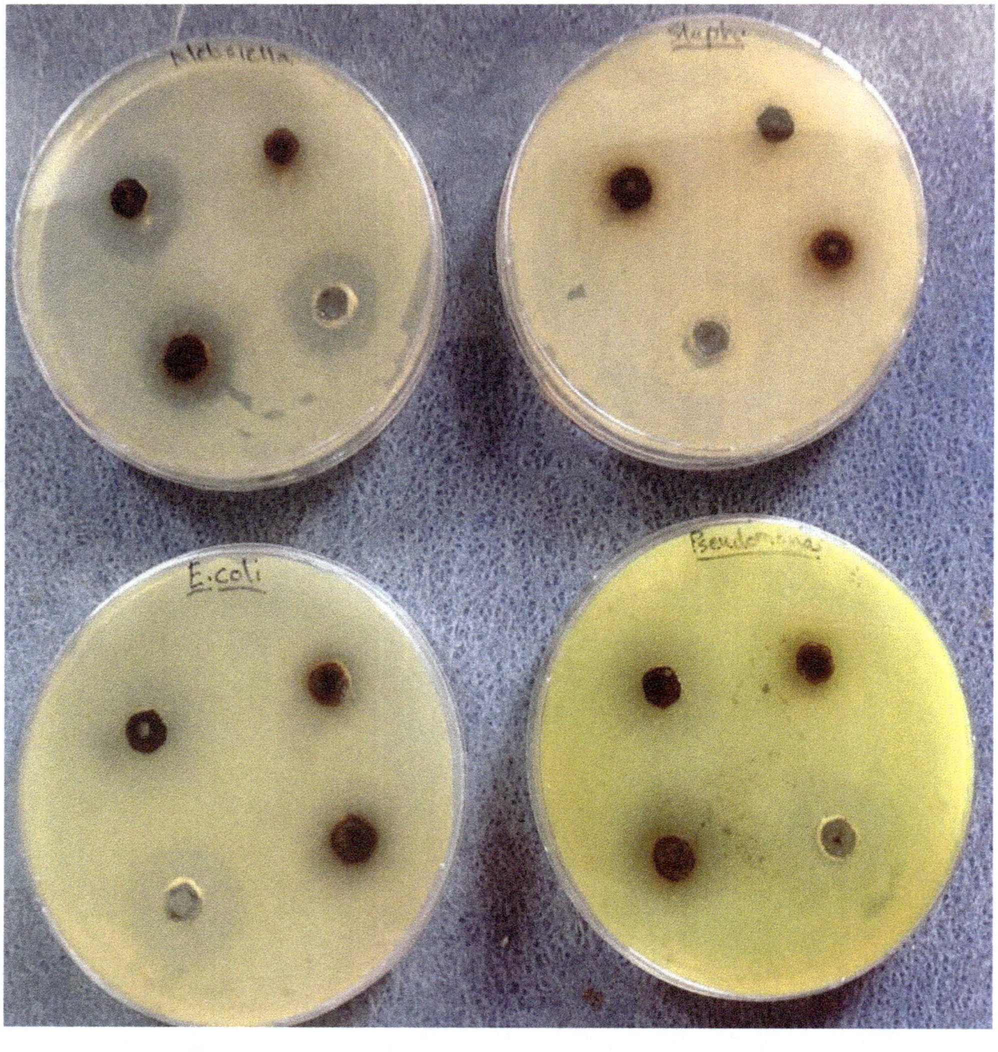

Figure 32. Antimicrobial activity of *P. expansum.*

Table 1. Bioactive chemical compounds identified in methanolic extract of *P. expansum*.

S/N	Phytochemical compound	RT (min)	Formula	Molecular weight	Exact mass	Chemical structure	MS Fragment- ions
1.	Levoglucosenone	3.230	$C_6H_6O_3$	126	126.031694	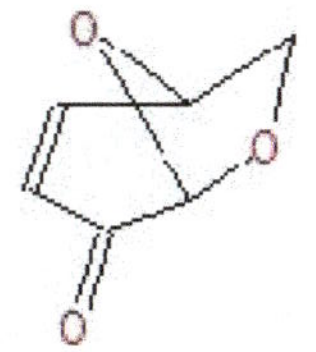	53,81,98,126
2.	Edulan II	3.613	$C_{13}H_{20}O$	192	192.151415	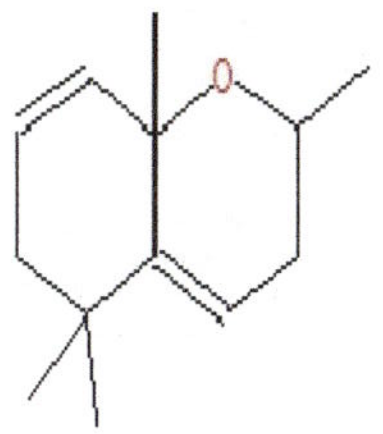	55,77,91,105,119,133,148,177,192
3.	4-[Dichloromethyl]-2-[[2-[1-methyl-2-pyrrolidinyl]ethyl]amino-6-trichloro	3.693	$C_{13}H_{17}Cl_{15}N_4$	403	403.989586	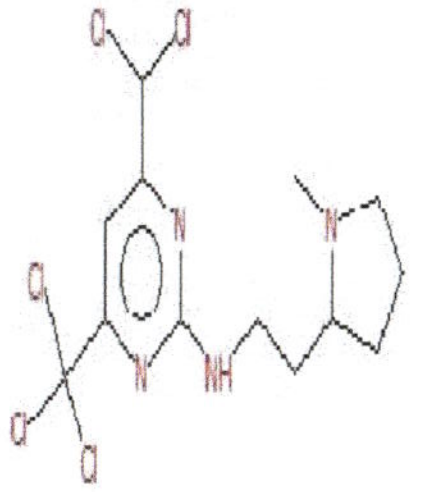	54,67,84,98,110,124,149,177,207,266
4.	1,2-Cyclopentanedione	3.750	$C_5H_6O_2$	98	98.0367794	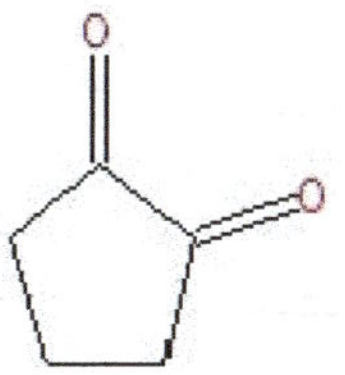	55,69,82,98

Table 1. Cont'd.

5.	Ethanethiol , 2-(5-(4-methyl-2-pyridyloxy)pentyl)amino-,hydrogen su	3.779	$C_{13}H_{22}N_2O_4S_2$	334	334.102098	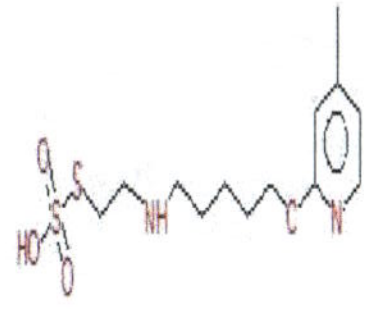	64,80,98,144,177,221,254,334
6.	Imidazole,2-amino-5-[(2-carboxy)vinyl]	3.859	$C_6H_7N_3O_2$	153	153.053826	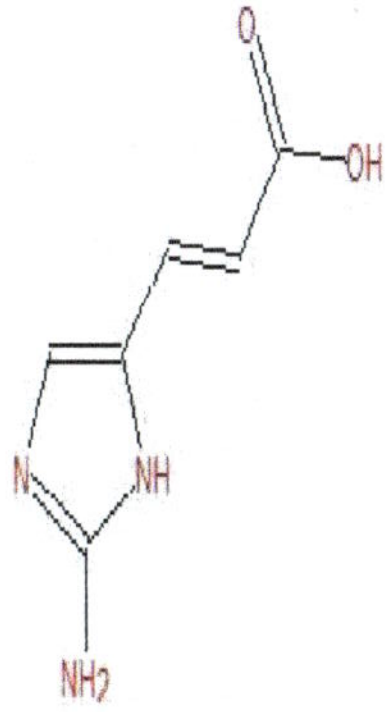	55,69,82,96,109,135,153
7.	D-Glucose,6-O-α-D-galactopyranosyl	3.997	$C_{12}H_{22}O_{11}$	342	342.11621	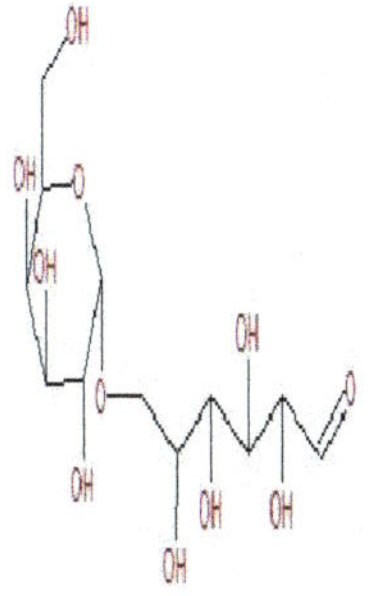	60,73,85,110,126,144,164,182,212,261
8.	Eicosanoic acid , phenylmethyl ester	4.546	$C_{27}H_{26}O_2$	402	402.349781	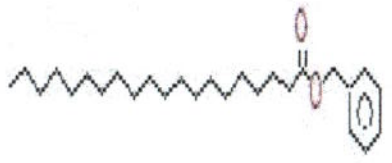	57,71,85,91,108,126,147,167,207,281

Table 1. Cont'd.

9.	Dodecanoic acid , 3- hydroxyl	4.626	$C_{12}H_{24}O_3$	216	216.1725445	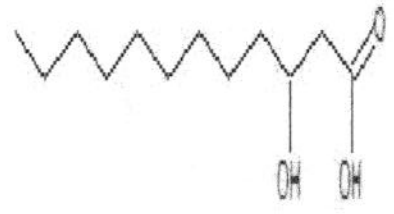	55,69,83,96,112,138,151,180,200
10.	DL-Leucine,N-glycyl	4.763	$C_8H_{16}N_2O_3$	188	188.116093	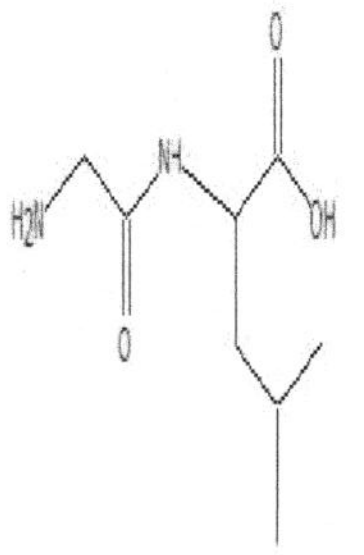	55,70,86,114,132,154,173
11.	Cyclohexene,1,5,5-trimethyl-6-acetylmethyl	5.124	$C_{12}H_{20}O$	180	180.151415	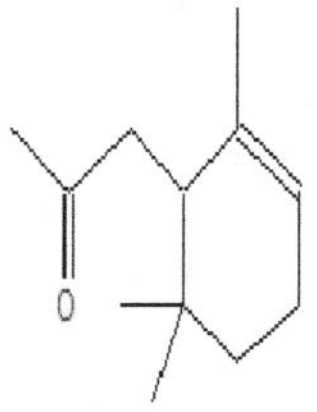	55,67,81,95,123,137,165,180
12.	1,2-Nonadecanediol	5.095	$C_{19}H_{20}O_2$	300	300.30283	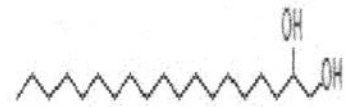	57,69,83,96,110,124,138,153,166,195,221,240,269,282
13.	Bicyclo[2.2.1]heptane-2-carboxylic acid isobutyl-amide	5.232	$C_{12}H_{21}NO$	195	195.162314	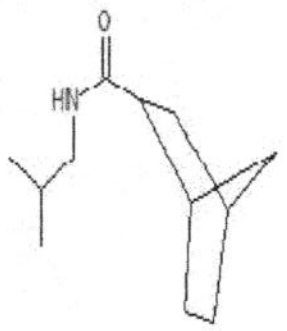	57,67,79,95,128,140,154,166,180,195

Table 1. Cont'd.

14.	6-Acetyl-ß-d-mannose	5.536	$C_8H_{14}O_7$	222	222.073953	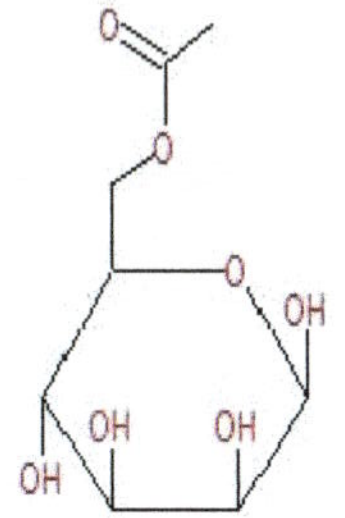	60,81,97,109,126,144,192
15.	α-D-Glucopyranoside,O-α-D-glucopyranosyl-(1.fwdarw.3)-ß-D-fruc	5.805	$C_{18}H_{23}O_{16}$	504	504.169035	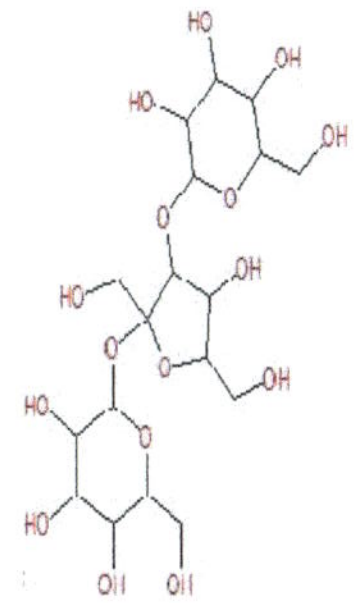	60,73,85,97,113,126,145,187
16.	Propanedioic acid , amino -, diethyl ester	5.862	$C_7H_{13}NO_4$	175	175.084458	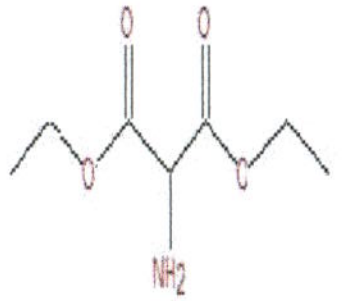	57,74,84,102,130,142,175
17.	4H-Pyran-4-one,2,3-dihydro-3,5-dihydroxy-6-methyl	5.942	$C_6H_8O_4$	144	144.042258	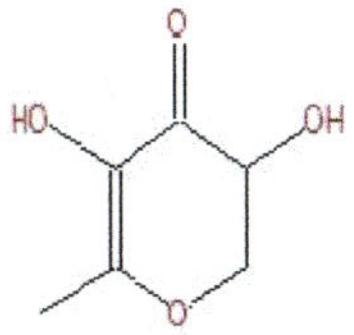	55,72,85,101,115,144
18.	Valeric acid , dodecyl ester	6.600	$C_{17}H_{34}O_2$	270	270.25588	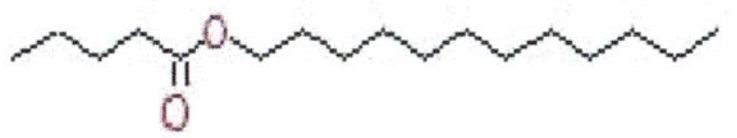	,1

Table 1. Cont'd.

19.	Deoxyspergualin	6.852	$C_{17}H_{37}N_7O_3$	387	387.295788	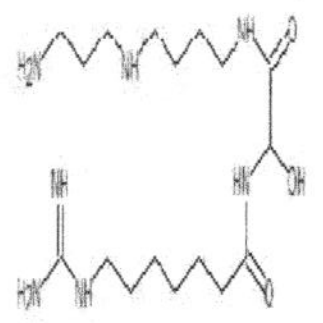	59,72,86,100,128,138,163,187,208,229,252
20.	l-Gala-l-ido-octonic lactone	6.766	$C_8H_{14}O_8$	238	238.068868	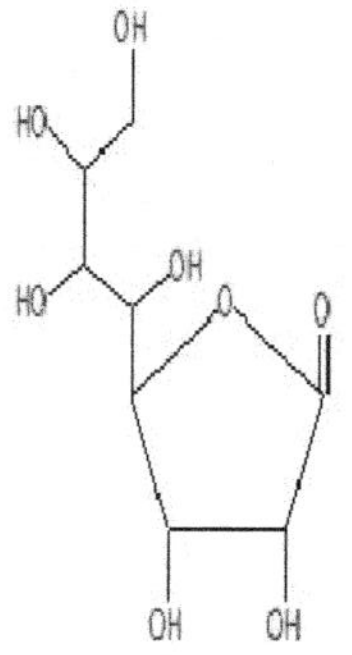	55,61,73,84,97,112,127,142,159,189,238
21.	5-Hydroxymethylfurfural	6.983	$C_6H_6O_3$	126	126.031694	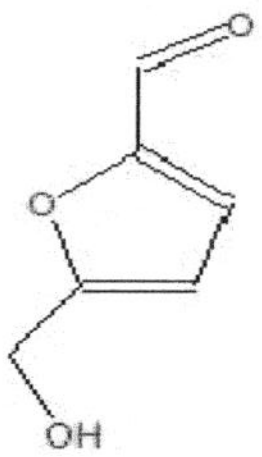	53,69,81,97,109,126
22.	Paromomycin	7.807	$C_{23}H_{45}N_5O_{14}$	615	615.296303	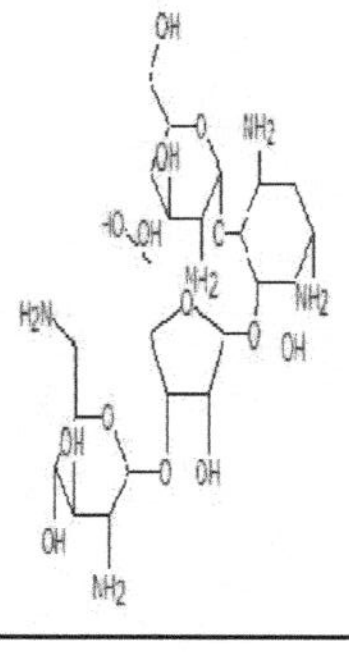	57,67,80,109,124,162,191,212,233,254,277,303,324

Table 1. Cont'd.

23.	16-Nitrobicyclo[10.4.0]hexadecane-1-ol-13-one	8.797	$C_{16}H_{27}NO_4$	297	297.194008	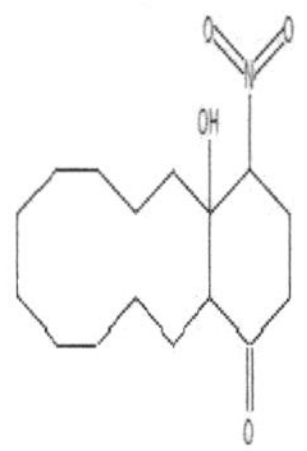	55,69,81,98,126,158,173,209,221,249,267,297
24.	cis-Vaccenic acid	10.085	$C_{18}H_{34}O_2$	282	282.25588	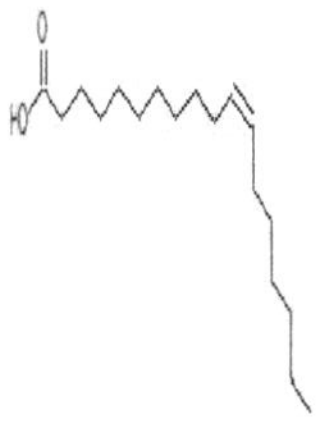	55,69,83,97,111,123,165,193,222,264,282
25.	2-Bromotetradecanoic acid	11.567	$C_{14}H_{27}BrO_2$	306	306.119442	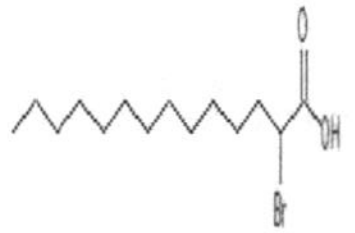	55,73,83,99,111,138,153,201,227,249,306
26.	Phthalic acid , butyl undecyl ester	14.279	$C_{23}H_{36}O_4$	376	376.26136	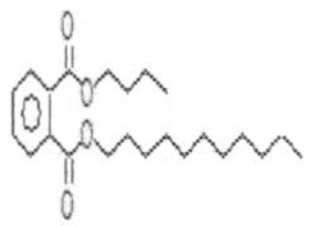	57,69,104,121,149,167,205,223,321
27.	Picrotoxin	14.582	$C_{30}H_{34}O_{13}$	602	602.19994	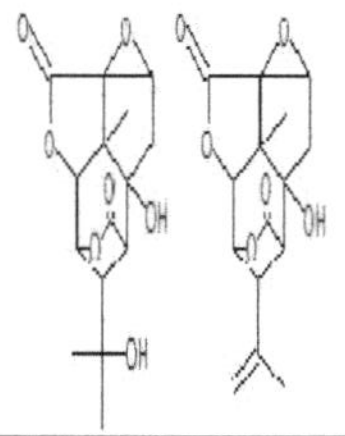	55,67,83,95,109,121,135,149,193,205,252,277,292

Table 1. Cont'd.

28.	D-Fructose , diethyl mercaptal , pentaacetate	15.046	$C_{20}H_{32}O_{10}S_2$	496	496.14369	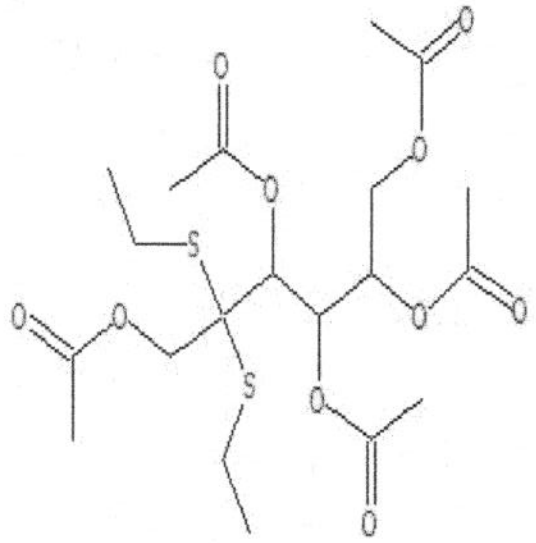	9,97,113,129,1 85,213,245,273

Table 2. FT-IR peak values of *P. expansum*.

No.	Peak (Wave number cm^{-1})	Intensity	Bond	Functional group assignment	Group frequency
1.	966.34	84.642	-	Unknown	-
2.	1028.06	80.509	C-F stretch	Aliphatic fluoro compounds	1000-10150
3.	1151.50	86.828	C-H	Tetiary amine, C-N stretch	1150-1207
4.	1205.51	88.792	C-H	Tetiary amine, C-N stretch	1150-1207
5.	1303.88	88.221	-	Unknown	-
6.	1377.17	86.934	-	Unknown	-
7.	2852.72	91.145	-	Methylene-CH. asym	2840-2860
8.	2924.09	89.745	-	Methylene-CH. asym	2915-2935

Table 3. Antibacterial activity of bioactive compounds of *Penicillium expansum* against bacterial strains.

Fungal products antibiotics	Zone of inhibition (mm)				
	Bacteria				
	K. pneumonia	*P. eurogenosa*	*S. aureus*	*P. mirabilis*	*E. coli*
Fungal products	5.94±0.491	3.88±0.913	7.01±0.141	5.64±0.203	5.97±0.192
Streptomycin	0.91±0.711	1.41±0.282	1.50±0.407	1.29±0.32	1.00±0.46
Kanamycin	0.93±0.162	0.49±0.500	0.70±0.195	0.50±0.097	0.90±0.204
Rifambin	1.10±0.303	1.09±0.201	0.99±0.496	0.78±0.41	0.76±0.300
Cefotoxime	1.29±0.502	0.91±0.310	1.40±0.203	0.98±0.841	1.47±0.180

Conclusion

This study showed that *P. expansum* produce many important secondary metabolites with high biological activities. Based on the significance of employing bioactive compounds in pharmacy to produce drugs for the treatment of many diseases, the purification of compounds produced by *P. expansum* can be useful.

ACKNOWLEDGEMENTS

The authors sincerely wish to thank Dr. Ali Al-Marzuqi from the Department of Biology for providing them with the opportunity to work on this project.

REFERENCES

Altameme HJ, Hameed IH, Kareem MA (2015). Analysis of alkaloid phytochemical compounds in the ethanolic extract of *Datura stramonium* and evaluation of antimicrobial activity. Afr. J. Biotechnol. 14(19):1668-1674.

Amiri A, Bompeix G (2005). Diversity and population dynamics of *Penicillium* spp. on apples in pre-and postharvest environments: consequences for decay development. Plant Pathol. 54:74-81.

Andersen B, Smedsgaard J, Frisvad JC (2004). *Penicillium expansum* : Consistent production of patulin, chaetoglobosins, and other secondary metabolites in culture and their natural occurence in fruit products. J. Agric. Food Chem. 52:2421-2428.

Baracat-Pereira MC, Valentim C, Muchovej JJ, Silva DO (1989). Selection of pectinolytic fungi for degumming of natural fibers. Biotechnol. Lett. 11:899-902.

Bracket RE, Marth EH (1979). Patulin in Apple Juice form Roadside Stands in Wisconsin. J. Food Prot. 42:862-3.

Bridge PD, Hawksworth DL, Kozakiewicz Z, Onions, AH, Paterson RR, Sackin MJ, Sneath PH (1989). Reappraisal of the terverticillate Penicillia using biochemical, physiological and morphological features. I. Numerical taxonomy. J. Gen. Microbiol. 135:2941-2966.

Frisvad JC (1992). Chemometrics and chemotaxonomy: a comparison of multivariate statistical methods for the evaluation of binary fungal secondary metabolite data. Chemometr. Intell. Lab. Syst. 14:253-269.

Frisvad JC, Filtenborg O (1989). Terverticillate penicillia: chemotaxonomy and mycotoxin production. Mycologia 81:837-861

Grassin C, Fauquembergue P (1996). Fruit juices. *In*: Godfrey, T., West, S. (eds). *Industrial Enzymology*. MacMillan, London pp. 225-264.

Hameed IH, Hussein HJ, Kareem MA, Hamad NS (2015a). Identification of five newly described bioactive chemical compounds in methanolic extract of *Mentha viridis* by using gas chromatography-mass spectrometry (GC-MS). J. Pharmacogn. Phytother. 7 (7):107-125.

Hameed IH, Ibraheam IA, Kadhim HJ (2015b). Gas chromatography mass spectrum and fourier-transform infrared spectroscopy analysis of methanolic extract of *Rosmarinus oficinalis* leaves. J. Pharmacogn. Phytother. 7(6):90-106.

Hameed IH, Jasim H, Kareem MA, Hussein AO (2015c). Alkaloid constitution of *Nerium oleander* using gas chromatography-mass spectroscopy (GC-MS). J. Med. Plant. Res. 9(9):326-334.

Hussein AO, Hameed IH, Jasim H, Kareem MA (2015). Determination of alkaloid compounds of *Ricinus communis* by using gas chromatography-mass spectroscopy (GC-MS). J. Med. Plant. Res. 9(10):349-359.

Imad H, Mohammed A, Aamera J (2014a). Genetic variation and DNA markers in forensic analysis. Afr. J. Biotechnol. 13(31):3122-3136.

Imad H, Mohammed A, Cheah Y, Aamera J. (2014b) Genetic variation of twenty autosomal STR loci and evaluate the importance of these loci for forensic genetic purposes. Afr. J. Biotech. 13:1-9.

Imad H, Muhanned A, Aamera J, Cheah Y (2014c). Analysis of eleven Y-chromosomal STR markers in middle and south of Iraq. Afr. J. Biotech. 13(38):3860-3871.

Jasim H, Hussein AO, Hameed IH, Kareem MA (2015). Characterization of alkaloid constitution and evaluation of antimicrobial activity of *Solanum nigrum* using gas chromatography mass spectrometry (GC-MS). J. Pharmacogn. Phytother. 7 (4):56-72.

Kareem MA, Hussein AO, Hameed IH (2015). Y-chromosome short tandem repeat, typing technology, locus information and allele frequency in different population: A review. Afr. J. Biotechnol. 14(27):2175-2178.

Massias M, Rebuffar S, Molho L, Chiaroni A, Riche C, Bodo B (1990). Expansolides A and B: tetracyclic sesquiterpene lactones from *Penicillium expansum.* J. Am. Chem. Soc. 112:8112-8115.

Mattheis JP, Roberts RG (1992). Identification of geosmin as a volatile metabolite of *Penicillium expansum*. Appl. Environ. Microbiol. 58:3170-3172.

Mohammed A, Imad H (2013). Autosomal STR: From locus information to next generation sequencing technology. Res. J. Biotechnol. 8(10):92-105.

Morales H, Sanchis V, Coromines J, Ramos AJ, Marin S (2008). Inoculum size and intraspecific interactions affects *Penicillium expansum* growth and patulin accumulation in apples. Food Microbiol. 25:378-385.

Murphy PA, Hendrich S, Landgren C, Bryant CM (2006). Food Mycotoxins: An update. J. Food Sci. 71:R51-R65.

Paterson RR, Kemmelmeier C (1989). Gradient high-performance liquid chromatography using alkylphenone retention indices of insecticidal extracts of *Penicillium* strains. J. Chromatogr. 483:153-168.

Pierson CF, Ceponis MJ, McColloch LP (1971). Market Diseases of Apples, Pears, and Quinces. Agricultural Handbook, US Department of Agriculture p 76.

Pitt JI, Hocking AD (1997). *Fungi and Food Spoilage*. Maryland, Aspen Publishers Inc., Maryland.

Rosenberger DA, Wicklow DT, Korjagin VA, Rondinaro SM (1991). Pathogenicity and benzimidazole resistance in *Penicillium* species recovered from flotation tanks in apple packinghouses. Plant Dis. 75:712-715.

Usha NS, Masilamani SM (2013). Bioctive compound produced by streptomycin strain. Int. J. Pharm. Pharm. Sci. 5(1):0975-14.

New pentacyclic triterpene ester and flavone glycoside from the biologically active extract of *Carduus pycnocephalus* L.

Wafaa H. B. Hassan[1]*, Hanan M. Al-Youssef[2], Latifa AL-Shammari[2] and Rehab H. Abdallah[1]

[1]Pharmacognosy Department, Faculty of Pharmacy, Zagazig University, Zagazig, Egypt.
[2]Pharmacognosy Department, Faculty of Pharmacy, King Saud University, Riyadh, Saudi Arabia.

Bioassay guided phytochemical investigation of petroleum ether, chloroform and butanol fractions obtained from biologically active total alcoholic extract of *Carduus pycnocephalus* led to isolation of two new compounds, 3-*O*-acetyl-ursolic acid-28-ethyl ester (compound 1) and diosmetin-7-*O*-*α*-L-arabinopyransyl (1```→4``)-*β*-D- glucopyranoside (compound 5) along with three known compounds, *bis* (2-ethylhexyl) benzene-1,2-dicarboxylate) (compound 2), 3α, 24 dihydroxyolean-12-en-28, 30-dioic acid dimethyl ester (compound 3) and kaempferol (compound 4). Their structures were established on the basis of spectroscopic methods (UV, MS, ^{1}H NMR, ^{13}C NMR, COSY, HSQC and HMBC) and by comparison with published data. Compounds 2 and 3 were isolated for the first time from genus *Carduus*. The cytotoxic, antioxidant, and antimicrobial activities of the ethanolic extract were evaluated and the extract showed variable degrees of activities. It showed significant cytotoxic activity against MCF-7, A-549 and HepG-2 cell lines with IC_{50}, 17.9, 17.5 and 21.8 µg, respectively. The extract displayed weak antioxidant activity by scavenging of DPPH with SC_{50} 554.2 µg. In agar diffusion assay, the extract exhibited strong antibacterial activities against Gram negative bacteria *Pseudomonas aeruginosa* and *Escherichia coli* and strong antifungal activity against *Syncephalastrum racemosum*.

Key words: *Carduus pycnocephalus* L.; new triterpene ester, flavonoidal glycoside, antioxidant, cytotoxic, antimicrobial activity.

INTRODUCTION

Genus *Carduus* which belongs to the family Asteraceae includes approximately 100 species worldwide (Chaudary, 2000) and is widely distributed around the Mediterranean. In Chinese folk medicine, the plants of genus *Carduus* are used for the treatment of various human diseases such as cold, stomach ache as well as rheumatism (Esmaieli, 2005). Genus *Carduus* was found to possess a wide range of biological activities such as liver tonic, anti-inflammatory, antispasmodic, anticancer, antiviral and antibacterial (Esmaeili, 2005; Jordon Thaden and Louda, 2003; Orhan and Ozcelik, 2009). Phytochemical studies on several *Carduus* species were

*Corresponding author. E-mail: wafbadr@yahoo.com; wafaabadr65@gmail.com.

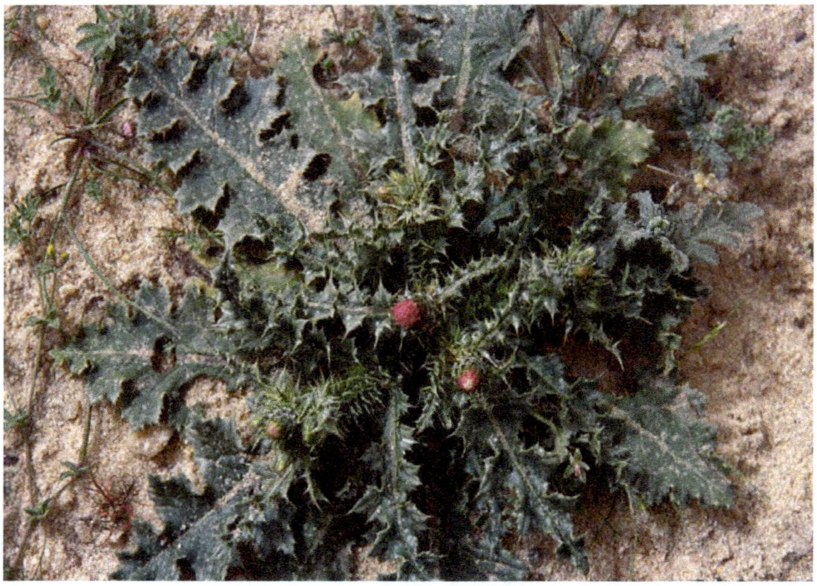

Figure 1. *Carduus pycnocephalus* L.

carried out and revealed that this genus is rich in secondary metabolites as lignans (Fernandez et al., 1991), flavonoids, flavonoidal glycosides (Jordon - Thaden and Louda, 2003; El-Lakany et al., 1995, 1997; Amer et al., 1985; Abdallah et al., 1989; Bain and Desrochers, 1988; Abdel Salam et al., 1982; Liu, et al., 2013), coumarins (Jordon Thaden and Louda, 2003; Cardona et al., 1992), alkaloids (Zanng, 2002), sterols and triterpenes (Abdel Salam et al., 1982, 1983). Concerning the phytoconstituents of *Carduus pycnocephalus*, the literatures survey revealed the presence of flavonoids (El-Lakany et al., 1995, 1997; Amer et al., 1985), essential oils (Esmaeili, 2005; Al-Shammari, 2012), sterols and triterpenes (Gallo and Sarachine, 2009). In our previous work on Saudi plant, the isolation of seven flavonoidal compounds were reported, apigenin, kaempferol-3-*O* *β* – D-glucoside, kaempferol-3- *O* – *α* – L- rhamnoside, kaempferol-7-methoxy-3- *O* – *α* – L- rhamnoside, diosmetin-7-O-*β*-D-xylosyl-(1```→6``)-*β*-D-glucopyranoside, diosmetin- 7- *O* - *α* – L- arabinosyl (1``` →6``) – *β* – D – glucopyranoside, kaempferol-3-*O*-*α*-L-rhamnosyl—(1``` →2``) -*α*-L rhamnoside, in addition to, lupeol, *β*-sitosterol and *β*-sitosterol-3-*O*-*β*-D- glucoside were isolated from the aerial parts of *C. pycnocephalus* L. Anti-inflammatory, antispasmodic and hypotensive activities were assessed for all extracts which showed variable activities (Al-Shammari, et al., 2012). In continuation of our phytochemical and biological studies on *C. pycnocephalus* which grows in Saudi Arabia, we report here the isolation and structure elucidation of two new compounds 1, 5 and three known compounds 2 to 4. Compounds 2 and 3 were reported for the first time from genus *Carduus*. In addition, the cytotoxic, antioxidant and antimicrobial activities for the total alcoholic extract of *C. pycnocephalus* L. were evaluated.

MATERIALS AND METHODS

General experimental section

Melting points were determined on a Mettler FP 80 Central Processor supplied with a Mettler FP 81 MBC Cell Apparatus, and were uncorrected. ^{1}H and ^{13}C NMR spectra were recorded in $CDCl_3$ and DMSO-d_6 on a Bruker Avance DRX – 500 instruments (Central Lab. at the College of Pharmacy, KSU) at 500 MHz for protons and 125 MHz for carbons using the residual solvent signal as an internal standard. All 1D and 2D spectra were obtained using the standard Bruker software; EI and FAB mass spectra on a Jeol JMS, Ax 500, 5890 series II (Tokyo, Japan), Ultraviolet spectra were obtained in methanol using the shifting reagents $AlCl_3$, NaOAc, NaOMe, and H_3BO_3 for flavonoids were obtained using a Hewlett-Packard HP-845 UV-Vis spectrophotometer. The ultraviolet lamp used in visualizing TLC plates was a Mineralight® device, multiband UV-254/366 nm obtained from UVP, Inc., USA. Column chromatography was performed on silica gel (60-230 mesh, Merck) and TLC was carried out with silica gel 60 pre-coated plates F-254 (Merck).

Plant

The fresh plant (Figure 1) was collected from Al-Hada (Saudi Arabia) on March, 2008 and was kindly identified by Dr. Jakob Thomas, Professor in College of Science, KSU. A voucher specimen (#15106) was deposited at the herbarium in the College of Pharmacy at King Saud University (KSU).

Extraction and isolation

The air dried aerial parts of *C. pycnocephalus* L. (2.0 kg) were exhaustively extracted with 95% ethanol. The concentrated ethanol extract (210 g) was suspended in methanol: water (1:9) and fractionated by extraction with petroleum ether (40 to 60°C), chloroform, ethyl acetate and water saturated butanol, each (0.5 L ×

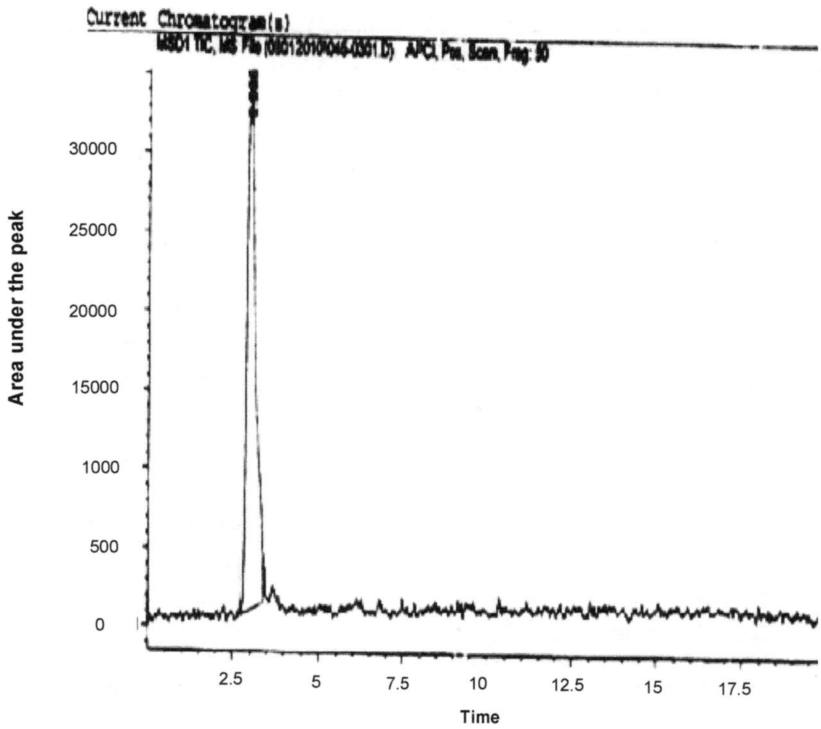

Figure 2. HPLC system used in isolation and chromatogram showing the purity of compound 5.

3), to give petroleum ether (47.3 g), chloroform (23.5 g), ethyl acetate (8.9 g), butanol (19.2 g) and aqueous (100 g) extracts.

Isolation of compounds 1 to 3 from petroleum ether extract

The petroleum ether extract (25 g) was subjected to silica gel column eluted with *n*-hexane and increasing the polarity with chloroform till 100% chloroform then with methanol, 60 fractions were collected (250 ml each), the important fractions were re-chromatographed using silica gel column eluted with *n*-hexane as eluent, then increasing the polarity by using chloroform and methanol to give compounds 1 (8 mg), 2 (1.37 g) and 3 (6 mg).

Isolation of compound 4 from chloroform extract

The chloroform fraction (2.5 g) was chromatographed on silica gel column. Elution was started with petroleum ether/chloroform (9:1) and the polarity was increased by methanol. Fifty fractions were collected, 100 ml each. The fractions were monitored by TLC and similar fractions were pooled together. From fraction 40 to 41 (120 mg) compound 4 (8 mg) was isolated by preparative TLC using chloroform: methanol (9.5:0.5) as solvent system.

Isolation of compound 5 from butanol extract

The butanol fraction (10 g) was chromatographed on silica gel column eluted with *n*-hexane/EtOAc (1:1) and increasing the polarity by ethyl acetate then by methanol. 70 Fractions were collected, 200 ml each. The fractions were monitored by TLC and similar fractions were combined together. Fractions 39 to 55 (750 mg) was subjected to preparative HPLC to yield 20 mg of highly pure compound 5 (Figure 2).

Acid hydrolysis of compound 5

Compound 5 (5 mg) was dissolved in MeOH (5 ml), to which an equal volume of 10% sulfuric acid was added. The mixture was refluxed on a boiling water bath for 3 h, and then cooled. The hydrolysate was shaken with ethyl acetate (3 × 50 ml). The combined extract was distilled off and subjected to TLC; the acidic mother liquor containing the sugar moiety (s) was neutralized with sodium carbonate, concentrated and separately spotted alongside with authentic sugars using chloroform:methanol (6:4) as solvent system and anisaldehyde sulfuric as spraying reagent. It showed the presence of *β*-D-glucose and *α*-L-arabinose as sugar moieties.

Compound 1: White powder (8 mg); R_f =0.59 [(*n*-hexane: $CHCL_3$) (2: 1)]; EI-MS *m/z* = 526 [M^+], 483 [M^+-$COCH_3$], 454 [M^+-$COCH_3$-C_2H_5], 411, 396, 382, 278, 248, 218; ^1H NMR and ^{13}C NMR (500 MHz, 125 MHz, $CDCl_3$, TMS) (Table 1).

Compound 2: Yellowish oily substance (1.37 g); ^1H NMR (500 MHz, $CDCl_3$, TMS) δ_H (ppm) 7.72 (2H, m, H-3, 6), 7.54 (2H, m, H-4, 5), 4.22 (4H, d, *J*= 6.4 Hz, H-3`, 3``), 1.70 (2H, m, H-4`, 4``), 1.35 (14H,m, H-5`, 5``, 6`, 6``, 7`, 7``), 0.88 (4H, m, H-8`, 8``), 1.35 (14 H, m, H-9`, 9``) and 0.90 (6H, t) H-10`, 10``); ^{13}C NMR (125 MHz, $CDCl_3$, TMS) δ_C 132.6 (s, C-1, 2), 129.0 (d, C-3, 6), 131.1 (d, C-4, 5), 167.9 (s, C-1`, 1``), 68.3 (t, C-3`, 3``), 38.9 (d, C-4`, 4``), 31.2 (t, C-5`, 5``), 29.6 (t, C-6`, 6``), 22.4 (t, C-7`, 7``), 14.4 (q, C-8`, 8``), 22.8 (t, C-9`, 9``) and 11.6 (q, C-10`, 10``); EI-MS: *m/z* = 390 [M^+,

Table 1. ^{1}H and ^{13}C NMR data of compound 1 in $CDCl_3$.

Position	δ_H	δ_C (DEPT)	Position	δ_H	δ_C (DEPT)
1	1.59, 1.0 (2H, m)	38.3 t	18	2.12 (1H, d, J=7.4 Hz)	55.3 d
2	1.57 (1H, m)	24.9 t	19	1.16 (1H, m)	40.9 d
3	4.45 (1H, t, *J* =7.0 Hz)	80.3 d	20	0.88 (1H, m)	39.8 d
4	-	37.8 s	21	1.36 (1H, m)	32.6 t
5	0.76 (1H, br)	55.3 d	22	1.26, 1.51 (2H, m)	31.9 t
6	1.32, 1.45 (2H, m)	18.3 t	23	0.80 (3H, s)	28.4 q
7	1.26, 1.46 (2H, m)	33.3 t	24	0.78 (3H, s)	16.8 q
8	-	39.8 s	25	1.25 (3H, s)	14.1 q
9	1.50 br	47.6 d	26	0.89 (3H, s)	16.8 q
10	-	37.1 s	27	1.08 (3H, s)	23.7 q
11	2.20 d, *J*= 7 Hz)	23.7 t	28	-	173.9 s
12	5.12 (1H, t, *J* =3.6 Hz)	121.7 d	29	0.90 (3H, d, *J*=5.5 Hz)	14.3 q
13	-	145.2 s	30	0.82 (3H, d, *J*=4.5 Hz)	23.5 q
14	-	41.7 s	31	-	173.7 s
15	1.62, 0.92 (2H, m)	26.1 t	32	2.20 (3H, s)	23.0 q
16	1.15, 1.50 (2H, m)	23.6 t	33	4.05 (2H, q, *J*=7.2 Hz)	60.1 t
17	-	47.2 s	34	1.20 (3H, t, *J*=5.0 Hz)	15.5 q

36%] , 149 [100%].

Compound 3: White powder (6 mg); ^{1}H NMR (500 MHz, $CDCl_3$, TMS) δ_H (ppm) 5.19 (1H, broad t, *J*= 7.6 Hz, H-12), 4.10 (1H, m, H-3), 3.50 (6H, s, two OCH_3- 31 and 32), 2.30 (1H, broad t , *J*=7.0 Hz, C-18), 1.26 (9H, s, for three methyl groups), 0.85 (6H, s, two methyl groups) ; ^{13}C NMR (125 MHz, $CDCl_3$, TMS) δ_C (ppm) 38.2 (C-1), 24.4 (C-2), 80.6 (C-3), 37.8 (C-4), 55.2 (C-5), 18.2 (C-6), 32.7 (C-7), 39.2 (C-9), 36.6 (C-10), 23.2 (C-11), 121.6 (C-12), 145.2 (C-13), 42.9 (C-14), 28.3 (C-15), 23.2 (C-16),46.7 9C-17), 37.8 (C-18), 41.8 (C-19), 47.2 (C-20), 31.1 (C-21), 34.7 (C22), 60.1 (C-23), 14.2 (C-24), 15.5 (C-25), 16.5 (C-26), 25.8 (C-27), 173.7 (CO-28), 50.3 (OCH_3-31), 29.7 (C-29), 174.0 (CO-30) and 50.3 (OCH_3-32). EI-MS: *m/z* 530 [M^+], 512, 470 and 247.

Compound 4: Pale yellow powder (8 mg); R_f =0.45 [$CHCl_3$:MeOH, 9:1]; UV λ max; MeOH (266, 338); ^{1}H NMR (500 MHz, DMSO-d_6, TMS) δ_H 6.05 (1H, *s*, H-6), 6.40 (1H, *s*, H-8), 6.85 (2H, *d*, *J* = 8.0 Hz, H-3`and 5`), 7.80 (2H, *d*, *J*= 8.0 Hz, H-2`and 6`), 5.50 (1H, s, OH-4`), 13.10 (1H, br s, OH-5); EI-MS: *m/z* = 286 [M^+], 134, 152.

Compound 5: Gray to greenish powder (20 mg); mp: 187-188 ^{0}C; R_f = 0.62 [butanol : acetic acid : water, 24:10:1]; UV λ_{max} MeOH: (nm) 269, 344; (NaOMe): 269 , 300 sh, 280; ($AlCl_3$): 273, 362, 390; ($AlCl_3$/HCl): 276, 297, 361, 383; (NaOAc): 271, 365 (NaOAc/H_3BO_3): 269, 348; ^{1}H NMR (500 MHz, DMSO-d_6, TMS); ^{13}C NMR (125 MHz, DMSO-*d*6, TMS) (Table 2); FAB-MS (Positive ion mode) *m/z* = 633 [M^++K] for $C_{27}H_{30}O_{15}$, 595 [M^++H], 463 [M^+-arab+H], 301 [M^+-glu-arab], 152.

Biological activities

All the biological activities were carried out at Regional Center for Mycology and Biotechnology (RCMB) at Al- Azhar University, Cairo, Egypt.

Cytotoxic activity

The cytotoxic effect of total alcoholic extract of *C. pycnocephalus* L. (Figure 6) was investigated at different concentrations, 50, 12.5, 6.25, 3.125, 1.56, 0.78 and 0.39 µg/ml. The tested cell lines, breast carcinoma (MCF-7), lung carcinoma (A-549) and hepatocellular carcinoma (HepG-2) were obtained from American Type Culture Collection (ATCC, Rockville, MD). The cells were grown as mono-layers in growth RPMI-1640 medium supplemented with 10% inactivated fetal calf serum and 50 µg/ml gentamycin. The monolayers of 10,000 cells adhered at the bottom of the wells in a 96-well microtitre plate incubated for 24 h at 37°C in a humidified incubator with 5% CO_2. The monolayers were then washed with sterile phosphate filtered saline (0.01 M, pH 7.2) and simultaneously the cells were treated with 100 µl from different dilutions of the test sample in fresh maintenance medium and incubated at 37°C. A control of untreated cells was made in the absence of the test sample. Six wells were used for each concentration of the test sample. Every 24 h, the observation under the inverted microscope was made. The number of the surviving cells was determined by staining the cells with crystal violet followed by cell lysing using 33% glacial acetic acid and read the absorbance at λmax 490 nm using ELISA reader (SunRise TECAN, Inc, USA) after well mixing. The absorbance values from untreated cells were considered as 100% proliferation. The number of viable cells was determined using ELISA reader as previously mentioned and the percentage of viability was calculated as:

$$[1- (ODt / ODc) \times 100\%]$$

where ODt: optical density of wells treated with the test sample. ODc: optical density of untreated cells. The IC_{50} value which reduces the cells number by 50%, was determined from dose response curve.

Antioxidant activity

Radical scavenging activity of total alcoholic extract of *C.*

Table 2. NMR data of compound 5 (500, 125 MHz, DMSO-d_6, TMS).

No.	δ_H (δ ppm)	δ_C (DEPT)	HSQC	HMBC	HHCOSY
2	-	164.7 s	-	-	-
3	6.84 s	104.3 d	C-3	4, 10	-
4	-	182.5 s	-	-	-
5	12.90 (OH, s)	161.6 s	-	-	-
6	6.48 (1H, d, *J*=2.0 Hz)	100.1 d	C-6	8, 10	8
7	-	163.4 s	-	-	-
8	6.81 (1H, d, *J*=2.0 Hz)	95.3 d	C-8	6, 10	6
9	-	157.5 s	-	-	-
10	-	105.9 s	-	-	-
1`	-	123.4 s	-	-	-
2`	7.46 (1H, d, *J*=8.8 Hz)	113.7 d	C-2`	4`, 6`, 2	6`
3`	9.24 (OH, s)	147.3 s	-	-	-
4`	OCH_3 3.87 (3H, brs)	151.8 s; 55.8 q	OCH_3	4`	-
5`	7.16 (1H, d, *J*=8.8 Hz)	112.7 d	C-5`	1`, 3`	6`
6`	7.58 (1H, dd, *J*=2.0, 8.8 Hz)	119.4 d	C-6`	2`, 4`	2`, 5`
1``	5.06 (1H, d, *J*=7.2 Hz)	100.4 d	C-1``	7	2``
2``	3.65 (1H, m)	75.9 d	C-2``	-	1``, 3``
3``	3.25 (1H, m)	76.7 d	C-3``	-	2``, 4``
4``	3.32 (1H, m)	78.9 d	C-4``	-	3``, 5``
5``	3.10 (1H, m)	76.1 d	C-5``	-	4``, 6``
6``	3.40 , 4.10 (2H, m)	60.1 t	C-6``	-	5``
1```	4.15 (1H, d, *J*= 4.8 Hz)	103.3 d	C-1```	-	2```
2```	3.33 (1H, m)	70.9 d	C-2```	-	1```, 3```
3```	3.24 (1H, m)	72.9 d	C-3```	-	2```, 4```
4```	3.60 (1H, m)	67.6 d	C-4```	-	3```, 5```
5```	3.20, 3.65 (2H, m)	64.5 t	C-5```	-	4```

pycnocephalus L. was determined at the Regional Center for Mycology and Biotechnology (RCMB) at Al- Azhar University by the DPPH free radical scavenging assay in triplicate and average values were considered (Figure 7).

DPPH radical scavenging activity (Yen and Duh, 1994): Methanol solution (0.004% w/v) of 2,2-diphenyl-1-picrylhydrazyl (DPPH) radical was freshly prepared and stored at 10°C in the dark. A methanol solution of the test extract was prepared. A 40 µl aliquot of the methanol solution was added to 3 ml of DPPH solution. Absorbance measurements were recorded immediately with a UV-visible spectrophotometer (Milton Roy, Spectronic 1201). The decrease in absorbance at 515 nm was determined continuously, with data being recorded at 1 min intervals until the absorbance reference compound ascorbic acid were also measured. All the determinations were performed in three replicates and averaged. The percentage inhibition (PI) of the DPPH radical was calculated according to the formula:

$$\text{DPPH scavenging activity \% [PI]} = [\{(AC- AT)/AC\} \times 100] \quad (1)$$

where *AC* = Absorbance of the control and *AT* = absorbance of the sample + DPPH.

Antimicrobial activity

Agar diffusion method (Perez et al., 1990): The total alcoholic extract of *C. pycnocephalus* L. was dissolved in DMSO and evaluated by agar diffusion method at a dose of 50 µg/ml and the results were reported as shown in Table 3. The tested fungi were *Asperagillus fumigates* (RCMB 02568), *Syncephalastrum racemosum* (RCMB 05922), *Geotricum candidum* (RCMB 05097) and *Candida albicans* (RCMB 05036); Gram positive bacteria *were Streptococcus pneumonia* (RCMB 010010) and *Bacillus subtillis* (RCMB 010067) while Gram negative bacteria were *Pseudomonas aeruginosa* (RCMB 010043) and *Escherichia coli* (RCMB 010052). Amphotericin B, ampicillin and gentamicin were used as standard antifungal and antimicrobial agents; the diameter of zone of inhibition was measured in mm. The microorganisms were obtained from Regional Centre of Mycology and Biotechnology, Al-Azhar University.

RESULTS AND DISCUSSION

Phytochemical results

Characterisation of the isolated compounds

Petroleum ether, chloroform and butanol extracts of air dried aerial parts of *C. pycnocephalus* L. were subjected to chromatographic separation followed by purification and gave five pure compounds 1 to 5. The identification

Table 3. Antimicrobial activity of total alcoholic extract of *C. pycnocephalus* L.

Microorganism	Inhibition zone diameter (mm) of	
	Total alcoholic extract	Standards
Fungi		**Amphotericin B**
Asperagillus fumigates	16.8 ± 0.58	23.7 ± 0.1
Syncephalastrum racemosum	15.2 ± 0.58	19.7 ± 0.2
Geotricum candidum	18.6 ± 0.63	28.7 ± 0.2
Candida albicans	***NA**	25.4 ± 0.1
Gram positive bacteria		**Ampicillin**
Streptococcus pneumonia	17.3 ± 0.63	23.8 ± 0.2
Bacillus subtilis	18.6 ± 0.72	32.4 ± 0.3
Gram negative bacteria		**Gentamicin**
Pseudomonas aeruginosa	15.3 ± 0.58	17.3 ± 0.1
Escherichia coli	17.2 ± 0.63	19.9 ± 0.3

*NA: No activity; Extract and used standards were tested at a dose of 50 µg.

of these compounds was carried out on the basis of spectroscopic methods (UV, IR, ^{1}H NMR, ^{13}C NMR, DEPT 135, COSY, HMBC, HSQC and MS spectroscopy).

Compound 1, [3-*O*-acetyl ursolic acid-28-ethyl ester]: The EI-MS of compound 1 exhibited a distinct molecular ion peak at *m/z* 526 [M^+] corresponding molecular formula $C_{34}H_{54}O_4$. The ^{13}C NMR and DEPT data of compound exhibited 34 carbons. These carbons are attributed to nine methyls, ten methylenes, seven methines and eight quaternary carbon atoms. The ^{1}H-NMR data, (Table 1), revealed the presence of nine methyl signals, six appeared as singlet at δ_H 0.80, 0.78, 1.25, 0.89, 1.08, 2.20 and connected, via HSQC to C-23 (δ_C 28.4), C-24 (δ_C 16.8), C-25 (δ_C 14.1), C-26 (δ_C 16.8), C-27 (δ_C 23.7) and C-32 (δ_C 23.0), respectively; and two doublets at δ_H 0.90 (3H, d, J=5.5 Hz) and 0.82 (3H, d, J= 4.5 Hz) as well as one triplet at δ_H 1.20 (3H, t, J= 5.0 Hz) and connected to C-29 (δ_C 14.3), C-30 (δ_C 23.5) and C-34 (δ_C 15.5), respectively. In addition, the ^{1}H-NMR data showed a triplet signal at δ_H 5.12 (1H, t, J= 3.6 Hz) connected via HSQC to C-12 (δ_C 121.7). These information along with the carbon chemical shift of C-12 and C-13 (δ_C 121.7/145.2 and proton shift of H-12 (δ_H 5.12) suggested that compound 1 was a triterpene carrying a $(\Delta^{12})^{13}$ double bond (Ahmad and Rahman, 1994).

The presence of two douplet methyl groups at 0.90 (3H, d, J =5.5 Hz) and 0.82 (3H, d, J=4.5 Hz) for CH_3-29 and CH_3-30, respectively suggested the presence of ursolic acid nucleus. This suggestion was further confirmed by HMBC experiment (Figure 4) in which there are three bond correlations between CH_3-29 with C-18 and C-20; CH_3-30 with C-19 and C-21. Further HMBC correlations were detected between methine proton at C-12 (δ_C 121.7) and C-9 (δ_C 47.6), C-14 (δ_C 41.7), and two bonds correlations with C-11 (δ_C 23.7). The methine proton at C-3 appearing at δ_H 4.45 (1H, t, J=7.0 Hz) showed two bond correlation with C-2 (δ_C 24.9) and C-4 (δ_C 37.8). Also the ^{1}H NMR spectrum showed extra signals, quartet signal appear at δ_H 4.05 (2H, q, J= 7.2 Hz) and triplet δ_H 1.20 (3H, t, J=5.0 Hz) connected to C-33 (δ_C 60.1, CH_2) and C-34 (δ_C 15.5, CH_3) in HSQC spectrum, respectively which indicated the presence of ethyl group. The position of it was established from HMBC correlation of methylene group at δ_H 4.05 (2H, q, J= 7.2 Hz) with C=O -28 at δ_C 173.9. Further confirmation was obtained from the upfield shift of carbonyl group at 28 position to 173.9 ppm compared to that of ursolic acid 180.1 (Babalola and Shode, 2013). Other extra ^{1}H NMR signal at δ_H 2.20 (3H, s) and two ^{13}C NMR signals at δ_C 23.1 and 173.7 were observed which indicated the presence of acetyl group. The position of acetyl group was proved through HMBC correlation by three bonds of H-3 (δ_H 4.45) with carbonyl (C-31) (δ_C 173.7). The EI-MS confirmed the presence of acetyl and ethyl moieties in compound 1 where it showed fragments at *m/z* 483 [M^+-$COCH_3$] and 454 [M^+-$COCH_3$-C_2H_5]. From the aforementioned data and through comparison with reported literatures for related compounds (Ahmad and Rahman, 1994), the structure of compound 1 was established to be 3-*O*-acetyl ursolic acid-28-ethyl ester and it is the first report of this compound from nature.

Compound 2, [Bis (2-ethylhexyl) benzene-1, 2-dicarboxylate]: Compound 2 (1.37 g), was isolated as pale yellow oil, R_f 0.7 [(10% EtOAc in *n*-hexane)]. The EI/MS spectrum displayed a pseudo molecular ion $[M]^+$ at *m/z* 390, which is in a good agreement with the molecular formula $C_{24}H_{38}O_4$ (Figure 3). ^{1}H NMR and ^{13}C NMR data

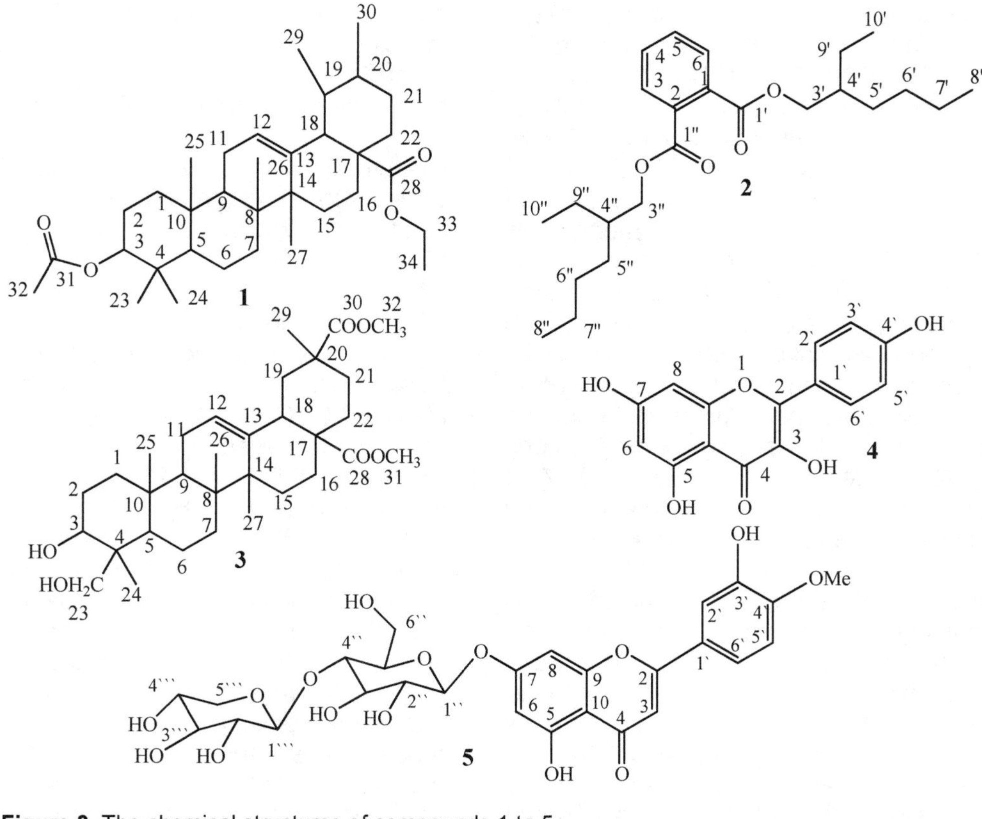

Figure 3. The chemical structures of compounds 1 to 5.

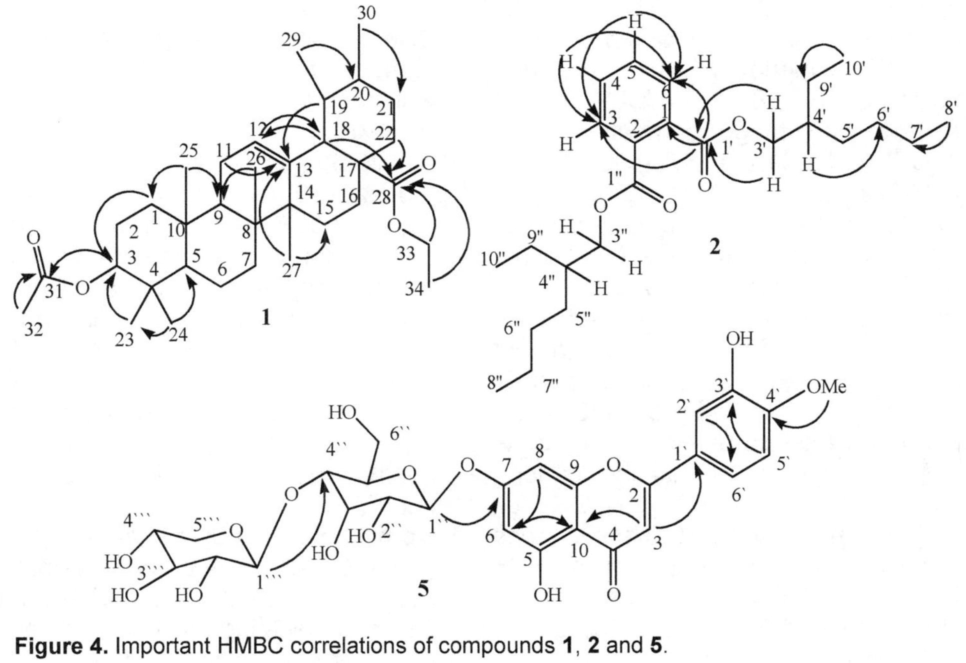

Figure 4. Important HMBC correlations of compounds **1**, **2** and **5**.

demonstrated the presence of 12 signals attributed to two methyls, five methylenes, three methines and two quaternary carbons indicated the symmetry of the compound since the number of carbons and protons measured by mass is 24 and 38, respectively. Two of the four quaternary carbons appeared at δ_C 167.9, indicated the presence of two esters carbonyl moiety in the compound. The ^{1}H NMR data exhibited two aromatic protons appeared at δ_H 7.72 (2H, *m*, H-3, 6) and 7.54 (2H, *m*, H-4, 5), two methylene protons at δ_H 4.22 (4H, *d*, *J* = 6.4 Hz, H-3`, 3``), two methine protons at $\delta_H$ 1.70 (2H, *m*, H-4`, 4``), four methyl resonances at δ_H 0.90 (4H, 10`, 10``) and 0.88 (4H, 8`, 8``). The spectrum also showed multiplets around δ_H 1.35 accounts for eight methylenes (16 H, 5`, 5``, 6`, 6``, 7`, 7``, 9`, 9``). Combined studies of 2D NMR experiments, notable COSY, HSQC and HMBC allowed to complete assignment of the spectral data. The existence of only two aromatic peaks in ^{1}H NMR spectrum (integrated to 2 protons each) suggested that the compound must have an *ortho*-disubstituted benzene ring bearing the same substituent in both positions (Silverstein et al., 1997). The aromatic protons at δ_H 7.72 (H-3/ H-6) showed direct coupling to a carbon at δ_C 129.0 in the HSQC experiment, in addition to long range HMBC correlations with carbons at δ_C 131.1, 132.6 and the carbonyl group at δ_C 167.9. Similarly, H-4/H-5 (δ_H 7.54) revealed direct coupling to carbon at δ_C 132.6 and long range correlations to carbons at δ_C 129.0. From the aforementioned correlations, the quaternary carbon at δ_C 132.6 was assigned as C-1/C-2 and the methine carbons at δ_C 131.1 and 129.0 to C-4/C-5 and C-3/C-6, respectively. The carbonyl quaternary carbon at δ_C 167.9 (C=O) showed correlation with H-3/ H-6. The methylene protons at δ_H 4.22 showed direct coupling to an oxygenated carbon at δ_C 68.3 and long range correlation with the carbonyl group at δ_C 167.9. Therefore, these protons were assigned as H-3'/H-3''. The multiplet (integrated for 2 protons) at δ_H 1.70 exhibited coupling with H-3'/H-3'' in COSY experiment which, in turn, showed direct coupling at δ_C 38.9 (C-4'/C-4'') in the HSQC experiment and long range correlations with carbons at δ_C 68.3 (C-3'/C-3''), 31.2 (C-5'/C-5''), 29.6 (C-6'/C-6''), 22.8 (C-9'/C-9'') and 11.6 (C-10'/C-10'') in HMBC (Figure 4). The methyls at δ_H 0.90 and 0.88 exhibited direct coupling to methyl carbons at δ_C 11.6 (C-10'/C-10'') and 14.4 (C-8'/C-8''), respectively. A common long range correlations by H-4'/H-4'' and the methyls at δ_H 0.88 (H-8'/H-8'') to δ_C 29.6 confirmed their assignment as C-6'/C-6''. These methyls were also connected to C-7'/C-7'' at δc 22.4. The other two methyl groups (δ_H 0.90, H-10'/H-10'') showed long range correlations to carbons at δ_C 38.9 (C-4'/C-4''). A multiplet at δ_H 1.35 showed long range correlations to C-10'/C-10'' (δ 11.6), C-4'/C-4'' (δ_C 38.9) and C-3'/C-3'' (δ 68.3). As a result, these protons must be H-9'/H-9'', which showed direct coupling with carbons at δ_C 22.8 (C-9'/C-9''). On the basis of the aforementioned data, compound 2 was identified as bis (2-ethylhexyl) benzene-1,2-dicarboxylate). This compound is a synthetic polypropylene derivative, which is used as a plasticizer for polyvinyl chloride (PVP) (Beeler et al., 1976). Bis (2-ethylhexyl) benzene-1,2-dicarboxylate) was previously isolated and reported as natural product from *Mentha longifolia* (Ertaş et al., 2015) and *Ziziphora persica* (Nadaf et al., 2013) and it showed larvicidal activity (Katadea et al., 2006). This is the first report to isolate *bis* (2-ethylhexyl) benzene-1, 2-dicarboxylate) from genus *Carduus*.

Compound 3, [3α, 24 -dihydroxyolean-12-en-28, 30-dioic acid dimethyl ester]: The ^{1}H NMR spectrum of compound 3 showed signals at δ (ppm) 1.26 (9H, s), 0.85 (6H, s) which in addition to the five ^{13}C NMR signals at δ_C 14.2 (C-24), 15.5 (C-25), 16.5 (C-26), 25.8 (C-27) and 29.7 (C-29) indicated the presence of five methyl groups in this compound. The other signal at δ_H 5.19 (1H, broad t, *J*= 7.6 Hz, H-12) in ^{1}H NMR spectrum with two signals at δ_C121.6 (C-12), 145.2 (C-13) in ^{13}C NMR spectrum revealed the presence of $(\Delta^{12})^{13}$ triterpenoidal compound (Ahmad and Rahman, 1994). The ^{1}H NMR signals at δ_H 4.10 (1H, *m*), 3.50 (6H, s), 2.30 (1H, broad t, *J*= 7.0 Hz) with ^{13}C NMR signals at 80.6, 50.3 and 37.8 were interpreted for CH-3, two OCH_3 groups at 31 and 32 and CH-18, respectively. The presence of CH_2OH was established from the ^{1}H NMR and ^{13}C NMR signals at δ_H 3.70 and 4.10 each for one proton with signal at δ_C 60.1 for CH_2OH at position 24 (Ahmad and Rahman, 1994). The aforementioned data with the remaining signals reported in experimental section and EI-MS spectrum at *m/z* 530, in addition to comparison with literature (Ahmad and Rahman, 1994) confirmed the structure of compound 3 as 3-*α*, 24- dihydroxyolean-12-en-28, 30-dioic acid dimethyl ester. This is the first report of this compound in genus *Carduus*.

Compound 4 [kaempferol]: The UV spectral data of compound 4 showed UV λ max; MeOH (266, 338 nm) which indicated the presence of flavonol compound. The ^{1}H NMR spectrum showed an A_2B_2 spin system for ring B at δ_H 6.85 (2H, *d*, *J*= 8.0 Hz, H-3`and 5`), 7.80 (2H, *d*, *J*= 8.0 Hz, H-2`and 6`). In addition, the presence of singlet signal at δ_H 6.40 for H-6, and other signal at δ 6.05 (1H, *s*, H-8) for H-8 indicated the presence of 3, 5, 7, 4` tetrahydroxy flavone nucleus. Also, the EI-MS spectrum showed a molecular ion peak at *m/z* 286 [M^+ , 100%] which are in a good agreement with the molecular formula $C_{15}H_{10}O_6$ from the aforementioned data and through comparison with literatures (Mabry et al., 1970; Markham et al., 1978) compound 4 was identified as kaempferol, it was previously reported in genus *Carduus*.

Compound 5 [Diosmetin- 7-*O* -*α*- L- arabinopyransyl - (1'''→ 4'') -*β* - D - glucopyranoside]: The UV spectral data of compound 5 showed absorption bands at 269 and 344 nm indicating the flavones nature of the compound. The different shifting reagents confirmed the presence of flavone nucleus with free hydroxyl group at 5 position and the absence of free hydroxyl group at 7 and 4` positions or presence of occupied ones. The FAB-MS spectrum(Figure 5), exhibited a molecular ion peak at *m/z* 633 [M^++ K] and *m/z* 595 [M^+ +H], which is in agreement

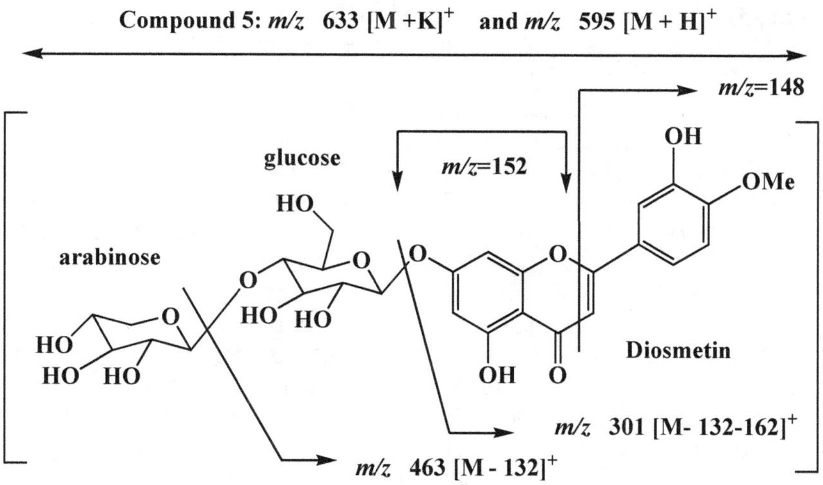

Figure 5. Fragmentation pattern of compound 5.

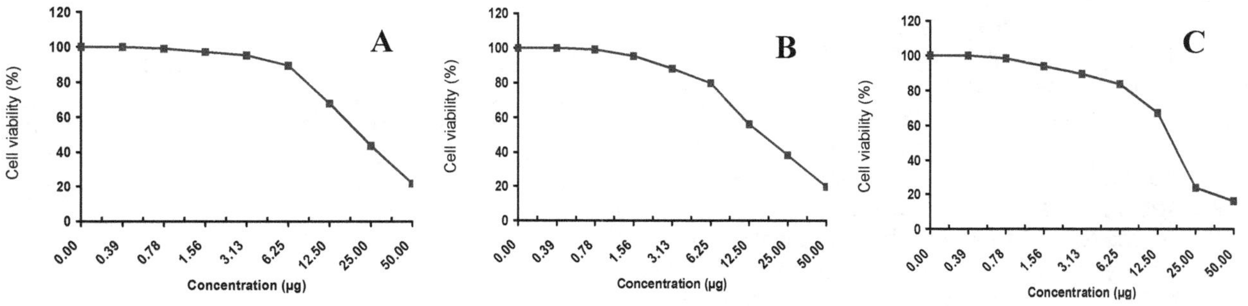

Figure 6. Cytotoxic effect of total alcoholic extract of *C. pycnocephalus* L. against HepG-2 (**A**), A-549 (**B**) and MCF-7 (**C**) cells.

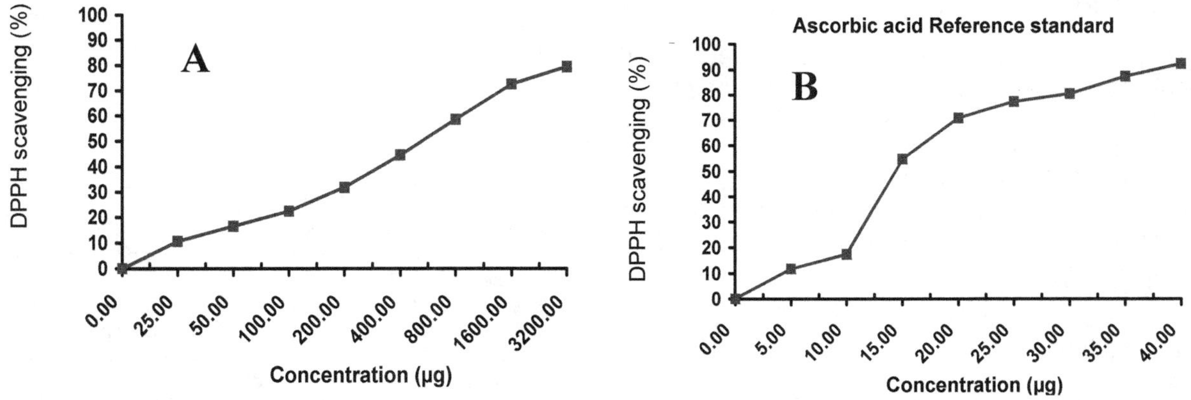

Figure 7. Antioxidant activity of total alcoholic extract of *C. pycnocephalus* (**A**) using DPPH free radical scavenging test and ascorbic acid as a reference compound (**B**).

with molecular formula $C_{27}H_{30}O_{15}$. The ^{1}H and ^{13}C NMR spectral data of compound 5 (Table 2) were close to that of compounds reported (El-Lakany et al., 1997; Saeidnia et al., 2011) suggesting that 5 had diosmetin as an aglycon. This was confirmed from the ^{13}C NMR spectral data of compound 5 which showed 27 carbons, 16 of which were very similar to those for diosmetin. Further confirmation for the presence of diosmetin was the ^{1}H NMR which showed the presence of methoxy group appeared as singlet signal at δ_H 3.88.

This methoxy group connected via HMBC correlation to C-4` at $\delta_C$ 151.8 (Figure 4). Furthermore, the $^{1}H$ NMR and H-HCOSY data showed ABX spin system for ring B appearing at $\delta_H$ 7.58 (1H, dd, *J* = 2.0, 8.8 Hz, H-6`), 7.46 (1H, d, *J* = 2.0 Hz, H-2`), 7.16 (1H, d, *J* = 8.8 Hz, H-5`). In addition to the presence of two meta coupled signals at δ_H 6.48 and 6.81 (*J* = 2.0 Hz) suggested the 5, 7-disubstituted A ring of flavonoid and assigned to H-6 and H-8, respectively. This was confirmed from the HMBC experiment that exhibited correlations of H-2' (δ_H 7.46) with C-2 (δ_C 164.7), H-6' at δ_H 7.58 with C-2 (δ_C 164.7) and C-4' (δ_C 151.8) and H-5' (δ_H 7.16) with C-1` (δ_C 123.4) and C-3' (δ_C 147.3). Further HMBC correlations of H-6 (δ_H 6.48) with C-10 (δ_C 105.9) and H-8 (δ_H 6.81) with C-6 (δ_C 100.1) and C-10 (δ_C 105.9) were detected. These data are in a good agreement with diosmetin (El-Lakany et al., 1997; Saeidnia et al., 2011). The remaining ^{1}H NMR signals and the other eleven ^{13}C NMR signals, with ^{1}H ^{1}H COSY spectrum (Table 2) of compound 5 suggested the presence of two sugar moieties (hexose and pentose), the sugar moieties were identified by acid hydroplysis of compound 5 as *β*-D-glucose and *α*-L-arabinose. The FABMS fragments at *m/z* 463 [M^+-ara] and *m/z* 301 [M^+- glu - ara + H] confirmed the presence of glucose and arabinose. The linkage of glucose moiety was found to be at C-7 from HMBC correlations (Figure 4), as the anomeric proton of glucose at δ_H 5.09 showed three bond correlation with C-7 (δ_C 163.4). The position of arabinose was deduced from the downfield shift of C-4`` ($\delta_C$ 78.9) of glucose and this confirmed the connection of arabinose moiety at C-4`` of glucose. From the earlier discussed NMR data, compound 5 was identified as diosmetin- 7-*O*-*α*-L- arabinopyransyl - (1'''→4'') -*β* - D - glucopyranoside. This is the first report of this compound in nature.

Cytotoxic activity

The cytotoxic effect of total alcoholic extract of *C. pycnocephalus* was assessed against breast carcinoma (MCF-7), lung carcinoma (A-549) and hepatocellular carcinoma (HepG-2) cell lines at different concentrations, 50, 12.5, 6.25, 3.125, 1.56, 0.78 and 0.39 µg/ml, and the extract showed strong activity against the tested cell lines with IC_{50} 16.9, 17.5 and 21.8 µg/ml, respectively as shown in Figure 6.

Antioxidant activity

The antioxidant effect of total alcoholic extract of *C. pycnocephalaus* using DPPH free radical scavenging method was measured at eight different concentrations and the extract showed weak antioxidant activity in comparison with ascorbic acid with SC_{50} 554.2 and 14.2 µg/ml, respectively as shown in Figure 7.

Antimicrobial activity

The antimicrobial activity against fungi, *A. fumigates* (RCMB 02568), *S. racemosum* (RCMB 05922), *G. candidum* (RCMB 05097), *C. albicans* (RCMB 05036); Gram positive bacteria, *S. pneumonia* (RCMB 010010), *B. subtillis* (RCMB 010067) and Gram negative bacteria *P. aeruginosa* (RCMB 010043) and *E. coli* (RCMB 010052) was evaluated using agar diffusion technique. The extract exhibited strong antifungal activity against *S. racemosum* with inhibition zone diameter of 15.2 mm compared to that of amphotericin B 19.7 mm. In addition, a wide range of inhibitory activity against Gram-negative bacteria was observed. The extract showed strong anti-bacterial activity against *P. aeruginosa* and *E. coli* with inhibition zone diameter of 15.3 and 17.2 mm compared to that of gentamicin 17.3 and 19.9 mm, respectively. The extract showed also variable activities against other tested microorganisms as shown in Table 3.

Conclusion

Conclusively, this work represented the isolation of two new compounds 1 and 5 from *C. pycnocephalus* extract with three known compounds 2 to 4. In addition, the plant extract showed highly significant anticancer and antimicrobial activity; so it is considered as a good source for strong anticancer and antimicrobial principles.

ACKNOWLEDGEMENTS

The authors would like to express their deep feeling of gratitude and indebtedness to Dr. Maher Al-Jabal, King Saud University, for NMR analysis. They are much thankful to Prof. Dr. Adnan Al-Rehaily for plant collection.

REFERENCES

Abdallah OM, Ramadan MA, El-Shanawany MA (1989). Phytochemical study of *Carduus nutans* L. (Asteraceae). Bull. Pharm. Sci. Assiut Univ. 18:69-76.

Abdel-Salam NA, Mahmond ZF, Abdel-Hamid R, Khafagy SM (1982). The flavonoid,steroid and triterpenoid constituents of *Carduus getulus* Pomel (Compositae). Egypt. J. Pharm. Sci. 23:199-203.

Abdel-Salam NA, Morelli I, Catalano S (1983). An unusual triterpene ester in a Compositaceous plant, *Carduus getulus* Pomel. Int. J. Crude Drug Res. 21:79-80.

Ahmad VU, Rahman AU (1994). Handbook of Natural products Data, Vol (2), Pentacyclic triterpenoids, Elsevir Publishing, Amesterdam-London-New York Tokyo. pp. 1038, 365.

Al-Shammari L, Hassan WHB, Al-Youssef HM (2012). Phytochemical and biological studies of *Carduus pycnocephalaus* L. J. Saudi Chem. Soc. In press.

Amer MMA, Salama OM, Omar AA (1985). Flavonoids of *Carduus pycnocephalus*. Fitoterapia 56:61-63.

Babalola IT, Shode FO (2013). Ubiquitous Ursolic Acid: A Potential PentacyclicTriterpene Natural Product. J. Pharmacogn. Phytochem. 2 (2):214-222.

Bain JF, Desrochers AM, (1988). Flavonoids of *Carduus nutans* and *C. acanthoides*. Biochem. Syst. Ecol. 16:265-268.

Beeler D (1976). New Tetraphthalate Plasticizer for PVC. Plastic Eng. 32:40-47.

Cardona L, Garcia B, Pedro JR, Preaz J (1992). 6-Prenyloxy-7-methoxycoumarin, A coumarin hemiterpene ether from *Carduus Tenuiflorus*. Phytochemistry 31:398-402.

Chaudary SA (2000). Flora of the Kingdom of Saudi Arabia, Ministry of Agriculture and Water, National Herbarium, National Agriculture and Water Research Center, Riyadh, KSA. Vol. 2, Part 3:117-202.

El-Lakany M, Abdel-Kader MS, Hammoda, HM, Ghazy NM, Mahmoud ZF (1995). Flavonoids from *Carduus pycnocephalus* L. Alexandria J. Pharm. Sci. 9:41-42.

EL-Lakany AM, Abdel-Kader MS, Hammoda, HM, Gazy NM, Mahmoud ZF (1997). A new flavone glycoside with antimicrobial activity from *Carduus pycnocephalus* L. Pharmazie 52:78-79.

Ertaş A, Gören AC, Haşimi N, Tolan V, Kolak U (2015). Evaluation of Antioxidant, Cholinesterase Inhibitory and Antimicrobial Properties of *Mentha longifolia* subsp. *noeana* and Its Secondary Metabolites. Rec. Nat. Prod. 9(1):105-115.

Esmaeili F, Rustaiyan A, Nadimi M (2005). Volatile constituents of *Centaurea depressa* and *Carduus pycnocephalus* L. two Compositae herbs growing wild in Iran. J. Essent. Oil Res. 17:539-541.

Fernandez I, Garcia B, Pedro JR, Vareae A (1991). Lignans and flavonoids from Carduus. Assoc. Phytochem. 30:1030-1032.

Gallo MBC, Sarachine MJ (2009). "Biological activities of Lupeol". Int. J. Biomed. Pharm. Sci. 3 (1):46-66.

Jordon-Thaden FE, Louda SM (2003), Chemistry of *Cirsium* and *Carduus*: a role in ecological risk assessment for biological control of weeds. Biochem. Syst. Ecol. 31:1353-1396.

Katadea SR, Pawarb PV, Tungikarb VB, Tambec AS, Kalalc KM, Wakharkarc RD, and Deshpande NR (2006). Larvicidal Activity of Bis (2-ethylhexyl) Benzene-1,2-dicarboxylate from *Sterculia guttata* Seeds Against Two Mosquito Species. Chem. Biodivers. 3:49-53.

Liu SK, Que S, Cheng W, Zhang QY, Ye M, Liang H (2013). Two new glycosides from *Carduus acanthoides*. J. Asian Nat. Prod. Res. 15(12):1243-1248.

Mabry TJ, Markham KR, Thomas MB (1970). The Systematic Identification of Flavonoids. Springer-Verlag Berlin – Heidelberg – New York.

Markham KR, Ternal B, Stanley R, Geiger H, and Mabry TJ (1978). Carbon- ^{13} NMR studies of flavonoids-III: Naturally occurring flavonoid glycosides and their acylated derivatives. Tetrahedron 34:1389-1397.

Nadaf M, Halimi M, Nasrabadi M (2013). Identification of Compounds Nonpolar Extract *Ziziphora persica* growing in Iran by GC-MS. World Appl. Sci. J. 28 (11):1723-1726.

Orhan I, Orhan D, Ozçelik B (2009). Antiviral activity and cytotoxicity of thelipophilic extracts of various edible plants and their fatty acids. Food Chem. 115: 701-705.

Perez C, Pauli M and Bazerque p. 1990. An antibiotic assay by agar diffusion method. Acta. Biol. Med. Expert. 15:113-115.

Saeidnia S, nourbakhsh MS, gohari AR, Davood A (2011). Isolation and identification of the main compounds of *Satureja sahendica* brown. Aust. J. Basic Appl. Sci. 5 (6):1450-1453.

Silverstein RM, Bassler GC. and Morrillv (1997). Spectrometric Identification of Organic Compounds, 6th ed. John Wiley & Sons, Singapore.

Yen GC, Duh, PD (1994). Scavenging effect of methanolic extracts of peanut hulls on free radical and active oxygen species. J. Agric. Food Chem. 42:629-632.

Zanng Q, Tu G, Zhao Y, Cheng T (2002). Novel bioactive isoquinoline alkaloids from *Carduus crispus*. Tetrahedron Lett. 58 (34):6795-6798.

Permissions

All chapters in this book were first published in JPP, by Academic Journals; hereby published with permission under the Creative Commons Attribution License or equivalent. Every chapter published in this book has been scrutinized by our experts. Their significance has been extensively debated. The topics covered herein carry significant findings which will fuel the growth of the discipline. They may even be implemented as practical applications or may be referred to as a beginning point for another development.

The contributors of this book come from diverse backgrounds, making this book a truly international effort. This book will bring forth new frontiers with its revolutionizing research information and detailed analysis of the nascent developments around the world.

We would like to thank all the contributing authors for lending their expertise to make the book truly unique. They have played a crucial role in the development of this book. Without their invaluable contributions this book wouldn't have been possible. They have made vital efforts to compile up to date information on the varied aspects of this subject to make this book a valuable addition to the collection of many professionals and students.

This book was conceptualized with the vision of imparting up-to-date information and advanced data in this field. To ensure the same, a matchless editorial board was set up. Every individual on the board went through rigorous rounds of assessment to prove their worth. After which they invested a large part of their time researching and compiling the most relevant data for our readers.

The editorial board has been involved in producing this book since its inception. They have spent rigorous hours researching and exploring the diverse topics which have resulted in the successful publishing of this book. They have passed on their knowledge of decades through this book. To expedite this challenging task, the publisher supported the team at every step. A small team of assistant editors was also appointed to further simplify the editing procedure and attain best results for the readers.

Apart from the editorial board, the designing team has also invested a significant amount of their time in understanding the subject and creating the most relevant covers. They scrutinized every image to scout for the most suitable representation of the subject and create an appropriate cover for the book.

The publishing team has been an ardent support to the editorial, designing and production team. Their endless efforts to recruit the best for this project, has resulted in the accomplishment of this book. They are a veteran in the field of academics and their pool of knowledge is as vast as their experience in printing. Their expertise and guidance has proved useful at every step. Their uncompromising quality standards have made this book an exceptional effort. Their encouragement from time to time has been an inspiration for everyone.

The publisher and the editorial board hope that this book will prove to be a valuable piece of knowledge for researchers, students, practitioners and scholars across the globe.

List of Contributors

Huda Jasim and Imad Hadi Hameed
Department of Molecular Biology, Babylon University, Hilla City, Iraq

Ameera Omran Hussein and Muhanned Abdulhasan Kareem
Babylon University, Centre of Environmental Research, Iraq

Abayomi S. Faponle, Adeleke Atunnise, Bukunola O. Adegbesan, Olugbenga O. Ogunlabi and Kuburat T. Odufuwa
Department of Biochemistry, Faculty of Basic Medical Sciences, Ikenne Campus, Obafemi Awolowo College of Health Sciences, Olabisi Onabanjo University, Ago-Iwoye, Nigeria

Emmanuel O. Ajani
Phytomedicine, Toxicology and Drug Development Laboratory, Department of Biosciences and Biotechnology, Kwara state University, Malete, P. M B. 1530, Ilorin, Nigeria

Sipamla, A. M. and Mtunzi, F. M.
Department of Chemistry, Vaal University of Technology, P. Bag 021, Vanderbijlpark, 1900, South Africa

Muleya, E.
Department of Chemistry, Vaal University of Technology, P. Bag 021, Vanderbijlpark, 1900, South Africa
Phytomedcine Programme, University of Pretoria, P. Bag X04, 0110, Onderstepoort, South Africa

Ahmed, A. S.
Phytomedcine Programme, University of Pretoria, P. Bag X04, 0110, Onderstepoort, South Africa

Mutatu, W.
Midlands State University, P. Bag 9055, Gweru, Zimbabwe

Florence Dushimemaria
Science, Technology and Innovation Division, Multidisciplinary Research center, University of Namibia, Private Bag 13301, 340 Mandume Ndemufayo Avenue, Pionier spark, Windhoek, Namibia

Davis R. Mumbengegwi
Science, Technology and Innovation Division, Multidisciplinary Research center, University of Namibia, Private Bag 13301, 340 Mandume Ndemufayo Avenue, Pionier spark, Windhoek, Namibia

Messaoudi Moussi I, Filali, H., Tazi and Hakkou, F.
Laboratory of Pharmacology and Taxicology, Faculty Of Medicine and Pharmacy of Casablanca, University Hassan II. Morocco

Huda Jasim Al-Tameme, Imad Hadi Hameed, Salah Ali Idan and Mohammed Yahya Hadi
Department of Biology, Babylon University, Hilla City, Iraq

J. S. Ashidi and O. J. Ojetola
Department of Plant Science and Applied Zoology, Olabisi Onabanjo University, Ago-Iwoye. Ogun State, Nigeria

P. I. Aziba
Department of Pharmacology, Obafemi Awolowo College of Health Sciences, Olabisi Onabanjo University, Sagamu, Ogun State, Nigeria

E. O. Ajaiyeoba
Department of Pharmacognosy, University of Ibadan, Ibadan, Nigeria

Zayneb Alami
Department of Pharmacy and Clinical Pharmacology, Mohammed VI University Hospital, Medical and Pharmacy School, Mohammed First University, Oujda, Morocco

Hayat Aynaou, Youssef Hdidou and Hanane Latrech
Department of Endocrinology and Metabolism, Mohammed VI University Hospital, Medical and Pharmacy School, Mohammed First University, Oujda, Morocco

Bouchra Alami
Department of Ophtalmology, Mohammed VI University Hospital, Medical and Pharmacy School, Mohammed First University, Oujda, Morocco

Erol Ayaz
Department of Medical Parasitology, Faculty of Medicine, Abant İzzet Baysal University Bolu, Turkey

Cengiz Gökbulut
Department of Medical Pharmacology, Balıkesir University Faculty of Medicine, Balıkesir, Turkey

Hamit Coşkun
Department of Psychology, Faculty of Art and Science, Abant İzzet Baysal University, Bolu, Turkey

Arzu Türker
Department of Biology, Faculty of Art and Science, Abant İzzet Baysal University Bolu, Turkey

Şeyda Özsoy and Kübra Ceylan
Department of Medical Microbiology, Faculty of Medicine, Abant İzzet Baysal University Bolu, Turkey

Huda Jasim Al-Tameme, Mohammed Yahya Hadi and Imad Hadi Hameed
Department of Biology, Babylon University, Hilla City, Iraq

Ismail Adamu Hassan, Amina Muhammed Malut, Ibrahim Abdulkadir S. and Audu Sani Ali
Faculty of Pharmacy, University of Maiduguri, PMB 1069, Maiduguri, Nigeria

Idris Abdullahi Nasiru
Department of Medical Microbiology, University of Abuja Teaching Hospital, PMB 228 Gwagwalada, Abuja Nigeria

Sara Bonavia and Claire Shoemake
Department of Pharmacy, University of Malta, Msida MSD 2080, Malta

Tshodi M. Ehata, Nsaka S. Lumpu, Kikweta C. Munduku, Mbenza A. Phuati and Kambu O. Kabangu
Faculty of Pharmaceutical Sciences, University of Kinshasa, Kinshasa XI, Democratic Republic of Congo

Cimanga R. Kanyanga
Faculty of Pharmaceutical Sciences, University of Kinshasa, Kinshasa XI, Democratic Republic of Congo
Department of Pharmaceutical Sciences, Laboratory of Natural Products and Food-Research and Analysis (NatuRa), University of Antwerp, Universiteitsplein 1, B-2610, Antwerp, Belgium

Cos, P. and Maes, L.
Faculty of Pharmaceutical Sciences, Biomedical and Veterinary Sciences, Laboratory of Microbiology, Parasitology and Hygiene, University of Antwerp, Universisteitsplein 1, B-2610 Antwerp, Belgium

Apers, S., Vlietinck, A. J. and Pieters, L.
Department of Pharmaceutical Sciences, Laboratory of Natural Products and Food-Research and Analysis (NatuRa), University of Antwerp, Universiteitsplein 1, B-2610, Antwerp, Belgium

Imad Hadi Hameed, Lena Fadhil Hamza and Sabreen A. Kamal
Department of Molecular Biology, Babylon University, Hilla City, Iraq

Abdelkrim Berroukche, Khaled Kahloula, Miloud Slimani, Imane Denai and Kheira Ammour
Laboratory of Biochemistry, Biology Department, Faculty of Sciences, Dr. Tahar Moulay University, Saida 20000, Algeria

Uthayashanker R. Ezekiel and Rita M. Heuertz
Department of Biomedical Laboratory Science,Doisy College of Health Sciences,Saint Louis University, 3437 Caroline Street, Saint Louis, USA

Azhar Abduameer Sosa and Suhaila Husaein Bagi
College of Education for Women, Al-Qadisyia University, Iraq

Imad Hadi Hameed
College of Nursing, Babylon University, Iraq

Lena Fadhil Hamza, Sabreen A. Kamal and Imad Hadi Hameed
Department of Biology, Babylon University, Hilla City, Iraq

Hanan M. Al-Youssef and Latifa AL-Shammari
Pharmacognosy Department, Faculty of Pharmacy, King Saud University, Riyadh, Saudi Arabia

Wafaa H. B. Hassan and Rehab H. Abdallah
Pharmacognosy Department, Faculty of Pharmacy, Zagazig University, Zagazig, Egypt

Index

A

Aliphatic Fluoro Compounds, 60, 70, 74, 109, 140, 144, 169, 188-189, 195, 206, 231

Alkaloid, 1-5, 36-38, 75, 78, 80, 110-111, 113, 115, 120-121, 129, 171, 205, 232

Alkaloids, 1-2, 5, 16, 34-36, 38, 61, 77-82, 97, 111-113, 115-118, 131-134, 138-139, 170, 173, 180, 234, 243

Alternative Medicine., 83, 189

Amaranthus Spinosus, 18-19, 21-24

Amaranthus Viridis, 24-25

Analgesia, 77-79

Anthraquinones, 34, 36-37, 78-79, 111, 113, 115, 131, 138

Anti-cancer, 34, 36, 39, 72, 185-186, 190, 192

Anti-hyperglycemic, 78

Anti-inflammatory, 26-27, 29, 32-33, 35, 37, 39, 56, 71-75, 77-82, 93, 96, 106, 108-109, 112, 118, 182-183, 186-187, 190, 192-195, 204, 233-234

Antibacterial, 1-2, 5, 16-17, 26-27, 29, 32-33, 37, 71-72, 81, 93, 107, 110, 115, 118-119, 140-141, 144, 190-191, 193, 206-207, 210, 231, 233

Antibacterial Activity, 1-2, 16, 29, 33, 115, 118, 140-141, 144, 191, 193, 206-207, 210, 231

Antibiotics, 1-5, 140-141, 170, 206, 231

Antidiabetic, 19, 56, 71, 135, 139

Antifungal, 16, 26-27, 29, 33, 56, 61, 95, 141-142, 144, 161, 170, 180, 191, 233, 237, 242

Antimalarial, 94-95, 112, 118, 134, 138-139

Antimicrobial, 1, 4-5, 16-17, 26-27, 29-33, 61, 72, 75, 106, 108, 110-111, 118-119, 139, 142, 144, 160, 171, 193, 204-206, 224, 232-234, 237-238, 242-243

Antimicrobial Activity, 1, 5, 16, 29, 31, 75, 110, 142, 160, 171, 205-206, 224, 232-233, 237-238, 242-243

Antioxidant, 19-20, 23-27, 29, 32, 34-40, 56, 61, 72, 75, 106, 108, 110, 119, 180-181, 186, 193, 204, 233-234, 236, 241-243

Antiprotozoal Activity, 130-132, 138-139

Antiviral, 24, 37, 56, 106, 190, 194, 233, 243

Apiaceae, 26-28, 33, 41, 87

Artemia Salina, 16

Ascaridole Epoxide, 188-189, 192, 199

Ascorbic Acid, 29, 36, 188-189, 193, 201, 237, 241-242

Asteraceae, 43, 83, 87-89, 233, 242

Atherogenic, 18, 20, 22-25

B

Bioactive Compounds, 39, 60, 138, 140, 170-171, 188, 206, 232

Biochemical Markers, 172

Breast Cancer, 35

Brucea Sumatrana, 130, 134, 139

C

Candida Albicans, 26, 28, 30-31, 33, 237-238

Cardiac Glycosides, 78, 115-116

Cardiovascular Risk, 18, 24-25, 84-85

Carduus Pycnocephalus L., 233-234, 243

Cassia Angustifolia, 204

Chemotaxis, 182-187

Chloroform Extract, 117-118, 235

Chromatography, 1-2, 34, 36-37, 60-61, 75, 96-97, 110-113, 131, 140-142, 171, 188-189, 204-207, 232

Crude, 5, 17, 26-32, 36, 39, 61, 78-79, 131, 139, 141-142, 170, 204, 207, 210, 242

Cytotoxic Activity, 130, 139, 233, 236, 242

Cytotoxic,, 134, 233-234

Cytotoxicity, 27, 119, 132, 243

D

Diabetes, 19, 22, 24-25, 34, 78, 83-90, 93

Diabetes Mellitus, 19, 22, 24-25, 83-84, 89-90

Diclofenac Sodium, 77-81

E

Ethnopharmacological Survey, 59, 90

Extract, 1-3, 5-16, 18-20, 22-30, 32-33, 36, 39, 60-62, 71, 74-82, 89-90, 92-98, 106, 1110, 112-113, 115-119, 130-140, 142-144, 161, 170-171, 173-174, 178-181, 187-190, 196, 204-210, 225, 232-238, 241-243

F

Flavonoid, 37-38, 79-80, 82, 111, 113, 242-243

Flavonoidal Glycoside, 233

Foeniculum Vulgare, 205

Foenum-graecum, 89-90

Fourier Transform Infrared, 141, 189, 205, 207

Fourier Transform Infrared Spectroscopy, 141, 207

G

Gallic Acid, 36

Gas Chromatography, 1-2, 60-61, 75, 96-97, 110, 140-142, 171, 188-189, 204-207, 232

Gas Chromatography-mass Specroscopy

(gc-ms), 1-2

H

Hepatoprotective Activity, 24, 172, 178, 180-181

Herbal Medicine, 18, 41, 90, 95, 129, 172

Herbal Medicines, 83-84, 90

High-fat Diet, 18

I

Ibuprofen, 77-81

Inflammation, 19, 25-27, 29, 32-33, 42, 77, 79-80, 82, 179, 182-183, 185-187, 189

L

Lamiaceae, 41, 43, 58, 60, 83, 87-88

Lipoprotein, 18, 22-25, 137

M

Malaria, 115, 119, 130-131, 138

Mass Spectrometry, 1, 60-61, 75, 96, 110, 140-142, 188, 204-207, 232

Medicinal Plants, 16, 25, 27, 32-35, 37-45, 47-48, 58-60, 77-78, 82-83, 87-88, 90, 92-93, 111, 118-119, 139, 144, 161, 173, 180, 204

Metabolites, 1-2, 58, 96, 115, 117-118, 140-142, 171, 178, 204, 206-207, 210, 232, 234, 243

Methanol, 1-3, 5, 20, 27-29, 32, 36-37, 39, 61, 76, 81-82, 94, 96-97, 109, 111-118, 130-135, 139, 141-142, 189, 207, 209, 234-235, 237

Methanolic Dried Galls Extract, 205

Minimum Inhibitory Concentrations, 26-27, 29

N

Namibia, 34-40

Neutrophils, 136, 182-187

Nigella Sativa, 39, 87, 110, 204

O

Obesity, 19, 22, 24, 187

Ocimum Basilicum, 56

Olea Europaea, 87

P

Palliative Care, 34-35, 37, 39-40

Phenolics, 118, 133, 180

Phytochemical, 3, 16-17, 27, 34, 36-40, 59-61, 71, 75, 77-82, 96, 106, 110-113, 115, 118-119, 131, 138, 161, 171, 183-184, 188-190, 204-205, 225, 232-234, 237, 242

Phytochemicals, 22, 36-39, 96, 110-111, 113, 118, 182-186

Phytotherapy, 24, 41, 48, 58, 83, 95

Polyphenols, 32, 35, 81, 173, 205

R

Rhamnaceae, 88, 172, 180

S

Solanum Nigrum., 1, 4-5

Streptozotocin, 89-90, 110

T

Thin Layer Chromatography, 34, 36-37, 111-113, 131

Toxicity, 5, 25, 40, 61, 130-132, 134-135, 137-139, 172, 178

Traditional Medicine, 2, 17, 27, 34-35, 37, 41, 60, 78, 82, 84, 88-89, 91-92, 95, 112, 118-119, 138-139, 172-173

Z

Zingiber Officinale, 82

CPSIA information can be obtained
at www.ICGtesting.com
Printed in the USA
BVHW010802300519
549552BV00014B/162/P

9 781632 428363